Oro-Facial Bone Grafts and Biomaterials

Scrivener Publishing
100 Cummings Center, Suite 541J
Beverly, MA 01915-6106

Publishers at Scrivener
Martin Scrivener (martin@scrivenerpublishing.com)
Phillip Carmical (pcarmical@scrivenerpublishing.com)

Oro-Facial Bone Grafts and Biomaterials

Edited by

Randa A. Alfotawi
Department of Oral and Maxillofacial Surgery, College of Dentistry, King Saud University, Riyadh, Saudi Arabia

Scrivener Publishing

WILEY

This edition first published 2026 by John Wiley & Sons, Inc., 111 River Street, Hoboken, NJ 07030, USA and Scrivener Publishing LLC, 100 Cummings Center, Suite 541J, Beverly, MA 01915, USA

For more information about Scrivener publications please visit www.scrivenerpublishing.com.

Wiley Global Headquarters
111 River Street, Hoboken, NJ 07030, USA

For details of our global editorial offices, customer services, and more information about Wiley products visit us at www.wiley.com.

The manufacturer's authorized representative according to the EU General Product Safety Regulation is Wiley-VCH GmbH, Boschstr. 12, 69469 Weinheim, Germany, e-mail: Product_Safety@wiley.com.

Library of Congress Cataloging-in-Publication Data

ISBN 978-1-394-39848-5

Front cover images courtesy of the Editor
Cover design by Russell Richardson

Set in size of 11pt and Minion Pro by Manila Typesetting Company, Makati, Philippines

Printed in the USA

10 9 8 7 6 5 4 3 2 1

Contents

Foreword

The new textbook on oro-facial bone grafts and biomaterials is to be commended for its comprehensive review of the topic. It provides thorough documentation and explanation of the various types of bone grafting for application in the maxillofacial region. The textbook updates the readers on the broad range of biomaterials and the contemporary biomimetic grafts for bone augmentation and oro-facial reconstruction.

The biological basis of osteogenesis and the osteo- intergeneration of the grafts are well described and provide a comprehensive reference to students and scholars. The textbook explains the complex signaling process for tissue engineering in a simplified manner which will appeal to those who are new to the field.

The anatomical consideration for bone reconstruction is an essential component of the textbook. This chapter explains the importance of understanding the morphological and radiographic characteristics of the orbital cavity as well as the maxillary and mandibular bones. It highlights the anatomical considerations for the successful reconstruction of the bony foundation. The textbook is a useful resource for the full range of autogenous grafts, the allografts, alloplastic materials and xenografts for bone augmentation and maxillofacial reconstruction.

I recommend the textbook as a comprehensive reference to researchers, dental and medical students, surgical trainees, as well as clinicians who are interested in tissue bioengineering.

Ashraf F. Ayoub
Professor of Oral & Maxillofacial Surgery, the University of Glasgow, UK

Preface

In the ever-evolving field of maxillofacial surgery, the role of bone grafts and biomaterials has become paramount in enhancing patient outcomes. This book provides an in-depth exploration of these critical components, drawing from the latest clinical evidence and technological advancements.

The book begins by addressing the pressing need for effective bone grafts in facial reconstruction and augmentation. Then it explores the advanced technologies that are shaping the future of these procedures, offering insights into the latest innovations.

Furthermore, this book illuminates the evidence-based practices surrounding facial rejuvenation and augmentation, providing a comprehensive review of various grafting techniques. Each method is examined through the lens of clinical evidence, weighing the pros and cons to guide practitioners in choosing the most suitable approach for their patients.

In closing, I wish to express my gratitude to everyone who supported this project, especially Martin Scrivener and the team at Scrivener Publishing for their effort in bringing it to publication.

May 2026

Acknowledgment

First and foremost, I extend my deepest gratitude to my family, whose unwavering support has been the cornerstone of my journey. To my beloved sons, Walid and Yazid, thank you for your patience and understanding during times when I was deeply engrossed in my work. You have been my source of strength and inspiration.

I dedicate this book to the memory of my father, who passed away two years ago. His belief in the value of education and his constant encouragement have been my guiding light. I always felt his presence and guidance, especially during challenging moments in my career. This book is a tribute to his enduring influence on my life and work.

I am also profoundly thankful to my co-authors, Dr. Manju Philip and Dr. Hourya Al-Nofaie, for their invaluable contributions and insights throughout the process of bringing this book to fruition.

Lastly, I want to express my heartfelt appreciation to all my friends and colleagues who have been part of this incredible journey. Your camaraderie and collaboration have made this endeavor not just successful but also immensely enjoyable.

1

Definitions

Randa A. Alfotawi

Department of Oral and Maxillofacial Surgery, College of Dentistry, King Saud University, Riyadh, Saudi Arabia

Abstract

This chapter summarises key definitions commonly used in the field of bone grafting and biomaterials within the craniofacial region. The terminology presented throughout this chapter is derived from current and authoritative literature and is intended to provide a conceptual framework for researchers, clinicians, and postgraduate students. Clear understanding of these definitions facilitates interpretation of biological mechanisms, material behaviour, and assessment parameters discussed in subsequent chapters, including those related to osteointegration, bone–implant contact (BIC), and radiostereometric analysis.

Keywords: Radiostereometric, alloplasts, allograft, graft, flap, bioactive material, bone–implant contact, biomimetic graft

1.1 Definitions

1.1.1 Allografts

Allografts are tissues harvested from one individual and transplanted into another genetically non-identical individual of the same species. In oral and maxillofacial applications, the most commonly used forms include demineralized freeze-dried bone allograft (DFDBA) and freeze-dried bone allograft (FDBA) [1].

Email: ralfotawei@ksu.edu.sa

Randa A. Alfotawi (ed.) Oro-Facial Bone Grafts and Biomaterials, (1–14) © 2026 Scrivener Publishing LLC

1.1.2 Alloplasts

Alloplasts are synthetic materials that contain some of the essential chemical constituents of normal bone and are used to promote bone regeneration. When it comes to osteoinduction and osteogenesis, the ideal alloplastic bone substitutes behave similarly to autologous bone [2].

1.1.3 Antibody

B-lymphocytes that are produced by bone marrow and have the capacity to develop into plasma cells produce the remarkable proteins known as antibodies. Antibodies are adaptor molecules that can attach to microorganisms, activate complement, and attach to phagocytic cells. The Fab end of the molecule, which binds microorganisms, is a specific recognition site for each antibody. The antibody molecule's Fc end has domains that can attach to phagocyte Fc receptors and bind and activate the first component of complement. There are five antibody subtypes: IgG, IgM, IgA, IgD, and IgE [3].

1.1.4 Antigen

Any type of molecule that may be identified by particular adaptive immune system receptors on T and B cells is considered an antigen. They can be proteins or protein peptide fragments, carbohydrates, lipids, nucleic acids (DNA or RNA), or even haptens. To be considered immunogenic, an antigen must be able to both activate the immune system and be recognized by the immune system (antigenic), usually as foreign body [4].

1.1.5 Autogenous

Autogenous grafts are tissues transferred from one site to another within the same individual. They are considered the most biologically effective graft material due to their osteogenic, osteoinductive, and osteoconductive properties and are widely regarded as the reference standard in bone regeneration procedures.

1.1.6 Bone–Implant Contact (BIC)

The BIC is the ratio of the overall length of the implant profile to the linear measurement of the surface of the implant that is in direct contact with bone. Previously, this interface was described as "a direct structural and functional connection between ordered, living bone and the surface of a load-carrying implant" made by highly differentiated tissue [6].

1.1.7 Bioactive Material

Bioactive materials are characterized by their ability to elicit a specific biological response at the interface with host tissue, resulting in the formation of a biologically active layer typically calcium phosphate that facilitates bonding between the material and surrounding bone.

1.1.8 Biodegradation

Biodegradation refers to the biologically mediated breakdown of a graft material through cellular and enzymatic processes within the host microenvironment.

1.1.9 Bioengineered Graft

Bioengineered grafts are advanced synthetic or hybrid constructs designed to replicate biological functions of autogenous grafts by incorporating regenerative biomaterials, cells, or bioactive molecules.

1.1.10 Bioinert Graft

Bioinert graft is a graft material that, when introduced into a biological tissue, does not initiate a response or interact with the tissue. It is a substance that elucidates minimal interaction with its surrounding tissue and/or does not trigger a response from the host immune system [10].

1.1.11 Biomaterials

Biomaterials are natural or synthetic materials specifically designed to interact with biological systems for therapeutic or diagnostic purposes.

1.1.12 Biomimetic Graft

A biomimetic graft is a graft material that is designed to imitate the biological characteristics of natural tissues. The aim of biomimetic graft is to address a number of intricate biological issues, including inadequate tissue perfusion, drug delivery in biomedical settings, and the characterization of nanostructured biohybrid materials. It also intends to improve the structure, function, or production of materials and substances produced by biological processes [12].

1.1.13 Bone Graft

Bone graft is a material used to regenerate, reconstruct, or replace lost natural bone. Autogenic, allograft, xenograft, or alloplastic materials can all be used as a graft. The goal is to restore the function and continuity of lost bone [9].

1.1.14 Bone Remodelling

Bone remodelling is a continuous physiological process involving coordinated bone resorption and formation.

1.1.15 Cell Surface Markers

Cell surface markers are molecules found on a cell's surface that are used to determine the type of cell. When these molecules bind to specific substances, they function as receptors that trigger a reaction or activity within the cell. They might also function as antigens, binding to specific antibodies [14].

1.1.16 Composite Bone Graft

A composite bone graft is a procedure that combines various graft materials to form a bone graft with the best biological characteristics and sufficient volume to support a prompt, effective bone repair response. These combinations can be made by combining two distinct biomaterials, natural and synthetic materials, or autogenous extracts such as growth factors, cytokines, and cells. Getting a synergistic effect in terms of biomimetics, optimal resorption time, and regeneration ability is the goal [15].

1.1.17 Cumulative Survival Rate (CSR)

The percentage of dental implants that remain functional over a given period of time is indicated statistically by the Cumulative Survival Rate (CSR). It is determined by dividing the number of surviving implants in a group by the total implants placed. This rate is a crucial dependability indicator that shows how well the implants work over time and aids in evaluating the implants' survival *in situ* [16].

1.1.18 Extracellular Matrix (ECM)

The extracellular matrix (ECM), a form of connective tissue present in the cell microenvironment, is crucial to tissue development. It is the non-cellular element present in every organ and tissue. In addition to providing the required physical scaffolding for the cellular components, it initiates critical biochemical and biomechanical signals required for tissue morphogenesis, differentiation, and homeostasis [17].

1.1.19 Graft

Tissue which is used to reconstruct a lost or damaged part is transferred from one site to another, depending on its revascularisation from the recipient site. This tissue can be from the same person, another human donor, an animal, or synthetic.

1.1.20 Gene Expression

Inducible gene expression is the term used to describe the quick activation of gene transcription that leads to the generation of new proteins as a result of external stimuli. In response to the same stimulus, it is frequently necessary for several genes to be synchronously activated so that the proteins needed to react to the stimulus are generated concurrently at the proper relative quantities. Similar to this, for the proper morphogenetic process to take place across a broad region of cells, several cells in an organism must react to develop signals in a coordinated manner [18].

1.1.21 Foreign Body Reaction

Following the implantation of biomaterials, host reactions known as foreign body reactions include granulation tissue development, fibrosis/fibrous capsule creation, acute and chronic inflammation, damage, blood–material interactions, and provisional matrix synthesis. Phases of the reaction include mast cells in the acute inflammatory phase and lymphocytes in the transient chronic inflammatory phase, which generate IL4 and IL3 and can cause monocyte/macrophage fusion to generate body giant cells [19].

1.1.22 Flap

Tissue which is used to reconstruct lost or damaged part is transferred from one site to another with its own blood supply. It depends on its revascularisation from its own blood vascular structure. This vascular pedicle tissue can be from the same person only. It is considered the gold standard for reconstructive surgery.

1.1.23 Immunohistochemistry

Immunohistochemistry is the gold standard of research techniques for identifying the presence of proteins (antigens). Based on a particular chemical interaction between antigens and antibodies, immunohistochemistry can identify individual antigens (proteins) in cells within a tissue segment. Either fluorescent or chromogenic immunostaining is typically used to visualize the antigen–antibody interaction [20].

1.1.24 Macrophages

Macrophages have significant immunological function and phenotypic heterogeneity, potentially changing into several cell subtypes upon encountering a variety of immune microenvironments. One essential macrophage activity for pathogenic host defence is autophagy. In addition to being additional stimulators and regulators of aging inflammation, tissue macrophages are key producers of inflammatory cytokines. Furthermore, macrophages are an essential component of the tumour microenvironment (TME) that subvert immune cells, which promotes the formation and progression of cancer cells with clinical significance [21].

1.1.25 Osteoblasts

The cells that comprise bone tissue are called osteoblasts. In order to regulate the ratio of calcium to phosphate ions in growing bone, they can produce and secrete bone matrix and take part in bone mineralization. Osteoprogenitor cells give rise to osteoblasts. Numerous factors, including different hormones and locally produced bioactive chemicals following fracture, influence the conversion of osteoprogenitors. These conditions allow osteoprogenitors to proliferate and start differentiating into osteoblasts, which perform osteogenic functions [22].

1.1.26 Osteocytes

In bone, osteocytes are the most common type of cell. Osteocytes regulate both bone production and resorption. The unmineralized matrix (osteoid) that surrounds the osteocytes, which are formerly osteoblasts, during bone formation traps the osteocytes in place and keeps them buried for the remainder of their lives. Given that they are arranged in networks, osteocytes can interact with other cells on the surface of bones as well as with one another [23].

1.1.27 Osteogenesis

Osteogenesis is the process by which mesenchymal stromal cells (MSCs) differentiate to become bone. Two distinct mechanisms are involved: either the skull's neural crest-derived mesenchymal cells proliferate and produce capillaries, or other cells transform into osteoblasts, committed bone precursor cells, and generate osteoid matrix. Sclerosome-derived cells are the alternative process, in which mesenchymal cells are dedicated to becoming cartilage cells and then convert into bone [24].

1.1.28 Osteoinduction

Osteoinduction is the process of attracting immature cells and stimulating their development into pre-osteoblasts. In other words, it is the process that promotes osteogenesis. This bio-stimulation process is brought on by the presence of cytokines, inflammatory substances, bone morphogenic proteins, or bioactive fourth-generation biomaterials [25].

1.1.29 Osteoconduction

Osteoconduction describes the ability of a graft material to serve as a scaffold that supports the ingrowth of bone.

1.1.30 Osteoclasts

Multinucleated large cells called osteoclasts resorb bone, which promotes the growth and ongoing remodelling of the skeleton and the bone marrow's hematopoietic niche. The discovery of the intracellular signals that mediate the cell's resorptive ability was made possible by the fact that the cell is hematopoietic and regulated by cytokines [26].

1.1.31 Osteointegration Graft

Osteointegration graft is a direct structural and functional bond between the surface of an implant or graft material and a living bone. It is the presence of an amorphous layer with an ultrastructure range of [2040–500] nm thick, composed of collagen and calcified tissue, near the bone–graft contact. This region is too small to be visible at the resolution of a light microscope. High biocompatibility is required for the graft material [27, 28].

1.1.32 Osteoid Matrix

Osteoid matrix is an extracellular organic matrix that is secreted by osteoblast bone cells, before the mineralized bone is formed. It is composed of a gelatinous material consisting of an organic glue called mucopolysaccharide and collagen, a fibrous protein [29]. The hardened substance known as mature bone is then formed by the subsequent deposition of inorganic salts.

1.1.33 Osteogenic Proteins

These polypeptides belong to the family of bone matrix and have been isolated from a range of mammalian species. These proteins belong to the superfamily known as transforming growth factor-beta. They are essential for triggering the differentiation of mesenchymal stem cells into osteoblasts, which promotes the growth of new bone. These proteins are known as bone morphogenic proteins 7 and 2 and bone sialoprotein BSP [30].

1.1.34 Radiostereometric Analysis

Radiostereometric analysis is the clinical evaluation of graft material integration. It is an accurate tool for measuring motion between supposedly rigid objects [31].

1.1.35 Regeneration

The act of replacing or regaining the complete function of injured or absent cells, tissues, organs, and even entire body parts is called regeneration. In order to maintain their tissues and organs, all living things, including plants and animals, have the capacity to regenerate to some extent [32].

1.1.36 Regenerative Medicine

Regenerative medicine is a multidisciplinary field focused on restoring, replacing, or regenerating human cells, tissues, or organs.

1.1.37 Reconstructions

The regeneration or augmentation of a damaged bodily part that was lost as a result of trauma, a degenerative body process, surgical resection, or a congenital imperfection is known as reconstruction. Both synthetic and biological biomaterials may be used for the reconstruction.

1.1.38 Rejuvenation

Rejuvenation is the act of reversing the aging-related alterations in soft tissue, which manifest as atrophic laxity that causes tissue descent. With a focus on lift vectors, this procedure seeks to red rape and reposition the tissues [34]. The mandibular region, the medial suborbital and pyriform regions of the maxilla, and the superomedial and inferolateral portions of the orbit are the sites of selective resorption associated with facial skeleton aging.

1.1.39 Reverse Torque Test

This is the maximum amount of force required to remove implants or the critical torque threshold where bone-implant contact is destroyed [35].

1.1.40 Scaffolds

A scaffold is a natural or artificial three-dimensional skeleton that aids in the growth of cells, the synthesis of extracellular matrix and other biological components, and the subsequent formation of functioning tissues or organs [36, 37].

1.1.41 Signalling System

The process by which cells interact with one another or with the outside world is known as cell signalling. Allosteric effects, chemical amplification, and feedback loops are some of the control mechanisms used by these complex chemical networks. Cell signalling occurs *via* a number of different mechanisms. Cell signalling is necessary in multicellular organisms to control several processes. Both intracellular and intercellular cell signalling are possible. The same cells that receive an intracellular signal also create it. Signals between cells circulate throughout the body. This makes it possible for particular glands to provide signals that affect several tissues [38, 39].

1.1.42 Tissue Engineering

Tissue engineering involves the application of engineering principles and life sciences to develop biological substitutes that restore, maintain, or improve tissue function.

1.1.43 Xenograft, Xenotransplantation

Xenograft involves the transplant of tissue or organ in which the recipient is a member of a different species and the donor is a member of another animal species.

Xenotransplantation or heterologous transplant is the process of transferring living cells, tissues, or organs from one species to another [41].

AI disclosure statement: The author acknowledges the use of AI-based tools for minor language editing or grammatical correction. However, all intellectual contributions, analyses, and conclusions presented in this chapter are entirely the author's own.

References

1. Moore, M.A., Samsell, B., McLean, J., Allograft Tissue Safety and Technology, in: *Biologics in Orthopaedic Surgery*, pp. 49–62, 2019, doi: 10.1016/B978-0-323-55140-3.00005-9. Epub 2018 Nov 26. PMCID: PMC7151900.1.
2. Bray, C.C., Walker, C.M., Spence, D.D., Orthobiologics in Pediatric Sports Medicine. *Orthop. Clin. North Am.*, 48, 3, 2017.
3. Seare, W.J. Jr., Alloplasts and biointegration. *J. Endourol.*, 14, 1, 9–17, 2000 Feb, doi: 10.1089/end.2000.14.9. PMID: 10735567.3.
4. Spiess, C., Zhai, Q., Carter, P.J., Alternative molecular formats and therapeutic applications for bispecific antibodies. *Mol. Immunol.*, 67, 2, 95–106, 2015 Oct 1.
5. Stewart, J., Immunological principles: Antigens and antigen recognition, in: *Medical Microbiology*, Eighteenth Edition, D. Greenwood, M. Barer, R. Slack, W. Irving (Eds.), pp. 98–108, Churchill Livingstone, 2012, ISBN 9780702040894.

6. Myeroff, C. and Archdeacon, M., Autogenous Bone Graft: Donor Sites and Techniques. *J. Bone Joint Surg.*, 93, 23, 2227–2236, 2011.
7. Sagirkaya, E., Kucukekenci, A.S., Karasoy, D., Akca, K., Eckert, S., Çehreli, M.C., Comparative assessments, meta-analysis, and recommended guidelines for reporting studies on histomorphometric bone-implant contact in humans. *Int. J. Oral Maxillofac. Implants*, 28, 5, 2013.
8. Zhao, X., Introduction to bioactive materials in medicine, in: *Woodhead Publishing Series in Biomaterials, Bioactive Materials in Medicine*, X. Zhao, J.M. Courtney, H. Qian (Eds.), pp. 1–13, Woodhead Publishing, 2011, ISBN 9781845696245.
9. Wei, S., Ma, J.X., Xu, L., *et al.*, Biodegradable materials for bone defect repair. *Mil. Med. Res.*, 7, 54, 2020, https://doi.org/10.1186/s40779-020-00280-6.
10. Das, S. and Hollister, S.J., Tissue Engineering Scaffolds, in: *Encyclopedia of Materials: Science and Technology*, K.H. Jürgen Buschow, R.W. Cahn, M.C. Flemings, B. Ilschner, E.J. Kramer, S. Mahajan, P. Veyssière (Eds.), pp. 1–7I, Elsevier Amsterdam, 2003.
11. Yamamuro, T., Bioceramics, in: *Biomechanics and Biomaterials in Orthopedics*, D.G. Poitout (Ed.), pp. 281–322, Springer, London, 2004.
12. Guarino, Raucci, M.G., Ronca, A., Cirillo, V., Ambrosio, L., Multifunctional scaffolds for bone regeneration, in: *Woodhead Publishing Series in Biomaterials, Bone Substitute Biomaterials*, K. Mallick (Ed.), pp. 95–117, Woodhead Publishing, Sawston, 2014.
13. Farag, M.M., Recent trends on biomaterials for tissue regeneration applications. *J. Mater. Sci.*, 58, 2, 527–58.10, 2023.
14. Eriksen, E.F., Cellular mechanisms of bone remodeling. *Rev. Endocr. Metab. Disord.*, 11, 219–227, 2010, https://doi.org/10.1007/s11154-010-9153-1.
15. Meyfour, A., Pahlavan, S., Mirzaei, M., Krijgsveld, J., Baharvand, H., Salekdeh, G.H., The quest of cell surface markers for stem cell therapy. *Cell. Mol. Life Sci.*, 78, 469–95, 2021.
16. Dhruvakumar, D. and Gupta, C., Role of combination therapy/composite graft in periodontal regeneration: A mini review. *Tanta Dent. J.*, 14, 4, 169–172, Oct–Dec 2017, DOI: 10.4103/tdj.tdj_19_17.
17. Nam, D.H., Kim, P.J., Koo, K.T., Seol, Y.J., Lee, Y.M., Ku, Y., Rhyu, I.C., Kim, S., Cho, Y.D., The cumulative survival rate of dental implants with microthreads: a long-term retrospective study. *J. Periodontal Implant Sci.*, 54, 1, 53, 2023.
18. Frantz, C., Stewart, K.M., Weaver, V.M., The extracellular matrix at a glance. *J. Cell Sci.*, 123, Pt 24, 4195–200, 2010, doi: 10.1242/jcs.023820. PMID: 21123617; PMCID: PMC2995612.
19. Weake, V. and Workman, J., Inducible gene expression: diverse regulatory mechanisms. *Nat. Rev. Genet.*, 11, 426–437, 2010.
20. Anderson, J.M., Rodriguez, A., Chang, D.T., Foreign body reaction to biomaterials. *Semin. Immunol.*, 20, 2, 86–100, 2008, doi: 10.1016/j.smim.2007.11.004. Epub 2007 Dec 26. PMID: 18162407; PMCID: PMC2327202.

21. Mikuni, T., Genome editing-based approaches for imaging protein localization and dynamics in the mammalian brain. *Neurosci. Res.*, 150, 2–7, 2020.
22. Chen, S., Saeed, A.F., Liu, Q., *et al.*, Macrophages in immunoregulation and therapeutics. *Sig. Transduct. Target. Ther.*, 8, 207, 2023.
23. Wlodarski, K.H., Properties and origin of osteoblasts. *Clin. Orthop. Relat. Res.*,® 252, 276–93, 1990.
24. Schaffler, M.B., Cheung, W.Y., Majeska, R., Kennedy, O., Osteocytes: master orchestrators of bone. *Calcif. Tissue Int.*, 94, 1, 5–24, 2014.
25. Chan, W.C., Tan, Z., To, M.K., Chan, D., Regulation and role of transcription factors in osteogenesis. *Int. J. Mol. Sci.*, 22, 11, 5445, 2021.
26. Albrektsson, T. and Johansson, C., Osteoinduction, osteoconduction and osseointegration. *Eur. Spine J.*, 10, Suppl 2, S96–101.12, 2001 Oct.
27. Jacome-Galarza, C.E., Percin, G.I., Muller, J.T., *et al.*, Developmental origin, functional maintenance and genetic rescue of osteoclasts. *Nature*, 568, 541–545, 2019, https://doi.org/10.1038/s41586-019-1105.
28. Stanford, C.M. and Keller, J.C., The Concept of Osseointegration and Bone Matrix Expression. *Crit. Rev. Oral Biol. Med.*, 2, 1, 83–101, 1991.
29. Albrektsson, T., Brånemark, P.I., Hansson, H.A., Ivarsson, B., Jönsson, U., Ultrastructural analysis of the interface zone of titanium and gold implants, in: *Adv Biomaterials*, vol. 4, pp. 167–177, 1982.
30. Bonewald, L.F., Osteocyte Biology, in: *Osteoporosis*, Fourth Edition, R. Marcus, D. Feldman, D.W. Dempster, M. Luckey, J.A. Cauley (Eds.), pp. 209–234, Academic Press, New York, 2013.
31. Cook, S.D. and Rueger, D.C., Osteogenic protein-1: biology and applications. *Clin. Orthop. Relat. Res.*,® 324, 29–38, 1996.
32. Shareghi, B., Johanson, P.E., Kärrholm, J., Clinical evaluation of model-based radiostereometric analysis to measure femoral head penetration and cup migration in four different cup designs. *J. Orthop. Res.*, 35, 4, 760–767, 2017, doi: 10.1002/jor.23177. Epub 2017 Mar 8. PMID: 26825861.
33. Tsukamoto, A., Abbot, S.E., Kadyk, L.C., DeWitt, N.D., Schaffer, D.V., Wertheim, J.A., Whittlesey, K.J., Werner, M.J., Challenging regeneration to transform medicine. *Stem Cells Transl. Med.*, 15, 1, 1–7, 2016.
34. Mason, C. and Dunnill, P., A brief definition of regenerative medicine. *Regener. Med.*, 13, 1, 1–5, 2008.
35. Mendelson, B. and Wong, C.H., Changes in the Facial Skeleton With Aging: Implications and Clinical Applications in Facial Rejuvenation. *Aesthet. Plast. Surg.*, 36, 753–760, 2012, https://doi.org/10.1007/s00266-012-9904-3.
36. Simeone, S.G., Rios, M., Simonpietri, J., "Reverse torque of 30 Ncm applied to dental implants as test for osseointegration"—a human observational study. *Int. J. Implant Dent.*, 2, 1–6, 2016.
37. Ma, P.X., Tissue Engineering, in: *Encyclopedia of Polymer Science and Technology*, 3rd Edition, J.I. Kroschwitz (Ed.), John Wiley & Sons, NJ, 2004.

38. Zhang, R. and Ma, P.X., Synthetic nano-fibrillar extracellular matrices with predesigned macroporous architectures. *J. Biomed. Mater. Res.*, 52, 2, 430–438, 2000.
39. Müller, P. and Schier, A.F., Extracellular movement of signaling molecules. *Dev. Cell*, 21, 1, 145–58, 2011 Jul 19.
40. Vunjak-Novakovic, G. and Kaplan, D.L., Tissue engineering: the next generation Tissue engineering. *Tissue Eng.*, 12, 12, 3261–3, 2006, doi: 10.1089/ten.2006.12.3261.
41. Lu, T., Yang, B., Wang, R., Qin, C., Xenotransplantation: current status in preclinical research. *Front. Immunol.*, 23, 10, 3060, 2020.

2

Anatomical Considerations of Facial Bone Reconstruction

Maryam Alhindi*, Mohammed Binsalah and Afnan AlJuaid

Oral and Maxillofacial Surgery Department, King Saud University, Riyadh, KSA

Abstract

Facial bone grafting is a cornerstone of contemporary oral and maxillofacial surgery, addressing osseous deficiencies resulting from trauma, congenital anomalies, oncologic resection, or alveolar atrophy. Such defects can significantly affect facial aesthetics, mastication, speech, and airway function. Successful reconstruction relies on a comprehensive understanding of regional anatomy, meticulous surgical planning, appropriate material selection, and patient-specific considerations. This chapter provides an anatomically driven, evidence-based overview of orbital, maxillary, and mandibular bone grafting, with emphasis on critical neurovascular structures, radiographic planning, surgical approaches, and potential complications

***Keywords*:** Orbital reconstruction, maxillary reconstruction, mandibular grafting, inferior alveolar nerve, graft materials, anatomical variations, bone augmentation

2.1 Orbital Bone Grafting

Defects of the orbital floor and walls may occur following high-energy trauma, tumour resection, or congenital deformity [1]. Orbital reconstruction is frequently considered challenging due to the complex anatomy of the orbit and its close relationship to vital ocular and neurovascular structures.

**Corresponding author*: mnoo2001@gmail.com

Randa A. Alfotawi (ed.) Oro-Facial Bone Grafts and Biomaterials, (15–34) © 2026 Scrivener Publishing LLC

Orbital reconstruction is always considered a challenge for oral and maxillofacial surgeons due to the unique anatomy of the orbit.

2.1.1 Orbital Wall Anatomy

The orbital floor is formed anteriorly by the maxilla, posteromedially by the palatine bone, and laterally by the zygomatic bone. The medial wall comprises contributions from the maxilla, ethmoid, sphenoid, and lacrimal bones. Accurate anatomical understanding is essential for defect assessment and reconstruction planning (Figure 2.1) [2].

The diagnosis of orbital fracture includes thorough clinical examination and radiographic evaluation. The radiographic examination will include plain radiographs such as Posteroanterior, Occipitomental, and Waters' view. Radiographic evaluation typically includes computed tomography (CT) with three-dimensional reconstruction, which provides detailed visualization of orbital anatomy and fracture extent [1].

Clinical signs and symptoms of orbital fracture include orbital swelling, raccoon's eyes, orbital dystopia, traumatic telecanthus, palpebral haemorrhage, restricted ocular movement, diplopia, and enophthalmos [1–4]. Many other signs and symptoms are associated with facial fractures, such as step deformity, facial depression, and elongated dish face [4, 5].

2.1.2 Classification of Orbital Bone Fracture

Trauma can result in isolated orbital fractures, which account for more than 40% of all craniofacial fractures [5]. Isolated orbital fractures comprise approximately 14–16% of facial fractures and about 30–55% when

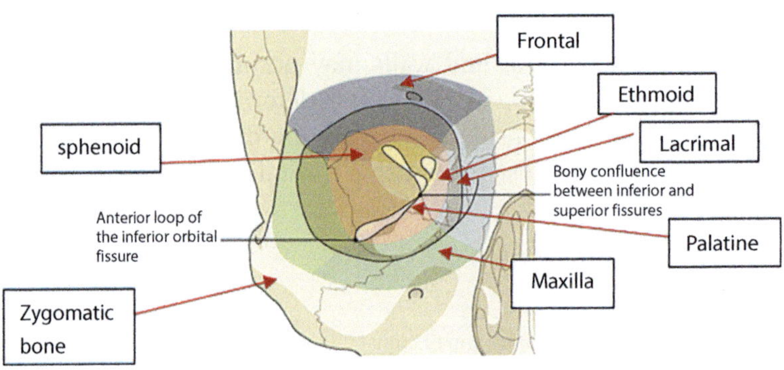

Figure 2.1 Diagrammatic illustration of the bony anatomy of the orbital walls and the orbital cavity.

associated with other facial fractures [6, 7]. Orbital fracture usually occurs medial to the infraorbital groove due to weak bone in this area [8].

The Arbeitsgemeinschaft für Osteosynthesefragen (shortened to AO) for craniomaxillofacial (CMF) has developed three levels of orbital fracture [9]. a) When the force is directed to the malar bone, the fracture occurs at the region of orbito-zygomatic; b) when the impact of force is directed to central upper midface, the fracture occurs at the region of naso-orbito-ethmoid; c) only orbital walls fracture as in case of a blow in or out. Finally, combined orbital wall and frame [9].

2.1.3 Reconstruction of the Orbit

Orbital reconstruction aims to restore the orbital floor, support the globe, restore the orbital shape, and maintain the normal vision in all directions [10]. Replacement of damaged and lost bone can be achieved using bone or soft tissue from a patient's own body, synthetic or natural substitute [11]. The orbit is a pyramidal structure that contains the eye and separates the upper and middle third of the facial bone. Orbital reconstruction aims to restore orbital volume, support the globe, re-establish normal contour, and preserve ocular motility and vision. Reconstruction is generally indicated for defects exceeding approximately 2 cm, persistent diplopia, clinically significant enophthalmos, or radiographic evidence of orbital asymmetry. Early intervention, typically within two weeks of injury, is associated with improved functional and aesthetic outcomes compared with delayed reconstruction [12, 13]. The approaches to orbital floor fractures can be accessed through infraorbital incision, transconjunctival, mid-lower eyelid, subciliary, or transantral using endoscopy [14]. All these approaches will give a clear surgical field with some limitations in each approach [16–18].

The principle of treatment of bone fractures includes exposure of all fractures, reduction, and fixation. The principle of plate fixation includes the use of minimum 4 screws, starting with the screws close to the fracture line. If the floor of the orbit is not indicated for fixation by the absence of enophthalmos and diplopia, then the lateral and infraorbital rim is to be fixed alone [15].

When the fixation of the orbital floor is indicated, the procedure typically starts with the orbital rim, encompassing the frontozygomatic suture, the infraorbital rim, and the zygomaticomaxillary buttress [16]. Reconstruction for the floor of the orbit using a mesh plate is very common, with care not to entrap the inferior rectus muscle with the test using the force ducting technique [5]. Autogenous bone graft, on the other hand,

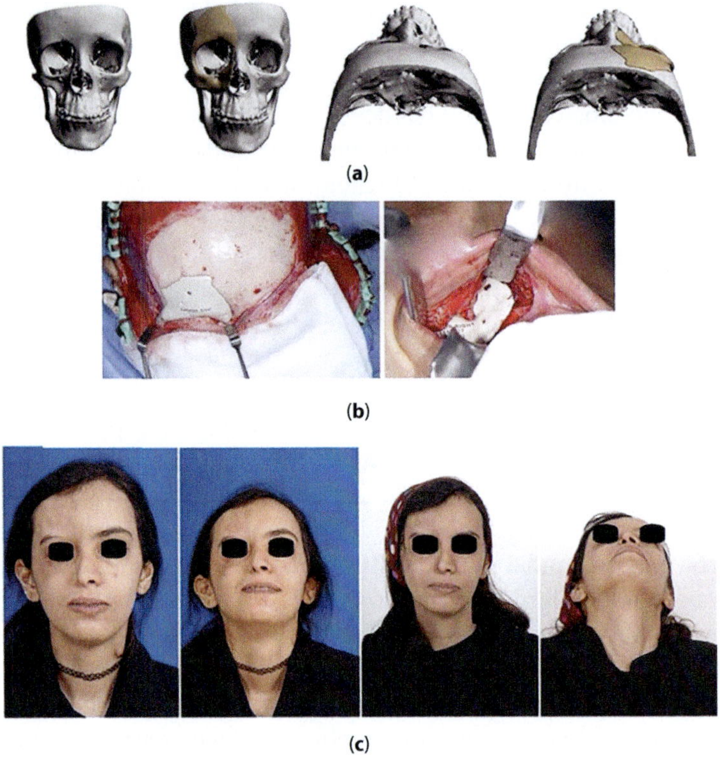

Figure 2.2 Patient-specific implant for orbital construction using peek the image id reprinted from publication: Maxillofacial plastic reconstruction surgery by Alasseri N, Alasaj A. Patient specific implants for maxillofacial defects: challenges and solution 2020;24(15), copyright (2020) with permission from Springer open.

is inexpensive with the disadvantages of increasing the operating time and donor site morbidity [3]. Porous polyethylene is widely used and easy to insert, but it is invisible in radiograph (Figure 2.2) [17]. Titanium with porous polyethene has the advantage of being stronger and visible in radiographs [18]. Preformed implants have the most compatible contour for the medial and floor of the orbit, which will make it easy for adaptation [16]. Nowadays, positive aesthetic result reaches 95.7% in orbital reconstruction using custom-made specific patient implants, using computer-aided design/computer-aided manufacturing (CAD/CAM) technologies [17, 19] (Figure 2.3). Orbital floor construction is not an easy task, and the need for a second surgery is possible if some complication persists.

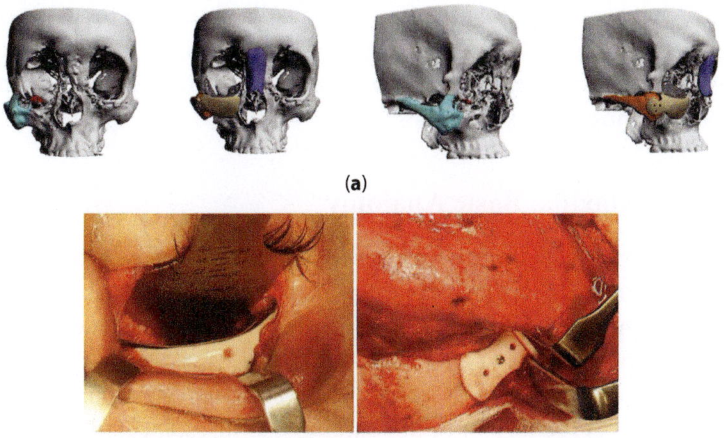

(a)

(b)

Figure 2.3 Patient-specific implant for orbital construction using peek the image ID reprinted from publication: Maxillofacial plastic reconstruction surgery by Alasseri N, Alasaj A. Patient specific implants for maxillofacial defects: challenges and solution 2020;24(15), copyright (2020) with permission from Springer open.

2.1.4 Complication of Orbital Reconstruction

Orbital deformities cause motor and sensory deficit, traumatic telecanthus, lacrimal apparatus injuries [1]. Moreover, more serious complication such as epiphora [20], Ectropion, Diplopia, Dysesthesia, Enophthalmos, extrusion, and iatrogenic vision loss [18]. Secondary revision surgery of orbital complications is mandatory in many cases.

2.2 Maxillary Bone Grafting

Maxillary bone grafting encompasses procedures ranging from alveolar ridge augmentation to complex orthognathic and reconstructive surgeries. The success of these procedures is strongly influenced by detailed anatomical knowledge, particularly of adjacent neurovascular structures and the maxillary sinus. Precise anatomical knowledge is critical not only for achieving optimal aesthetic and functional outcomes but also for minimizing the risk of complications such as nerve damage, oroantral communication haemorrhage, or airway obstruction.

The key anatomical considerations in maxillary surgery focusing on the bony structures, neurovascular elements, maxillary sinus, and surrounding soft tissues will be covered. Each component must be well known during surgical planning and execution.

2.2.1 The Maxilla: Basic Anatomy

The maxilla is a paired bone which made the maxilla and contributes to the structure of the nasal cavity, orbit, and hard palate. It articulates with the nasal bone, zygomatic bone, and palatine bone, playing an essential role in facial function and form [21].

Key features of the maxilla include the following: Maxillary sinus—the maxillary sinus is the largest of the paranasal sinuses, located laterally and inferiorly to the nasal cavity. It plays a critical role in different maxillary surgical procedures, including sinus lift and bone grafting [22]. Alveolar ridge—the maxilla houses the upper alveolar ridge, which supports the upper teeth and acts as a critical structure in surgeries like dental implant insertion and orthognathic surgery [23]. Zygomatic process—this bony extension articulates with the zygomatic bone, contributing to the prominence of the cheek and serving as a crucial landmark. It holds a prominent role in shaping the bony contour of the midface [24]. Hard palate—the anterior part is formed by the maxilla, which is important in procedures such as cleft palate repair [25].

2.2.2 Neurovascular Considerations

A robust understanding of the neurovascular structures surrounding the maxilla is essential to avoid the risk of complications like nerve damage and excessive bleeding. The infraorbital nerve is a branch of the maxillary division of the trigeminal nerve (CN V2), which provides sensation to the lower eyelid, upper lip, and part of the nasal cavity. The infraorbital foramen, situated just below the orbital rim, is the point through which the nerve exits the skull. Damage to this nerve during procedures like orthognathic surgery or sinus procedures may result in sensory disturbances like paraesthesia or numbness [26].

The infraorbital nerve, anterior superior alveolar nerve, and posterior superior alveolar nerve are critical structures that must be preserved during maxillary surgery. Sensory disturbances are uncommon but may occur if these nerves are compromised. Injuries to these nerves rarely occur during procedures like dental extractions or insertion of dental implants.

The maxillary artery gives off multiple branches, including the inferior alveolar and superior alveolar arteries [27]. The pterygoid venous plexus, which receives venous blood from the maxilla and surrounding regions, is another structure that must be carefully considered in maxillary orthognathic surgery. Damage to these vessels during surgery can result in significant haemorrhage [28].

2.2.3 The Pterygopalatine Fossa

The pterygopalatine fossa contains the pterygopalatine ganglion, the maxillary nerve, and branches of the maxillary artery. Understanding the anatomy of the pterygopalatine fossa is critical for procedures such as maxillary osteotomies and bone grafting [29].

2.2.4 The Maxillary Sinus

The maxillary sinus plays a central role in posterior maxillary reconstruction. Lateral antrostomy techniques, as traditionally described by Tatum, and crestal approaches, as advocated by Summers, remain widely used depending on residual bone height and implant planning.

The most common technique for sinus lift is Tatum's classic lateral antrostomy (Figure 2.4). The second most common technique indicated for atrophic maxilla is advocated by Summers, which is a more conservative crestal technique that allows placement of an implant [30].

2.2.5 Key Considerations

Sinus exposure: Precise dissection is mandatory to avoid puncturing the sinus membrane, which can lead to complications such as oroantral communication or sinus infections [31].

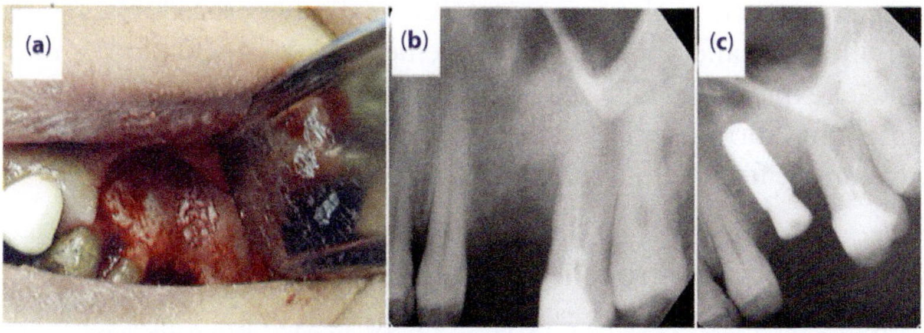

Figure 2.4 (a) Clinical photograph for classic lateral antrostomy for sinus lift. (b) Radiographic assessment after sinus lift. (c) Implant insertion in grafted area.

Sinus septa: Septa could be found within the maxillary sinus, which may complicate access during procedures like sinus grafting [32]. Communication with the nasal cavity: The maxillary sinus communicates with the nasal cavity through the ostium, situated in the middle meatus of the nasal passage. Any disruption of this communication could lead to chronic sinusitis or other sinus-related complications after maxillary sinus grafting [33].

2.2.6 Soft Tissue Considerations

Maxillary surgery involves not only the underlying bone but also the adjacent soft tissues. During maxillary surgery, these tissues must be carefully handled to avoid scarring, altered sensation, or functional impairment.

2.2.6.1 The Buccal Fat Pad

The buccal fat pad located in the cheek is an important consideration in maxillary surgery, especially for aesthetic surgery. Displacement or disruption of this pad could affect facial aesthetics [34].

Muscles of Mastication

The muscles of mastication, including the masseter, temporalis, and pterygoid muscles, should be preserved during maxillary surgery to keep normal jaw function. These muscles have intimate anatomical relationships with the maxilla, and dissection must be done carefully to avoid muscles ptosis of the lower lip, e.g., mentalis muscle in genioplasty [35].

2.2.6.2 Facial Expression Muscles

The levator labii superioris, which lifts the upper lip, and the zygomaticus major, which contributes to smiling, could be affected during surgery. Buccinator muscle is also important during dimple procedures. Injecting facial filler may affect the muscle movement (Myo modulation) and thus the facial expression (Figure 2.5) [36]. Their preservation is essential for maintaining normal facial aesthetics and function postoperatively. With aging, muscle fibres are stretched as skin sags.

2.2.7 Surgical Approaches to the Maxilla

Maxillary surgery can be performed through different approaches, depending on the procedure being performed. Some of the most common approaches include the following.

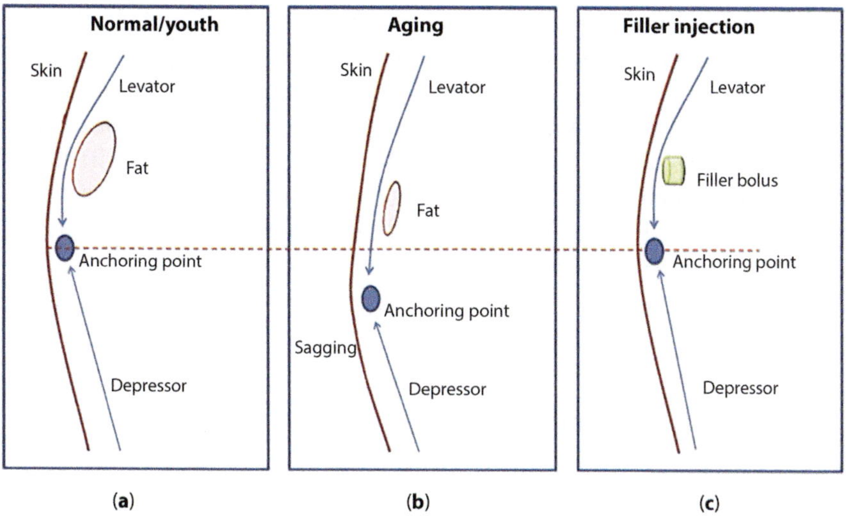

Figure 2.5 The location of levator labii superioris affected with aging, and with injection (Myo modulation) of filler. Levator: levator labii superioris; Depressor: Depressor labii inferiors.

Transoral approach: Used for procedures such as cleft palate repair. This approach allows access to the maxilla with minimal external scarring [37]. Keen approach: It is also a transoral approach through the vestibule used in multiple surgeries like Le Fort osteotomy technique, which is categorized into Le Fort I, II, and III types, and is used in orthognathic surgery in the reposition of the maxilla. Careful attention to the neurovascular structures is essential to avoid complications like nerve damage or bleeding [38]. Endonasal approach: Commonly used for accessing the maxillary sinus, nasal cavity, and for endoscopic sinus surgeries.

2.3 Mandibular Bone Grafting

Mandibular bone grafting is frequently required to address defects resulting from trauma, pathology, or alveolar atrophy, particularly in the posterior mandible. A substantial proportion of patients undergoing implant therapy may require augmentation to achieve adequate bone volume [1]. The dense cortical structure of the mandible and proximity to the inferior alveolar nerve necessitate careful surgical planning to minimize neurosensory complications and ensure graft stability [39].

Approximately 30% of patients undergoing dental implant therapy require augmentation, with the posterior mandible being the most affected due to horizontal and vertical atrophy [40]. Since the 1980s, surgical techniques have evolved from conventional onlay autografts to hybrid solutions involving allogenic materials, guided bone regeneration (GBR), and computer-assisted navigation [41]. This section aims to provide a region-specific and anatomically guided framework for mandibular grafting. It incorporates surgical planning strategies, material considerations, procedural protocols, and complication management, grounded in current evidence and best practices.

2.3.1 Surgical Anatomy of the Mandible

The mandible comprises the symphysis, body, angle, ramus, and condyles. The inferior alveolar canal, housing the IAN and artery, in dentate patients, lies approximately 2.4–2.9 mm from the buccal cortex and 9.4–14.8 mm from the inferior border [42]. The mental foramen (MF) is typically located between the first and second premolars and lies 12.0 +/- 1.67 mm to the most apical portion of the lower cortex of the mandible and the mean distance from the MF to cemento-enamel junction MF-CEJ = 15.2 +/- 2.37 mm in dentate patients [43]. Edentulism can reduce this vertical distance, increasing the risk of nerve exposure during surgical procedures. Anatomical variants such as anterior loops have a high prevalence of 88% [43], and accessory mental foramina (AMF) (up to 6.4–10%) demands precise radiographic identification to avoid postoperative paraesthesia; it was estimated at distance of 12.68 ± 4.10 mm to the alveolar ridge [43].

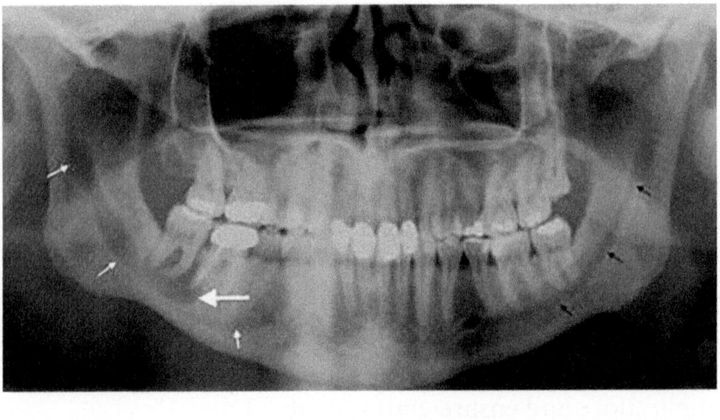

Figure 2.6 Widening of inferior alveolar canal on the right side denoted with white arrows.

The frequency of presence of bifid mandibular canal is in the range of 9.8–66.5% [44], which usually is present in the posterior part of the mandibular canal and may originate from the mandibular canal along its entire course [44]. Widening of the canal is a rare variant of anatomy or part of pathology like neurofibromatosis or lymphoma (Figure 2.6) [45].

The submandibular fossa or lingual concavity poses a risk during posterior grafting. Its depth varies; the average depth of the fossa was 6.9 mm, which significantly decreased with increased age and dental health deterioration, with males and posterior sites exhibiting more pronounced concavities [46]. Perforation of the lingual plate in this region can lead to haemorrhage or graft dislodgement [46].

The lingual vasculature, primarily the sublingual, submental, and facial arteries, provides vital perfusion to the periosteum and floor of the mouth. Inadvertent injury to these vessels during flap elevation or lingual drilling may result in haematoma or airway compromise [47].

2.3.2 Regional Considerations

2.3.2.1 Posterior Mandible

The posterior mandible features thicker cortical bone and prominent undercuts. Lingual concavities are classified as follows: Type U (deep)—highest risk of lingual perforation; type V (moderate) and type flat (shallow) [10]. Thus, CBCT is mandatory to assess concavity depth and canal trajectory. Bone density in this region averages 850–1000 Hounsfield units (HU) [48].

2.3.2.2 Anterior Mandible

The symphysis offers a predictable graft site with dense cortical and cancellous bone. Harvesting should avoid the mental foramen and root apices, preserving a 5-mm safety zone [49]. Prominent genial tubercles may obstruct harvesting but also serve as useful landmarks.

2.3.2.3 Ramus Region

The ramus is ideal for harvesting cortical bone blocks with low morbidity and aesthetic invisibility. The donor site lies between the external oblique ridge and the lingula, staying superior and lateral to the mandibular canal with average available volume: 1.5–3.0 cc [50].

2.3.3 Radiographic and Surgical Planning

Cone-beam computed tomography (CBCT) with recommended protocols include the following: voxel size of ≤0.2 mm for canal visualization, field of view (FOV) focused on the graft site, and adjacent anatomical structures are the modality of choice [51]. CBCT identifies mandibular canal location and variations, lingual concavity depth, and mental foramen position and anterior loop presence and bone volume thickness [52]. Radiopaque markers (e.g., gutta-percha, stents) enhance surgical guide accuracy. On other hand, software such as DTX Studio™, SimPlant™, or Blue Sky Plan™ enables virtual planning and 3D printing of surgical guides [53]. Dynamic navigation systems like X-Guide® provide real-time visualization, improving safety in complex cases and near critical structures [54].

Composite grafts (e.g., autograft + xenograft at 30:70 ratio) combine biological activity with scaffold stability. The addition of platelet-rich fibrin (PRF) or collagen membranes enhances angiogenesis and graft retention [56]. Table 2.1 summarizes the common graft material used for bone regeneration.

2.3.4 Graft Material Selection

Table 2.1 Summary of the types of bone graft which are reported for ridge augmentation and resorption rate.

Material	Resorption time	Osteogenic	Clinical indication	Ref.
Autograft	4–6 months	Yes	Primary reconstruction, vertical defects	[55]
Allograft	6–12 months	No	Ridge preservation, minor horizontal loss	[57]
Xenograft	>12 months	No	Volume maintenance, sinus lifts	[58]
Alloplast	Variable	No	Small, non-load-bearing sites	[59]

2.3.5 Anatomically Driven Surgical Techniques

Onlay grafting: Used to correct horizontal and vertical deficiencies. Autografts are shaped and secured with titanium screws above the canal to prevent compression. Periosteal release is essential for tension-free closure [60].

Interpositional grafting: Requires segmental osteotomy with vertical displacement and graft interposition. Reserved for severe vertical atrophy. Minimum 5-mm residual bone above the canal is required [61].

Symphysis and ramus harvesting: Use piezosurgical instrumentation to minimize IAN trauma. Avoid the midline tubercles, mental foramen, and lingual during flap design and osteotomy [62].

Nerve Protection

Require visualization of the inferior alveolar nerve *via* CBCT and map anterior loop with virtual planning, and utilize dynamic navigation or neurosurgical probes in complex cases [54].

2.3.6 Complications and Anatomical Basis

The possible complications that may occur on the basis of the anatomy of mandible are provided in Table 2.2.

2.3.7 Paediatric and Geriatric Considerations

Paediatrics growth centres must be protected. Avoid harvesting from condyles or near developing dentition. Costochondral or iliac grafts are preferred for large reconstructions [66]. Whereas in geriatrics, bone is often

Table 2.2 Summary of the potential complication for surgery in lower jaw related to the anatomy of the mandible.

Complication	Prevalence	Aetiology	Prevention	Ref.
Mental, inferior alveolar nerve injury	5–10%	Inaccurate depth control	CBCT, use of short screws	[63]
Lingual haemorrhage	<2%	Fossa perforation, vessel laceration	Shallow drilling, fossa mapping	[46]
Flap dehiscence	15–20%	Excess tension, poor closure	Periosteal scoring, collagen membrane	[64]
Graft resorption	Variable	Instability, poor vascularization	Rigid fixation, decortication	[65]

osteoporotic with reduced vascularity. The IAN may be closer to the crest, especially in resorbed ridges. Prefer slow-resorbing materials and allow extended healing periods [67].

2.3.8 Clinical Pearls

- Always perform CBCT for IAN, mental foramen, and lingual undercut assessment [52].
- Maintain ≥5 mm clearance from root apices and neurovascular bundles [43, 44].
- Use piezosurgery in high-risk anatomical zones [62].
- Rigidly fix grafts to prevent resorption.

Use tension-free flaps and PRF to reduce wound complications [64].

2.4 Conclusion

In general, the faciomaxillary surgery is complex and delicate, which requires a thorough understanding of anatomy and its surrounding structures. A careful knowledge of the bony, vascular, and neural anatomy, along with the soft tissue structures, is essential to minimize complications and achieving optimum outcomes. Precision in anatomical knowledge, patient-specific planning, and technical execution determines success in faciomaxillary grafting. Digital imaging, guided surgery, and biologically active materials have improved outcomes. Future advancements in navigation and regenerative materials will further enhance predictability and safety.

AI disclosure statement: The author acknowledges the use of AI-based tools for minor language editing or grammatical correction. However, all intellectual contributions, analyses, and conclusions presented in this chapter are entirely the author's own.

References

1. Gadre, K.S., Kumar, B., Gadre, D.P., Panfacial Fractures, in: *Oral and Maxillofacial Surgery for the Clinician*, K. Bonanthaya, E. Panneerselvam, S. Manuel, V.V. Kumar, A. Rai (Eds.), Springer, Singapore, 2021, https://doi.org/10.1007/978-981-15-1346-6_60.

2. Audigé, C.K.L., Cornelius, C.-P., Buitrago-Téllez, C.H., Rudderman, R., Prein, J., The Comprehensive AOCMF Classification System: Orbital Fractures - Level 3 Tutorial. *Craniomaxillofac. Trauma Reconstr.*, 7, Suppl 1, S092–102, 2014.
3. Malhotra, S., Ahuja, V., Pandey, A.K., Management of Pan-Facial Trauma & Orbital Floor Reconstruction with Iliac Crest Bone Graft. Case report, SIPS Superspeciality Hospital & Trauma Centre, Lucknow (U.P.) India, 2019.
4. He, Blomquist, P.H., Ellis, E., Association Between Ocular Injuries and Internal Orbital Fractures. *J. Oral Maxillofac. Surg.*, 65, 4, 713–20, 2007, doi: 10.1016/j.joms.2006.09.006.
5. Emam, H.A. and Krishnan, D.G., Orbital and Ocular Trauma, in: *Peterson's Principles of Oral and Maxillofacial Surgery*, M. Miloro, G. Ghlia, P. Larsen, P. Waite (Eds.), p. 707, Springer Nature, Cham, Swizerland, 2022.
6. Kim, H.S. and Jeong, E.C., Orbital Floor Fracture. *Arch. Craniofac. Surg.*, 17, 3, 111–118, Sep. 2016, doi: 10.7181/acfs.2016.17.3.111.
7. Mc, M., *et al.*, Topographical CT-data analysis of the human orbital floor. *Int. J. Oral Maxillofac. Surg.*, 36, 1, 45–53, 2007.
8. Chodankar, N.U., Dhupar, V., Vijay, V., Classifications and Theories of Orbital Fractures: A Review of Literature. *Med. Res. Chronicles*, 10, 4, 248–260, 2023.
9. Cornelius, C.P., Audigé, L., Kunz, C., Buitrago-Téllez, C.H., Rudderman, R., Prein, J., The Comprehensive AOCMF Classification System: Midface Fractures - Level 3 Tutorial. *Craniomaxillofac. Trauma Reconstr.*, 7, Suppl 1, S068–91, 2014 Dec, doi: 10.1055/s-0034-1389561. PMID: 25489392; PMCID: PMC4251725.
10. Bahr, W., Bagambisa, F., Schlegel, G., Schilli, W., Comparison of transcutaneous incisions used for the exposure of the infraorbital rim and orbital floor: A retrospective study. *Plast. Reconstr. Surg.*, 90, 585–91, 1992, doi: 10.1097/00006534-199210000-00006.
11. Burnstine, M.A., Clinical recommendations for repair of orbital facial fractures. *Curr. Opin. Ophthalmol.*, 14, 236–240, 2003, doi: 10.1097/00055735-200310000-00002.
12. Levin, L.M. and Kademani, D., Clinical considerations in the management of orbital blow-out fractures. *Compend. Contin. Educ. Dent.*, 18, 593–602, 1997.
13. Dutton, J.J., Management of blow-out fractures of the orbital floor. *Surv. Ophthalmol.*, 35, 279–280, 1991, doi: 10.1016/0039-6257(91)90048-k.
14. Lee, M.J., Kang, Y.S., Yang, J.Y., Lee, D.Y., Chung, Y.Y., Rohrich, R.J., Endoscopic transnasal approach for the treatment of medial orbital blow-out fracture: A technique for controlling the fractured wall with a balloon catheter and Merocel. *Plast. Reconstr. Surg.*, 110, 417–426, 2002, doi: 10.1097/00006534-200208000-00006. [DOI] [PubMed] [Google Scholar].
15. Gadkari, N., Bawane, S., Chopra, R., Bhate, K., Kulkarni, D., Comparative evaluation of 2-point vs 3-point fixation in the treatment of zygomaticomaxillary complex fractures–a systematic review. *J. Craniomaxillofac. Surg.*, 47, 10, 1542–50, 2019 Oct 1.

16. Goh, *et al.*, Surgical management of naso-orbito-ethmoidal fractures: a systematic review. *Oral Maxillofac. Surg.*, 138, 1, 9–20, July 2024.
17. Alasseri, N. and Alasseri, A., Patient-specific implant for maxillofacial defect: challenges and solutions. *Maxillofac. Plast. Reconstr. Surg.*, 42, 15, 2020, https//doi.org/10.1186/s40902-02000262-7.
18. Harris, G.J., Avoiding complications in the repair of orbital floor fractures. *JAMA Facial Plast. Surg.*, 16, 4, 290–5, 2014 Jul 1.
19. Chepurnyi, Y., Chernogorskyi, D., Petrenko, O., Kopchak, A., Reconstruction of Post-Traumatic Orbital Defects and Deformities with Custom-Made Patient-Specific Implants: Evaluation of the Efficacy and Clinical Outcome. *Craniomaxillofac. Trauma Reconstr. Open*, 3, 1, 2020, doi: 10.1055/s-0039-1685505.
20. Boulos, P., Harris, G., Frenette, G., Long term complications of orbital floor fracture repair. *Can. J. Plast. Surg.*, 9, 5, 183–192, 2001.
21. Shendge, V., Anatomical Considerations in Maxillofacial Surgery and Rehabilitation, in: *Prosthetic Rehabilitation of Head and Neck Cancer Patients*, pp. 5–61, Elsevier, Amesterdam, Netherland, 2024.
22. Anand, R.S., Gopinath, A., Ramasamy, S., Maxillary sinus and its role in maxillary surgery. *J. Oral Maxillofac. Surg.*, 77, 2, 155–160, 2019.
23. Jung, S.I., Choi, J.S., Lee, S.K., Maxillary alveolar ridge anatomy and its implications for implant surgery. *Clin. Implant Dent. Relat. Res.*, 19, 6, 1000–1006, 2017.
24. Hwang, C.H. and Lee, M.C., Revision malarplasty guided by strategic categorization. *J. Plast. Reconstr. Aesthet. Surg.*, 72, 2, 322–334, 2019.
25. Chigurupati, R., Heggie, A., Bonanthaya, K., Cleft lip and palate: an overview, in: *Oral and Maxillofacial Surgery*, pp. 945–72, Wiley-Blackwell, Oxford, 2010.
26. Kim, Y.K., Complications associated with orthognathic surgery. *J. Korean Assoc. Oral Maxillofac. Surg.*, 43, 1, 3–15, 2017 Feb.
27. Otake, I., Kageyama, I., Mataga, I., Clinical anatomy of the maxillary artery. *Okajimas Folia Anat. Jpn.*, 87, 4, 155–64, 2011.
28. Peysakhov, D. and Ferneini, A., Vascular Injuries as a Complication of Maxillofacial Surgery, in: *Perioperative Assessment of the Maxillofacial Surgery Patient: Problem-based Patient Management*, pp. 691–707, Springer International Publishing, Cham, 2017 Nov 10.
29. Roberti, F., *et al.*, The pterygopalatine fossa: an anatomic report. *J. Craniofac. Surg.*, 183, 586–90, 2007, doi: 10.1097/scs.0b013e31805343c2.
30. Woo, I. and Le, B.T., Maxillary Sinus Floor Elevation: Review of Anatomy and Two Techniques. *Implant Dent.*, 13, 1, 28–32, 2004, DOI: 10.1097/01.ID.0000116369.66716.12.
31. Timmenga, N.M., *et al.*, Maxillary sinus floor elevation surgery. A clinical, radiographic and endoscopic evaluation. *Clin. Oral Implants Res.*, 14, 3, 322–8, 2003, doi: 10.1034/j.1600-0501.2003.140310.x.

32. Malec, M., Smektała, T., Trybek, G., Sporniak-Tutak, K., Maxillary sinus septa: prevalence, morphology, diagnostics and implantological implications. Systematic review. *Folia Morphol.*, 73, 3, 259–66, 2014.
33. Saibene, A.M., Wallace, S.S., Scaini, R., Maxillary Sinus Grafting Complications: Diagnosis, Management, Patient Outcomes, and Role of Multidisciplinary Care. *Clin. Implant Dent. Relat. Res.*, 27, 2, e13420, 2025 Apr.
34. Brown, K., McCoskey, M., Nakra, T., Complications of facial autologous fat grafting. *Plast. Aesthet. Res.*, 11, 7, 2024.
35. Avelar, R.L.S., Esses, C.D.L., Becker, D.F.S., Soares, O.E., de Oliveira, E.C.S., Belle, R., Unusual Complication After Genioplasty. *J. Craniofac. Surg.*, 25, 2, e180–e182, March 2014, DOI: 10.1097/SCS.0000000000000618.
36. de Maio, M., Myomodulation with Injectable Fillers: An Innovative Approach to Addressing Facial Muscle Movement. *Aesthet. Plast. Surg.*, 42, 798–814, 2018, https://doi.org/10.1007/s00266-018-1116-z.
37. Pucci, R., Cassoni, A., Weyh, A., Mangini, N., Della Monaca, M., Battisti, A., Fernandes, R., Valentini, V., Transoral versus transfacial surgical approach to maxillary tumors: evaluation of outcomes and perspectives. *Int. J. Oral Maxillofac. Surg.*, 53, 2, 101–8, 2024 Feb 1.
38. Gill, D.S., Naini, F.B., Koudstaal, M., Soft tissue effect of Orthognathic Surgery, in: *Orthognathic surgery: Principles and practice*, F.B. Naini and D.S. Gill (Eds.), pp. 341–347, Wily Blackwell, Hoboken, New Jersey, USA, 2017.
39. Greenstein, G. and Tarnow, D., The mental foramen and nerve: clinical and anatomical review. *J. Periodontol.*, 77, 12, 1933–1943, 2006.
40. Urban, I.A., Monje, A., Lozada, J.L., Wang, H.L., Long-term outcomes of vertical bone augmentation: a systematic review. *J. Periodontol.*, 88, 12, 1220–1228, 2017.
41. Block, M.S. and Emery, R.W., Static and dynamic navigation for dental implant placement: accuracy and clinical implications. *J. Oral Maxillofac. Surg.*, 74, 2, 269–277, 2016.
42. Kim, S.T., Hu, K.S., Song, W.C., *et al.*, Location of the mandibular canal and measurement of the thickness of the mandibular cortex using CBCT in Koreans. *J. Oral Maxillofac. Surg.*, 68, 2, 283–289, 2010.
43. Neiva, R.F., Gapski, R., Wang, H.L., Morphometric analysis of the mental foramen using CT scan. *J. Periodontol.*, 75, 10, 1231–1238, 2004.
44. von Arx, T. and Lozanoff, S., Bifid mandibular canals: literature review and case report. *J. Oral Maxillofac. Surg.*, 69, 10, 2668–2671, 2011.
45. Vartiainen, V.M., *et al.*, Widening of the inferior alveolar canal: a case report with atypical lymphocytic infiltration of the nerve. *Oral Surg. Oral Med. Oral Pathol. Oral Radiol. Endod.*, 106, 4, e35–9, 2008.
46. Watanabe, H., Mohammad, A.R., Hassan, B., *et al.*, Morphometric analysis of the submandibular fossa using CBCT. *Clin. Implant Dent. Relat. Res.*, 12, 1, 100–104, 2010.

47. Flanagan, D., Complications of mandibular implant surgery. *J. Oral Implantol.*, 38, 3, 233–241, 2012.
48. Kainulainen, V.T., Suuronen, R., Lindqvist, C., Hemorrhage from lingual vessels after dental implant surgery: case report and literature review. *J. Oral Maxillofac. Surg.*, 56, 12, 1441–1445, 1998.
49. Gungormus, M. and Celik, H.H., Evaluation of the shape and depth of the mandibular lingual concavity in relation to implant placement. *J. Nihon Univ. Sch. Dent.*, 41, 1, 23–26, 1999.
50. Mangano, C., Mangano, F., Piattelli, A., Histologic evaluation of human bone taken from the mandible using trephine. *J. Periodontol.*, 82, 3, 379–385, 2011.
51. Cordaro, L. and Torsello, F., Harvesting autogenous bone from the symphysis: a 5-year clinical and radiographic follow-up. *Clin. Oral Implants Res.*, 17, 3, 289–296, 2006.
52. Jacobs, R. and Quirynen, M., Dental cone beam CT: justification for use in planning oral implant placement. *Clin. Oral Implants Res.*, 24, Suppl A100, 131–138, 2013.
53. D'haese, J., Ackhurst, J., Wismeijer, D., *et al.*, Current state of the art of computer-guided implant surgery. *Periodontol. 2000*, 73, 1, 121–133, 2017.
54. Emery, R.W., Merritt, S.A., Lank, K., Gibbs, J.D., Accuracy of dynamic navigation for dental implant placement–model-based evaluation. *J. Oral Implantol.*, 42, 5, 399–405, 2016.
55. Chiapasco, M., Casentini, P., Zaniboni, M., Bone augmentation procedures in implant dentistry. *Int. J. Periodontics Restor. Dent.*, 29, 4, 377–385, 2009.
56. Wallace, S.S. and Froum, S.J., Effect of maxillary sinus augmentation on the survival of endosseous dental implants. *Ann. Periodontol.*, 8, 1, 328–343, 2003.
57. Le, B.T. and Borzabadi-Farahani, A., Simultaneous implant placement and bone grafting with particulate mineralized allograft in sites with buccal wall defects, a three-year follow-up and review of literature. *J. Craniomaxillofac. Surg.*, 42, 5, 552–9, 2014 Jul 1.
58. Schlegel, K.A. and Donath, K., Bio-Oss® as a bone substitute in sinus augmentation. *J. Long-Term Eff. Med. Implants*, 8, 3–4, 201–209, 1998.
59. Subash, P., Nerurkar, S.A., Krishnadas, A., *et al.*, Patient Specific Alloplastic Implant Reconstruction of Mandibular Defects–Safe Practice Recommendations and Guidelines. *J. Maxillofac. Oral Surg.*, 22, Suppl 1, 28–36, 2023, https://doi.org/10.1007/s12663-023-01881-.
60. De Groot, R.J., Oomens, M.A., Forouzanfar, T., Schulten, E.A., Bone augmentation followed by implant surgery in the edentulous mandible: a systematic review. *J. Oral Rehabil.*, 45, 4, 334–43, 2018 Apr.
61. Marconcini, S., Covani, U., Giammarinaro, E., Velasco-Ortega, E., De Santis, D., Alfonsi, F., Barone, A., Clinical success of dental implants placed in posterior mandible augmented with interpositional block graft: 3-year results from a prospective cohort clinical study. *J. Oral Maxillofac. Surg.*, 77, 2, 289–98, 2019 Feb 1.

62. Vercellotti, T., Technological characteristics and clinical indications of piezoelectric bone surgery. *Minerva Stomatol.*, 53, 5, 207–214, 2004.
63. Bartling, R., Freeman, K., Kraut, R.A., The incidence of altered sensation of the mental nerve after mandibular implant placement. *J. Oral Maxillofac. Surg.*, 57, 12, 1408–1412, 1999.
64. Von Doering, M., Longoni, S., Gonzalez-Martin, O., *et al.*, Flap management techniques for peri-implant plastic surgery. *Int. J. Oral Maxillofac. Implants*, 36, 1, e1–e12, 2021.
65. Simion, M., Baldoni, M., Zaffe, D., Jawbone resorption after vertical ridge augmentation with membranes and different grafts. *Clin. Oral Implants Res.*, 5, 1, 22–29, 1994.
66. Eppley, B.L., Use of costochondral grafts in pediatric mandibular reconstruction. *J. Oral Maxillofac. Surg.*, 60, 9, 1031–1036, 2002.
67. Atwood, D.A., Reduction of residual ridges: a major oral disease entity. *J. Prosthet. Dent.*, 13, 5, 810–824, 1963.

3

Bone and Bone Substitutes Grafts Resorption Rate

Raniah Abdullah Al Eid

Department of Oral and Maxillofacial Surgery, College of Dentistry, King Saud University, Riyadh, Saudi Arabia

Abstract

Bone graft resorption is a critical biological process that influences the stability, volume maintenance, and long-term performance of grafted sites in oral and maxillofacial reconstruction. Understanding the resorption behaviour of different graft materials is essential for anticipating clinical outcomes, optimizing treatment planning, and selecting materials appropriate to specific anatomical and functional requirements. The chapter begins with an introduction to the significance of bone grafting in various surgical contexts, highlighting the limitations of autografts, such as donor-site morbidity and availability, while discussing alternatives like allografts and synthetic materials. It outlines the mechanisms of bone graft healing and remodeling, emphasizing the roles of osteogenesis, osteoinduction, and osteoconduction. The chapter categorizes different types of bone grafts: autografts, allografts, xenografts, and synthetic materials, detailing their resorption rates and factors influencing these rates, including patient-related, material properties, and graft site factors. It presents examination techniques for assessing bone healing and graft integration, such as histological analysis, immunohistochemistry, radiographic evaluation, and microcomputed tomography. The discussion extends to strategies for prolonging structural support of grafts, including the use of slowly resorbing materials and surface modifications. The chapter concludes by underscoring the importance of understanding the resorption rates of various graft materials to optimize clinical outcomes in bone regeneration. Future advancements in tissue engineering and biomaterials are anticipated to enhance the integration and effectiveness of bone substitutes, aiming for an ideal balance between stability and biological integration.

Email: dr.raniahaleid@hotmail.com

Randa A. Alfotawi (ed.) Oro-Facial Bone Grafts and Biomaterials, (35–72) © 2026 Scrivener Publishing LLC

***Keywords*:** Resorption rates, remodeling, graft integration, controlled resorption

3.1 Introduction

Bone grafting and bone substitutes are pivotal in modern bone surgery, particularly for addressing bone defects in trauma, oncology, and arthroplasty revision. Although autogenous bone grafts are considered the gold standard, they come with notable drawbacks—mainly the potential complications at the donor site and the limited supply of usable bone. Alternatives such as allografts and synthetic substitutes have been explored to mitigate these challenges, but each presents its own set of advantages and drawbacks.

Autogenous bone grafts excel due to their unparalleled osteogenic, osteoinductive, and osteoconductive properties. However, complications arise from donor site harvesting and limited supply. They also demonstrate up to 50% resorption, sequestration, and insufficient integration [1]. Allografts offer convenience and reduced donor-site morbidity but are hindered by a risk of immune responses, infection, and diminished osteogenic potential due to sterilization and storage processes. On the other hand, their resorption rates vary but are slower than autografts due to the absence of living cells [1].

Synthetic bone substitutes like ceramics such as hydroxyapatite and tricalcium phosphate stand out for their structural similarity to natural bone and osteoconductive properties. However, their mechanical brittleness and variable biodegradation rates limit their applications in load-bearing sites. Regarding resorption, hydroxyapatite (HA) reported long resorption time up to 6 years [2]. The biodegradability of HA is influenced by several material properties, including the sintering temperature, overall porosity, and the diameter of its pores, all of which play a crucial role in determining how the material interacts with biological environments [2]. Meanwhile, advanced materials like calcium phosphate cement show promise with their injectability and potential for minimally invasive procedures. Bone remodeling occurred synchronously with the resorption of the graft material in a creeping substitution process [3]. An ideal graft must strike a balance between stability and biological integration resorbing slowly enough to maintain structural support, yet quickly enough to allow natural bone remodeling.

Clinicians must carefully consider factors such as defect size, site-specific mechanical requirements, infection risks, and economic implications when selecting graft materials. Moreover, advancements in tissue engineering and biomaterial science hold promise for developing next-generation bone substitutes that integrate osteogenesis, osteoinduction, and osteoconduction, exhibiting an ideal resorption rate while minimizing complications. Future developments should focus on optimizing biocompatibility, enhancing mechanical strength, optimizing the graft resorption rate matching bone formation, and thus improving integration with host tissues. Understanding the nuanced properties of existing bone grafts and substitutes remains integral to achieving successful clinical outcomes. This chapter focuses on a crucial parameter for bone regeneration and integration, which is the resorption rate of different graft material with up-to-date literature support.

3.2 Examination Techniques of Bone Healing, Remodeling, and Graft Integration

3.2.1 Histological and Histomorphometric

Histological and histomorphometric analyses provide detailed insight into cellular response, new bone formation, and residual graft material at the microscopic level. These methods are widely regarded as reference techniques for evaluating graft integration and tissue response in both experimental and clinical studies. Histological analysis provides a qualitative information on bone healing, whereas histomorphometric analysis emphasizes quantitative information [20].

3.2.2 Immunohistochemistry (IHC)

It is a popular biological technique that integrates biochemical, anatomical, physiological and immunological features. IHC, which originated from the antigen-antibody complex, is a method for visualizing the distribution and localization of specific antigens or cellular components in separated tissues or tissue slices [4].

3.2.3 Radiographic Evaluation

Radiographic assessment, including panoramic radiography, computed tomography (CT), and cone-beam computed tomography (CBCT), is routinely employed to evaluate graft volume changes and structural stability over time. While radiographic methods are valuable for longitudinal monitoring, their accuracy varies according to imaging modality, resolution, and anatomical site. A technetium-99 scan employs radiolabeled diphosphonates, such as technetium-99m-methyl diphosphonate (99mTc-MDP) and technetium-99m-hydroxymethylene diphosphonate (99mTc-HMDP), to assess bone activity. In addition, fluorine-18 sodium fluoride is used as a tracer for both bone perfusion and turnover. Once administered intravenously, these bone-seeking radiotracers primarily localize by adsorbing onto or within the crystalline structure of hydroxyapatite. In circulation, 99mTc-MDP demonstrates progressive protein binding, increasing from approximately 25% at the time of injection to nearly 50% after four hours. Only the unbound portion of the tracer is available for uptake into bone. The interaction of extravascular 99mTc-diphosphonates with bone is primarily driven by physicochemical adsorption (chemisorption) onto hydroxyapatite in bone tissue [5].

3.2.4 Microcomputed Tomography (μCT)

Microcomputed tomography (μCT) is a non-invasive imaging technique that produces high-resolution, three-dimensional (3D) visualizations of hard tissues, with spatial resolutions reaching up to $6 \times 6 \times 6\ \mu m^2$. Given its ability to accurately depict the three-dimensional architecture of bone with morphometric detail comparable to conventional histomorphometry, μCT is well suited for evaluating the remodeling process of bone substitute materials after healing, particularly in the context of the human jaw [6].

Computed tomography (CT) offers a reliable and reproducible method for measuring bone density, providing standardized values on the Hounsfield unit (HU) scale—a quantitative measure of radiodensity. In contrast, alternative imaging techniques like cone-beam computed tomography (CBCT) and intraoral radiographs lack the precision required for accurate bone density assessment [7]. CT imaging is also instrumental in evaluating changes in bone graft volume, as it enables the reconstruction and analysis of graft dimensions using volumetric data [8]. Alternative methods, including linear measurements using calipers and periodontal probes or through radiographic techniques, fail to yield three-dimensional data regarding bone graft volume.

3.3 Mechanism of Bone Graft Healing

The process of bone healing is dependent on mechanical stability, revascularization, osteogenesis, osteoinduction, and osteoconduction. The process of osteoinduction entails encouraging the differentiation of pluripotent stem cells into cells capable of producing bone. Some grafts integrate into the body quickly, while others take longer. Inflammation and rejection can occur with some of the transplants, while there are grafts that do not show any biological effect (BIOINERT). The three key components that aid in bone repair are osteoprogenitor cells, an osteoconductive collagen matrix made of hydroxyapatite, and bone matrix protein [9]. Bone grafts facilitate wound healing and new bone development by acting as a scaffold. To support new bone formation, graft materials also act as a reservoir for essential minerals. A wide range of bone graft types and substitutes exist, originating from various sources. While the use of bone grafting dates back over three centuries, the underlying biological mechanisms that contribute to its role in promoting bone healing have been increasingly elucidated over the past 30 years through ongoing research [10]. Three primary pathways are involved in the stimulation of osteogenesis by fresh autogenous bone transplant [10, 11]. Introducing osteogenic progenitor cells into the site is the initial step. The process of cell differentiation into new bone-producing cells requires these cells. Secondly, autogenous bone graft provides a framework within which osteoblasts can connect, and osteoconductivity provides a matrix over which supporting cells can adhere. Thirdly, osteoinduction is a term that describes the bone graft's capacity to attract localized mesenchymal cells and guide their development into cells capable of producing bone and cartilage. Autografts contain a rich array of bone growth factors that facilitate the formation of new blood vessels to nourish the graft and attract bone-forming cells to the site of injury [11]. Beyond their biological role, bone grafts also provide critical structural support. The healing process involves several stages—induction, inflammation, soft callus formation, hard callus development, and remodeling—all of which occur in conjunction with the integration of the graft material.

There is a strong relationship between the morphology and the mechanical circumstances surrounding the defect. Chamay A and Tschantz P postulated that during bone remodeling, compression-electronegative regions would enhance bone production. Bone resorption is accelerated in tension-electropositive regions [12]. For the defect to repair, mechanical stability is crucial [13]. Endosseous wound healing progresses through distinct stages, beginning with hematoma formation, followed by clot resorption and the migration of osteogenic cells to the injury site, ultimately leading to new bone formation. The bone healing phase includes three key processes: osteoconduction, which relies on the recruitment and guided migration of bone-forming cells to the implant surface; osteogenesis, where new bone is generated; and finally, osseous remodeling, which refines and strengthens the newly formed bone structure. Serum proteins adhere immediately post-implantation, while mesenchymal cells attach and multiply throughout the initial three days.

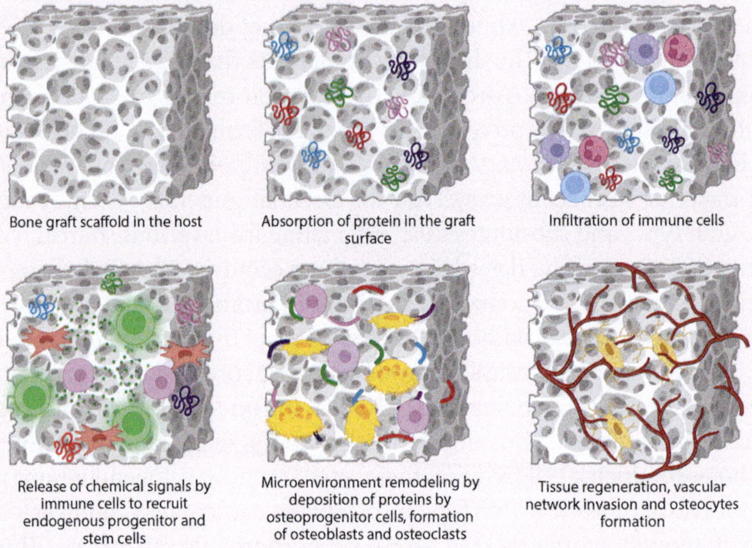

Figure 3.1 Bone graft implantation into the host: which indicates initial protein incorporation inside the graft followed by inflammatory cells infiltration, then release of chemicals from the inflammatory cells that recruit stem cells and endogenous progenitor cells, differentiation of osteoprogenitor cells into osteoblasts and osteoclasts that start process of remodeling of the graft, then finally tissue regeneration after vascular invasion and subsequent formation of osteocytes.

Osteoid development takes six days, while matrix calcification transpires by fourteen days. Remodeling commences in three weeks [14].

A bone graft's rate of disintegration and resorption might vary greatly based on the graft type and the patient's biological milieu [15]. The duration of time that the graft material sustains the healing process before being replaced by native bone is determined by these rates, which are critical success criteria for bone grafting surgeries. Stages of bone graft scaffold integration are illustrated (in Figure 3.1).

3.4 Bone Remodeling

Bone remodeling is a dynamic process involving the resorption of damaged or necrotic bone by osteoclasts, followed by the formation of new bone by osteoblasts, all aimed at repairing skeletal injury. Once new bone is formed, it is maintained and reshaped through two distinct but complementary processes: modeling, which alters bone structure in response to mechanical forces, and remodeling, which renews bone tissue. Both mechanisms play essential roles in the healing of fractures and other bone injuries [16]. Bone remodeling is a continuous physiological process that starts during early fetal development and remains vital throughout life. It plays a key role in maintaining skeletal integrity by consistently replacing old or damaged bone tissue with newly formed bone, thereby ensuring optimal bone function and strength.

Bone repair is unique among tissues as it reflects the developmental processes that transpire during embryonic skeletal formation. This procedure enables the entire restoration of the impaired organ to its pre-injury composition, architecture, and functionality [17].

Bone healing can be classified based on several influencing factors, one of which is the extent of tissue loss. This and other criteria help determine the nature and progression of the repair process [43]. The remodeling of the graft is a complex process influenced by anatomical, metabolic, genetic, and biomechanical aspects [18, 19]. The components fluctuate among individuals, and the diverse contributions from various elements explain the disparities in remodeling between them [20]. Bone grafts typically experience significant remodeling and resorption within the initial year post-surgery; thus, identifying characteristics of the grafts that may predict their resorption is very important. Some researchers suggest that the resorption rate of bone grafts may be linked to their embryologic origin. Specifically, grafts derived from membranous bone—such as those harvested from the calvaria or mandible—tend to show greater resistance to resorption compared to grafts obtained from endochondral bone sources, like the iliac crest [21, 22, 43]. Additionally, other studies have found that cancellous bone grafts resorb more rapidly than cortical bone grafts, leading to the conclusion that resorption is primarily determined by the structural and microarchitectural characteristics of the grafts [23–25]. The density of bone grafts may correlate with their resorption rates, in which high-density grafts have less resorption compared to low-density grafts [26]. The relationship between graft density and the rate of bone resorption may play a pivotal role in understanding the underlying mechanisms that influence the biological performance and longevity of bone grafts.

3.5 Types of Bone Grafts and Their Resorption Rates

3.5.1 Autografts

These grafts are derived from the patient's own body. They have variable resorption rates but tend to integrate well. Autografts assimilate and undergo remodeling throughout time when they are substituted by new bone. These grafts demonstrate minimal degradation and are widely considered the gold standard for bone healing due to their combined osteogenic, osteoconductive, and osteoinductive properties. They can exhibit up to 50% resorption, along with risks of sequestration and poor integration with the surrounding bone [1]. The pursuit of alternatives to bone autografts, prompted by the scarcity of donor sites and the risk of donor-related complications, has been a persistent emphasis [27]. The effectiveness of bone grafts is largely influenced by the presence of osteocompetent cells within the graft material, the vascular accessibility of the recipient site, and the lack of an adverse immune response [28]. It is recommended to use autografts instead of allografts or xenografts.

3.5.1.1 Source

Bone taken from the patient himself is the source of autografts. When it comes to osteogenesis, the area from which autografts are extracted is equally crucial. Sources include both intraoral and extraoral locations. Common intraoral donor sites include the mandibular symphysis, retromolar region, and maxillary tuberosity, while extraoral options include the iliac crest, calvarium, fibula, tibia, and ribs. Bypassing the need for a new set of veins allows for the autologous transplant of tissue from the same donor, eliminating the risk of infection. Not only that, it creates a source of live cells that the body does not reject. Because "creeping substitution" develops significantly more quickly in autografts, they are favored, especially when osteogenesis is the main goal. During revascularization, the porous and open nature of spongious bone facilitates the dilation of newly created blood vessels. Blood is supplied to the graft early with microanastomoses; however, vascular invasion can be prevented by using a bone graft that is more compact. Haversian channels are the sole means by which blood can enter the blood vessels. The surface area of spongious bone is larger than that of compact bone; therefore, more osteoprogenitor cells are present; osteogenesis and callus development are also easier [22, 29].

Once the graft is well established, the formation of a pool of mesenchymal stem cells by the new capillaries in the transplanted microcavities is the first thing that is noticed. These cells can potentially develop into cell lines that are osteogenic, chondrogenic, or fibrogenic.

3.5.1.2 Resorption Rate

3.5.1.2.1 Cancellous Autografts

Cancellous autografts are the most commonly used form of autologous bone grafting. Although only a small number of osteoblasts and osteocytes survive the transplantation process, a significant population of mesenchymal stem cells (MSCs) remains viable despite ischemic conditions, thereby maintaining the graft's osteogenic capacity and its ability to generate new bone [23]. The large surface area of cancellous grafts further facilitates rapid revascularization and promotes effective integration with the surrounding host bone. The proteins produced from the graft, responsible for its osteoinduction, are retained and present when the autografts are properly processed [1, 22]. In the early phase of autograft transplantation, bleeding and inflammation rapidly set in, triggering the recruitment of mesenchymal stem cells that contribute to the formation of fibrous granulation tissue. At the same time, macrophages begin clearing necrotic graft material, while new blood vessels start to form. As the graft integrates, osteoblasts deposit osteoid along the necrotic surfaces, and hematopoietic cells within the graft contribute to new bone formation. The complete resorption and replacement of the graft by native bone typically occurs over a period of 6 to 12 months [29, 30, 32].

3.5.1.2.2 Cortical Autografts

Cortical autografts offer enhanced structural strength and mechanical stability, largely due to their dense composition and relatively low content of osteoprogenitor cells [24, 33]. Unlike cancellous autografts, the integration of cortical grafts occurs predominantly through osteoclast-mediated resorption, following the rapid onset of hematoma and inflammation during the early stages of healing. The dense architecture of cortical bone impedes both revascularization and remodeling, delaying these processes compared to cancellous grafts. Typically, revascularization of cortical grafts takes at least 1–2 months—approximately twice the time required for cancellous grafts [34]. Consequently, cortical graft incorporation primarily occurs through appositional bone formation on the surface of the necrotic graft core after osteoclastic resorption has taken place [23, 24]. The duration of this procedure may extend over several years, contingent upon the size of the graft and the place of implantation [34].

Most autografts have a certain extent of resorption, leading to a reduction in volume over time. Particularly endochondral grafts frequently experience erratic resorption rates. The resorption of autologous bone grafts presents a significant challenge and must be carefully considered when planning reconstructive procedures, as it can compromise long-term stability and clinical outcomes [34]. This resorption is varied and contingent upon numerous parameters, including the sample and recipient locations [35]. On average, onlay bone grafts harvested from the iliac crest have been reported to undergo approximately 15% resorption [35]. Grafts obtained from the mandibular ramus and parietal bone exhibited no significant difference in postoperative resorption after a 4-month period. Both sites demonstrated an average resorption rate of approximately 25%, regardless of the variables assessed [34].

Similar bone resorption rates have been reported in the literature. Gultekin *et al.* observed that grafts harvested from the mandibular ramus exhibited resorption rates ranging between 5% and 28% [29]. Cordaro *et al.* conducted a prospective study involving 18 ramus grafts in 15 patients and reported resorption rates ranging from 23% to 42% over a 4-month healing period [36]. In a separate study, Iizuka *et al.* (2004) observed a 16.2% resorption rate after 6 months in 13 parietal bone grafts [37]. Similarly, Smolka *et al.* reported a resorption rate of 19% after one year in a cohort of 51 grafts [38].

The study by C. Fourcade *et al.* reported slightly higher resorption rates for parietal bone grafts; however, it concluded that the location of the bone defect does not significantly affect the postoperative resorption rate [34]. In contrast, a 2006 literature review by Chiapasco *et al.* highlighted the anatomical origin of the bone graft as the key determinant influencing postoperative bone resorption [39]. Consequently, a graft derived from the iliac region undergoes greater resorption than a graft sourced from cranial or intraoral regions. Zins JE and Whitaker LA (1983) demonstrated that bones of membranous origin, such as cranial bone, exhibit reduced resorption compared to those of endochondral origin, such as iliac bone [33]. The mandibular ramus shares a membranous embryological origin with the parietal bone, which partly explains their frequent selection as donor sites in dental pre-implant bone reconstruction. A key factor influencing post-transplant resorption rates is the graft's structural composition—particularly the ratio of cancellous to cortical bone. Cortical bone, being less permeable to revascularization, contributes to variations in resorption outcomes following transplantation.

A healing period of approximately 4 months is generally sufficient for grafts of membranous origin, such as those from the ramus or parietal bone. In contrast, grafts derived from endochondral bone, like the iliac crest, typically require a minimum of 6 months for adequate integration [40]. As a result, the use of iliac bone grafts has declined in pre-implant oral bone reconstruction. Interestingly, Chappuis *et al.* demonstrated that the recipient site has minimal influence on the rate of post-transplant bone resorption [41].

3.5.1.3 *Resorption Duration*

Generally, autogenous bone graft resorbs concurrently with new bone formation; no notable "degradation" occurs while they are reshaped by the recipient. Initially, osteoclastic resorption activity is elevated, leading to diminished graft porosity and longevity. Cancellous bone undergoes revascularization within a brief duration of 2–3 days owing to its open architecture. In contrast, the revascularization of cortical bone may extend for a duration of up to 2 months. In cortical bone grafts, the resorption of necrotic bone is often insufficient, which hinders the full integration of viable and nonviable bone components and limits their direct interaction with the underlying cancellous bone [31].

3.5.1.4 *Cellular and Molecular Cascades Following Bone Autograft*

Autografts possess strong osteogenic capabilities, allowing for rapid revascularization and effective integration into the host site. While their mechanical strength may be limited, this is offset by the early initiation of new bone formation. By the fourth week after implantation, active osteogenesis and osteoclastic activity are commonly evident, supporting the graft's incorporation and remodeling. During the secondary healing phase, osteoblasts begin depositing layers of osteoid around the necrotic bone core.

As previously discussed, the key distinction between cortical and cancellous autografts lies in their vascularization dynamics and osteoinductive capacity. Cortical grafts, characterized by their dense structure and limited number of endosteal cells, exhibit delayed vascular ingrowth and a lower osteoinductive capacity compared to more porous graft types [42].

Successful osseointegration requires adequate vascular supply from the recipient bed to sustain graft cells through nutrient diffusion until revascularization is established. This neovascularization enables the ingrowth of capillaries into the graft, forming a long-lasting vascular network. Surgical trauma triggers the initiation of the osteogenic cascade by stimulating the release of various bone-regenerative cytokines. Key among these are bone morphogenetic protein-2 (BMP-2), platelet-derived growth factor (PDGF), transforming growth factor-beta (TGF-β), and vascular endothelial growth factor (VEGF), all of which play crucial roles in promoting bone formation and vascularization [43–45].

Woven bone formation originates from trauma-exposed bone margins, where osteoblastic progenitors are activated by matrix exposure and provided a surface for cellular adhesion [46]. When a graft containing viable endosteal osteoblasts is placed at the recipient site, it creates a localized microenvironment that is hypoxic (with oxygen tension between 3 and 10 mmHg), acidic (pH 4.0–6.0), and rich in lactate. Osteoblasts can survive the crucial early period of 3–5 days after transplantation, primarily due to their peripheral positioning within the graft and their capacity to absorb nutrients from the surrounding tissue environment [45, 46].

Within hours of implantation, platelets trapped in the fibrin clot begin to degranulate, releasing platelet-derived growth factor (PDGF) in response to the local oxygen gradient within the graft. This release stimulates the proliferation of osteocompetent cells and initiates angiogenesis. Capillary sprouting generally starts within 72 hours, with a fully functional vascular network typically established between days 10 and 14 post-implantation. As healing progresses, PDGF activity is gradually supplanted by growth factors derived from macrophages and other mesenchymal stimulators, particularly those belonging to the transforming growth factor-beta (TGF-β) superfamily [42].

Minimal osteoid deposition is evident during the first postoperative week; however, once vascularization is established, improved oxygen and nutrient delivery accelerates the bone healing process. The biochemical and cellular events during the first 3–4 weeks promote graft consolidation and scaffold formation, setting the stage for osteoconduction [46].

This early phase of bone repair, marked by cellular proliferation and disorganized woven bone formation resembling fracture callus, is referred to as Phase I regeneration. Incorporation of exogenous growth factors—such as PDGF, recombinant human BMP (rhBMP), TGF-β, and insulin-like growth factor (IGF)—can significantly enhance both the rate and extent of bone regeneration.

Phase I bone is gradually resorbed and remodeled into Phase II bone, which is characterized by increased mineralization, reduced cellularity, and an organized lamellar structure. This remodeling process is initiated by osteoclasts, which enter the graft through the newly established vascular channels, beginning the resorption of necrotic bone and paving the way for new bone formation [42].

3.5.2 Allografts

Allografts are bone grafts obtained from a donor of the same species; these are primarily osteoconductive, with limited osteoinductive capacity. Resorption rates vary but are slower than autografts due to the absence of living cells [1, 47].

The first documented use of an allograft in the medical literature was reported by Sir William MacEwen in 1879, marking the early exploration of bone transplantation between individuals of the same species [48].

Allografts are porous structures that contain various chemical domains capable of supporting the attachment and retention of progenitor and endothelial cells. They also house growth factors embedded within the bone matrix, which are released during osteoclastic resorption. Although the concentration of bone morphogenetic proteins (BMPs) in allografts is relatively low, they contribute to the graft's osteoinductive potential. Demineralization of allograft bone enhances the bioavailability of these growth factors and further reduces the risk of viral transmission, including HIV [49]. It was previously shown that several demineralized bone allografts exhibited heterogeneity in osteoinductive and osteopromotive properties.

3.5.2.1 Source

Bone from a human donor, common forms include freeze-dried bone or demineralized bone matrix and osteoallogenic morphogenetic protein (OsteoAMP).

Osseous Repositories: The ideal age range for bone graft donors in tissue banks is typically between 16 and 65 years, as this range is considered to provide grafts with suitable biological and mechanical properties for clinical use. Donors should be excluded if they have a history of acute or fatal chronic infections, radiation exposure in the relevant donor site, malignancies, hepatitis, AIDS, HIV infections, drug abuse, chronic steroid therapy, osteoporosis, chronic insulin-dependent diabetes, immune complex diseases, connective tissue disorders, or recent history of vaccines. Donors can exist in a cadaveric state. Living donors necessitate a thorough physical examination and comprehensive medical history, while a meticulous autopsy is essential for cadavers [49, 50].

3.5.2.1.1 Demineralized Bone Matrix (DBM)

Extraction of DBM from humans was pioneered in 1975. In 1980, it was first used in the field of orthopedics. During the processing of allografts, key biological components such as type I collagen within the cortical bone matrix and non-collagenous proteins—including bone morphogenetic proteins (BMPs), transforming growth factor (TGF), insulin-like growth factor (IGF), and fibroblast growth factor (FGF)—are retained. However, this preservation often comes at the expense of the graft's mechanical strength, which may be significantly reduced. Despite the removal of bone minerals from allogenic bone, DBM can still serve as a scaffold in three dimensions due to the preservation of the original tissues' fibrous collagen structure.

3.5.2.1.2 Frozen or Cancellous Allografts

These aid in the process of osteogenesis. To protect against compression, they offer mechanical support. Freezing and vacuum packaging are the processes that are used to prepare them. Allograft bone can be used to smooth bone surfaces in periarticular metaphyseal fractures and to fill voids left after the curettage of bone cysts, aiding in structural support and promoting bone regeneration.

3.5.2.1.3 Allografts from the Cartilage and the Cortex

In cases involving extensive bone and joint loss, allografts are typically harvested from major weight-bearing bones such as the pelvis, femur, tibia, and fibula. Additionally, they offer mechanical and structural support. Osteoconductive properties are conferred upon them.

Resorption rate: Allografts degrade slower than autografts and provide a scaffold for new bone formation. However, the exact rate depends on the processing methods (e.g., demineralized, freeze-dried).

Resorption time: 6–12 months or longer, depending on the material's treatment [51].

Studies have indicated that at 6 months, CT scans showed that both the autogenous bone and fresh frozen bone grafts experienced significant resorption, with the FFB grafts losing a lot more volume than the AB grafts. Nevertheless, there was a great deal of variation in the rate of FFB resorption, with varying degrees of graft volume change ranging from nearly nonexistent to total resorption. The results demonstrate that graft volume resorption is not very predictable, which is consistent with findings from multiple studies [23, 27, 47, 48]. The rate of graft resorption is directly proportional to the initial density of the FFB. Grafts with a higher density showed less graft resorption than those with a lower density. Possible factors contributing to their resorption include density-based categorization for bone quality based on cortical and cancellous composition, which was found to be independent of graft embryologic origin.

Orsini observed contrasting findings, including the presence of small, newly formed blood vessels within the marrow spaces, grafted bone closely opposed to new bone, and well-integrated corticocancellous grafts within the recipient sites [52]. All things considered, cortical grafts are tough and impermeable to blood vessels, but they deteriorate over time due to degeneration and stay mixed with healthy and dead bone for a long time after they are fully integrated. In contrast, cancellous grafts generally undergo greater resorption; however, they benefit from faster remodeling and revascularization compared to cortical grafts.

After 5 months of recovery, Aslan and colleagues found that, on average, 5.4% of the vertical graft remained after using a cortical block allograft to increase the alveolar ridge [53]. According to Pereira and colleagues, the average horizontal bone resorption of corticocancellous fresh-frozen allogeneic bone blocks between augmentation and implant re-entry was approximately 7.1% [25]. Spin-Neto and colleagues reported that 6 to 8 months after placement of corticocancellous fresh-frozen block bone allografts, the average horizontal graft resorption rate was 8.3%. In comparison, freeze-dried cancellous allogeneic bone blocks exhibited a resorption rate of 2.0%, while cortical autogenous bone blocks showed a rate of 3.1%. Their histomorphometric analysis also revealed a high proportion of nonvital tissue within fresh-frozen allogeneic cortical bone blocks [54]. Conversely, studies have demonstrated excellent new bone formation and rapid remodeling in cancellous allogeneic bone blocks [27, 55, 56]. According to Ciszyński M., vertical bone augmentations with heights around 5 mm tend to exhibit significantly higher resorption rates [57].

3.5.2.1.4 Immunity and Allografts

At the time of allograft implantation, donor cells are completely eliminated, leaving the bone matrix to serve solely as a structural scaffold. Fresh bone allografts trigger both humoral and cellular immune responses, allowing the recipient's immune system to recognize and react against the transplant. This immune activation leads to antibody production, which causes cell destruction and vascular injury, ultimately resulting in graft rejection. The likelihood of rejection depends largely on the degree of antigenic mismatch between the donor tissue and the recipient [58]. Rejection of vascularized bone allografts typically occurs around the third postoperative day, with the initially affected cells identified as osteocytes and vascular endothelial cells. The use of cyclosporine can help mitigate this rejection response. Unlike autografts, allografts elicit a distinct immune reaction in the recipient, and their integration is characterized by slower vascular invasion and diminished perivascular osteogenesis. The dimensions of the graft and the environment for allograft storage add to the factors influencing the magnitude of the immune reaction to the transplant [59].

The increased immunogenicity and higher failure rates observed in allografts compared to autografts are believed to result from the activation of major histocompatibility complex (MHC) antigens. These antigens are found in osteogenic and hematopoietic cells, leukocytes, blood vessels, nerves, and connective tissue matrices within the graft, triggering a secondary immune response [60]. This immune reaction, along with the infiltration of inflammatory cells, rapidly surrounds the newly formed blood vessels, leading to the destruction of osteoprogenitor cells and compromising the initial osteoinductive phase essential for successful graft integration [60]. There is still much mystery surrounding the immune response during bone transplant integration; however, research has shown that reducing immunogenicity by making adjustments to the allograft to limit histocompatibility discrepancies improves allograft acceptance [58]. If allografts are devoid of their cellular components, they are safeguarded against immunological responses. Herndon *et al.* have demonstrated that the immunological response to frozen allografts diminishes, leading to their extensive utilization. Focus has transitioned to approaches for preserving allografts [61]. Cadaveric bones are utilized as osteoconductive scaffolds through the process of decellularization [62]. Consequently, the transmission of the disease between individuals is inhibited. The employed procedures include irradiation, debridement, ultrasonic cleaning, liquid nitrogen, ethylene oxide, and cryopreservation [62]. Allografts are processed and stored in tissue banks to ensure safety and availability. Freeze-dried bone grafts, in particular, demonstrate reduced immunogenicity toward both humoral and cellular immune responses. However, these processing methods also decrease the osteoinductive potential of the graft and alter its mechanical properties [2]. The development and widespread use of bone banks have been crucial in advancing these techniques, leading to their establishment in numerous regions around the world [2].

3.5.2.1.5 Cellular and Molecular Cascades After Allograft

Autograft promotes bone repair more than cancellous allograft. When compared to cortical transplants, allografts integrate more quickly. In this way, they facilitate the attachment of host bone. Because they are never entirely absorbed, they get stuck in the host bone [30]. The process of bone creation begins at the edges of the defect and works its way within. Demineralized freeze-dried bone allografts (DFDBAs) appear as spherical or cylindrical deposits, measuring approximately 3–5 μm in diameter, which form along the interface between the mineralized woven bone and the demineralized matrix. These mineral deposition sites were observed in an animal study conducted on minipigs around four weeks post-implantation [53]. Demineralized freeze-dried bone allografts (DFDBAs) can only undergo recalcification in regions where fresh, mineralizing bone matrix has recently been deposited. In contrast, areas of the graft surface in direct contact with bone marrow typically do not mineralize. Twelve weeks after implantation, the defect site is largely filled with new bone, although a substantial amount of the transplanted material remains. This newly formed bone consists of a combination of partially recalcified DFDBA, woven bone, and lamellar bone deposits present at the graft surface. Osteoclastic resorption begins and progresses along bone surfaces and recalcified DFDBA particles when remodeling begins. It was shown that there is diversity in the degradation and resorption rates of DFDBA particles. The lack of osteoclast activity in degrading DFDBA particles within the femoral defect model suggests that alternative degradation pathways are involved. This occurs despite the fact that DFDBA particles typically retain less than 2% mineral content following their preparation and processing [53]. Decalcified freeze-dried bone allografts may have a dearth of osteoclasts due to the little amount of calcified tissue present, and the primary cells seen around DFDBA particles in the investigation were primarily macrophages [61].

In less than 10% of instances, fibrous tissue formed around the graft, delaying osteointegration [27]. And even after years of rejection, the allografts are never fully absorbed. Mechanical rigidity is imparted by cortical allografts. Just like with autogenous transplants, creeping substitution is required prior to the inclusion of cortical allografts. Osteoclastic resorption often starts the process, and then osteoconduction causes the random production of new appositional bone [25, 29].

3.5.3 Xenografts

Bone graft taken from different species (e.g., bovine), these primarily provide osteoconductivity. They are slowly resorbing due to extensive processing, which reduces immunogenicity but also reduces osteoinductive potential [63]. It resorbs at a slower rate, making them suitable for cases requiring extended support.

Since allograft is a costly way, researchers have examined bones from different animal species. In 1632, van Meek'ren conducted the first officially recorded xenograft in Amsterdam. A canine calvarium successfully healed a skull defect in a Russian soldier [64].

Source: Bone derived from a different species, most commonly bovine.
Example: Natural bone mineral (NBM), commercially known as Bio-Oss (Geistlich, Wolhusen, Switzerland), is a highly purified inorganic bone matrix obtained from cattle and has been widely used as a grafting material for many years. Bone reconstruction procedures including dental implants frequently make use of this material due to its high levels of biocompatibility and osteoconductivity. In addition, when compared to using either NBM or enamel matrix derivative (EMD) alone, the combination of the two may potentially result in even better bone regeneration. One such product is Emdogain, manufactured by Straumann in Basel, Switzerland [65].

3.5.3.1 Resorption Rate and Time

Resorption rate: These tend to have very slow resorption rates. They often remain in the site for extended periods, acting as a long-term scaffold. **Resorption time**: Can persist for years, and some xenografts may never fully resorb [63].

3.5.3.2 Cellular and Molecular Cascades After Xenograft

In an animal study, defects grafted with compact coral-derived hydroxyapatite (HA) granules showed uniform distribution throughout the defect site, which was infiltrated by dense fibrous tissue and developing bone trabeculae. The pores lining the granules, as well as their outer surfaces, were coated with thin layers of woven bone. The density of the bone filling of pores and interspaces increases significantly at 12 weeks. Woven bone, which is strengthened by lamellar and parallel-fibered bone, still makes up half of the freshly created bone. But basically, there is not much renovation going on. By 24 weeks, the only noticeable difference in the coralline filler and bony regenerate composite is the fully developed bone structure. Enhanced remodeling primarily affects the bone compartment, substituting lamellar bone for woven bone, and does not penetrate the neighboring coralline material [66].

Jensen S.S. and colleagues conducted a qualitative and quantitative evaluation of bone formation and graft resorption using two different bone substitutes commonly employed in orthopedic and oral surgery. In their animal model, they created three standardized bone defects in the mandibular angles of twelve mature minipigs. These defects were then repaired using either autografts, anorganic bovine bone (ABB), or synthetic β-tricalcium phosphate [28]. Histologic and histomorphometric studies were performed at 1, 2, 4, and 8 weeks of grafting. At 2 weeks, autograft resulted in greater new bone growth compared to ABB and β-TCP. After 4 weeks, β-TCP did not significantly differ from the other two materials. Defects transplanted with ABB showed reduced bone growth compared to autograft. At 8 weeks post-implantation, defects treated with autograft and β-tricalcium phosphate (β-TCP) exhibited significantly greater bone formation compared to those grafted with anorganic bovine bone (ABB). No significant difference in bone growth was observed between β-TCP and autograft groups. Notably, β-TCP was almost completely resorbed by 8 weeks, whereas ABB maintained a stable volume throughout the period. Both bone substitutes appeared to slow early bone repair relative to autografts. However, all defects eventually healed with new bone and developing marrow, demonstrating full osseous integration of the graft materials. These findings suggest that both substitutes have potential roles in reconstructive surgery, particularly when different rates of biodegradability are therapeutically desired. Overall, the results indicated that ABB performed less effectively, especially at 2 and 8 weeks, showing reduced bone growth compared to autograft and β-TCP [28].

The fact that natural bone mineral (NBM) particles did not degrade was one of the most glaring findings from Koerdt S *et al.*'s investigation [67]. This agrees with other *in vivo* investigations that showed that bovine-derived NBM is almost never absorbed in both animal and human trials [68–70]. Recent research in a pig calvaria augmentation model found that deproteinized bovine bone mineral (DBBM, Bio-Oss) completely resorbs, despite the fact that other publications suggest little surface resorption [71]. The researchers note that they observed an increase in osteoclastogenesis and a decrease in partial bone breakdown when they combined NBM with EMD. Enamel matrix derivative (EMD) significantly increases osteoclast numbers, upregulates receptor activator of nuclear factor kappa-B ligand (RANKL) expression, and enhances tartrate-resistant acid phosphatase (TRAP) staining around natural bone mineral (NBM) particles. These findings support previous research demonstrating that EMD can stimulate both bone resorption and formation during periodontal tissue regeneration. Notably, Otsuka and colleagues were the first to demonstrate that EMD induces osteoclast production through RANKL expression in studies involving mouse bone marrow osteoblastic cells. Their findings imply that EMD might control the processes of bone creation and bone resorption during the regeneration of periodontal tissues [72]. Clinical studies have demonstrated that enamel matrix derivative (EMD) supports periodontal tissue regeneration. Additionally, evidence suggests that EMD interacts with the receptor activator of nuclear factor kappa-B ligand (RANKL) to activate signaling pathways such as extracellular signal-regulated kinase (ERK) and p38 MAPK. This activation promotes the differentiation of osteoclasts in RAW 264.7 cells, which are monocyte/macrophage-like cells commonly used as a model for osteoclastogenesis [72]. Scientists are currently trying to pin down the exact proportion of EMD that triggers the separate cell pathways that lead to the formation of osteoblasts or osteoclasts [78].

Neither of the DFDBA bone grafts lasted nearly as long as the NBM particles, which is not surprising. Osteotech DFDBA particles showed a limited number of osteoclasts in and surrounding them, while having a significantly faster disintegration rate compared to all other modalities as reported by Shuang Yang [70].

An intriguing question has arisen, challenging the common assumption that bone particles exhibiting the fastest degradation rates would necessarily be associated with a greater number of osteoclasts.

The interface between natural bone and graft tissue undergoes a complicated process that includes 5 phases: activation, resorption, reversal, formation, and resting. The activation phase is stimulated by a set of cytokines, growth factors, and hormones. The osteoblasts differentiated from mesenchymal stem cells in stages of maturation into preosteoblasts and then mature osteoblasts. The multinucleated osteoclasts originate from hematopoietic precursors of the monocytes or macrophages. Osteoclastogenesis is controlled by RANK and RANKL. The activated osteoclasts start resorbing the surface of bone graft by the creation of a resorbing channel making a cutting cone that leads to scalloped resorption lacunae (Howship's lacunae). As the preosteoblasts differentiate into osteoblasts, they start to deposit a thin coating of cement on the area of resorption; this cement is a noncollagenous matrix protein called the reversal line. Then a mineralized layer will be formed in the process of new bone formation [73] (Figure 3.2).

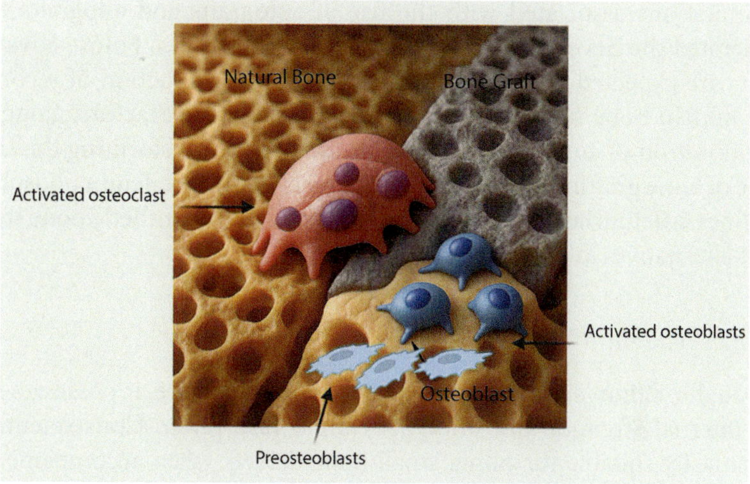

Figure 3.2 Bone graft or bone substitute and natural bone interface.

3.5.4 Alloplastic Materials or Synthetic Grafts

Alloplastic materials consist of components not derived from any living being. Alloplastic grafts can be either man-made chemicals or from natural sources, such as minerals or elements. Sometimes they are a mix of the two. Examples include calcium phosphates, hydroxyapatite (HA), and tricalcium phosphate (TCP).

3.5.4.1 Hydroxyapatite (HA)

Bone deficiencies that were once repaired with autogenous bone grafting are now regularly filled with synthetic porous hydroxyapatite (HA). Conventional wisdom holds that HA does not break down once implanted and instead stays in the body. On the other hand, other writers have found that the implanted HA blocks or granules absorb their own margin during long-term follow-up, which might mean that HA is biodegradable. In a patient case where full-thickness bone was harvested for grafting, the iliac bone defect was found to be filled with newly formed bone six years and seven months following the implantation of synthetic hydroxyapatite (HA) blocks, which had undergone substantial resorption. This finding supports the conclusion that HA is biodegradable. Moreover, the extent of HA biodegradation appears to be influenced by factors such as sintering temperature, porosity, and pore size [3].

Limitations associated with the use of autografts and allografts have accelerated the development of bioceramic technologies. Future advancements are expected to enhance the isolation and production of recombinant human bone morphogenetic proteins and growth factors, alongside the utilization of autologous stem cells, ultimately transforming the landscape of bone grafting procedures [74]. Bioactive glass, calcium phosphate, ceramics, calcium sulfate, or a mix of these and other synthetic bone transplant alternatives are available.

3.5.4.2 Calcium Sulfate (CS)

Although calcium sulfate lacks a macroporous structure, it possesses limited internal strength and undergoes rapid resorption. Consequently, it is primarily suitable for filling small bone defects when accompanied by rigid internal fixation, as graft resorption occurs in tandem with new blood vessel and bone ingrowth [75]. In spinal arthrodesis, Niu *et al.* observed that the accelerated breakdown of calcium sulfate during the early stages of bone regeneration, compared to the rate of new bone formation, resulted in suboptimal fusion rates [75].

Calcium phosphate ceramics: Synthetic osteoconductive materials having a composition comparable to bone. Depending on the kind of bone, natural bone often replaces TCP in 3–24 months, since it resorbs more quickly. Granules or blocks of porous calcium phosphate are on the market. Exactly how these molecules work in living organisms is still up for debate. Chemical dissolution and osteoclastic resorption are the mechanisms that cause resorption to occur [76]. Similar in chemical composition to the mineral phase of calcified tissues, calcium hydroxyapatites are the building blocks of calcium phosphate ceramics. The absorption rate and mechanical characteristics of CaP ceramics are two important factors that are directly correlated with the Ca/P ratios. Another important consideration when selecting CaP ceramics is their crystal and porous structure. Ever since Albee originally described it in 1920, the rhombohedral ß-form of tricalcium phosphate (TCP), ß-tricalcium phosphate (ß-TCP), and other calcium phosphate ceramics have been the subject of intense research. Because of its lower Ca/P ratio of 1.5 compared to hydroxyapatite, ß-TCP, which has the molecular formula $Ca_3(PO_4)_2$, may have a faster breakdown and absorption rate [77]. While TCP's increased number of linked pores can improve fibro-vascular invasion and bone replacement, it can reduce mechanical characteristics [77] and is similar to HAp in other respects. Thermodynamically unstable physiological pH causes some TCP to convert to hydroxyapatite after implantation, which slows down its destruction to some extent [77], most of which is reabsorbed by phagocytosis between 6 and 24 months after implantation, and some of that remains for years [63]. This characteristic makes β-tricalcium phosphate (TCP) effective for filling bone defects caused by trauma and benign tumors; however, its unpredictable biodegradation profile limits its recommendation as a reliable bone graft substitute.

3.5.4.3 Calcium Phosphate Cements (CPCs)

They may be easily injected into different shaped flaws and then solidified by combining with an aqueous phase using isothermic reaction. Theoretically, they are less conducive to ingrowth of neo-vascular and bone tissue than other CaP ceramics that support interconnected macroporosity because they can only degrade layer by layer according to the predetermined dissolution in physiological conditions and osteoclast resorption activity [79]. The composition has a significant impact on the rate of biodegradation.

3.5.4.4 Bioactive Glass

Bioactive glass, a synthetic silicate-based ceramic first developed in the 1970s, primarily consists of silica dioxide (SiO_2), sodium oxide (Na_2O), calcium oxide (CaO), and phosphorus pentoxide (P_2O_5) [80]. To enhance its stability, additional components such as potassium oxide (K_2O), magnesium oxide (MgO), and boric oxide (B_2O_3) were later incorporated. Silicate remains the principal component, accounting for approximately 45–52% of the glass's overall composition [81]. Bioglass and host bone form a strong physical connection due to the optimized constitutions. Bioactivity, as a phenomenon, was initially discovered on BGS [82]. The bone-binding ability of bioglass is believed to result from the leaching and accumulation of silicon ions when the material is exposed to body fluids after implantation, which subsequently leads to the formation of a hydroxyapatite layer on its surface [80]. Proteins are absorbed by this thin hydroxyapatite layer, which also attracts cells that can produce new bone. Furthermore, with long-term implantation, bone gradually substitutes for this biological apatite layer [81]. New blood vessels can develop into the implant site after the new bone has been deposited because of the implant's porosity and the relatively rapid rate of resorption in the initial two weeks after implantation [82, 83]. There is minimal inflammatory response and total resorption of bioglass fiber scaffolds after six months *in vivo*, according to one study [83]. Reports indicated that bioglass's mechanical qualities were weak and brittle, similar to those of conventional ceramics. Thus, when coupled with growth factors, it has mostly been used for the restoration of face deformities [82]. Lately, bioactive silica carbide was proven to integrate with underlying native bone, which may carry potential application for facial augmentation [84, 85].

3.5.4.5 *Poly(Methyl Methacrylate) (PMMA) Bone Cement*

Despite being the most commonly used synthetic material in clinical settings, polymethylmethacrylate (PMMA) cannot serve as a bone substitute because it is neither biodegradable nor resorbable. Orthopedic surgeons first introduced PMMA approximately 60 years ago [86]. The two-component, self-polymerizing PMMA bone cement has been widely employed in total joint replacements to secure implant components, valued for its excellent mechanical strength and ease of use [87].

3.5.4.6 *Magnesium Barrier Membranes (NOVAMag®)*

They are another well-known example of synthetic biodegradable metallic membranes composed of magnesium that fully dissolve in the human body. It offers great mechanical stability, space maintenance, and bioactivity with the added benefit of being resorbable over a predetermined period, combining the best features of both non-resorbable and resorbable membranes. There is enough time for bone rebuilding using magnesium membranes because their resorption duration is 8–16 weeks [88]. Because of this, a second operation to remove the membrane is not necessary. Biomaterials were proven to be safe and resorbable after healing. The membranes were held in place during the bone regeneration procedure using the resorbable fixation screws [88].

3.5.5 Molecular and Cellular Cascades After the Alloplast

For graft materials derived from calcium phosphate, their dissolution, composition, topography, and surface energy are shared characteristics of calcium phosphate that might influence cellular function [78]. Bone resorption occurs when osteoclasts colonize the substrate, after recruitment of monocytes and macrophages during the inflammatory response that follows surgery. Similar to how osteoclasts break down bone mineral, they cling tenaciously to the substrate-sealing zone when breaking down calcium phosphate ceramics. Their H+ secretion causes a local pH of 4–5 in the middle of the sealing zone [89]. By making room for new bone to grow, osteoclasts help break down calcium phosphate ceramics into minerals that may be used for bone regeneration in living organisms. The year 12 Minipigs with β-tricalcium phosphate (β-TCP) grafted defects had some new bone growth at 4 weeks, but it was not as extensive or mature as the bone growth observed with autograft. Additionally, bone had nearly completely replaced graft particles. By 8 weeks, the trabecular bone has filled in completely, and the β-TCP has been almost resorbed by dissolving instead of cellular resorption [28].

3.6 Factors Influencing Resorption and Degradation

Resorption and degradation of graft materials are influenced by patient-related factors, including systemic health and local biological conditions, as well as material-specific properties such as porosity, surface chemistry, and mechanical strength.

3.6.1 Patient-Related Factors

Age, health, and systemic conditions impact healing and graft resorption. Patients with lower bone density and smokers had higher resorption rates. Smoking negatively impacts bone graft outcomes through multiple biological mechanisms [90]. Nicotine and other harmful chemicals in tobacco stimulate osteoclastic activity, leading to accelerated bone resorption and faster breakdown of the graft material. At the same time, smoking impairs angiogenesis, reducing blood supply to the graft site. This restriction limits the delivery of oxygen and nutrients needed for new bone formation, resulting in a faster resorption rate without adequate replacement. In addition, smoking decreases osteoblast proliferation and activity, further reducing the body's capacity to form new bone to replace the resorbed graft, which can ultimately lead to premature graft loss and poor bone regeneration. Compounding these effects, smoking interferes with vascularization and tissue healing, preventing the proper integration of the graft with the surrounding bone and contributing to higher failure rates in dental, orthopedic, and craniofacial procedures. Furthermore, smoking weakens the immune response, increasing the risk of infection at the graft site, which can further compromise graft stability and bone healing [91].

3.6.2 Material Properties

Porosity, size, and composition influence degradation rates. A significant limitation of bone block graft surgery is the resorption that takes place during the initial phases of healing.

Table 3.1 Bone graft resorption comparison.

Graft type	Resorption rate	Resorption duration
Autograft (cortical)	Low	6–18 months
Autograft (cancellous)	High	3–6 months
Allograft (freeze-dried)	Moderate	6–12 months
Allograft (fresh-frozen)	Low to moderate	6–18 months
Demineralized bone matrix (DBM)	Moderate to high	3–9 months
Xenograft (e.g., bovine)	Low	12–36+ months
Synthetic (e.g., β-TCP)	High	3–9 months
Synthetic (e.g., HA)	Very low	36+ months
Bioactive glass	Moderate	6–12 months

A study comparing graft resorption rates of corticocancellous and cancellous allogeneic blocks was conducted on 28 patients. The study involved preoperative CT and 4 months postoperative CT, with 93 implants placed in 28 patients. Results showed a 100% survival rate in both groups after 24 months follow-up [25, 54]. Cancellous bone grafts had a higher resorption rate than corticocancellous grafts (see Table 3.1).

A retrospective cohort study compared the stability of vertical onlay bone grafts harvested from the iliac crest and the calvarium for the reconstruction of severe maxillary or mandibular bone atrophy. Bone resorption was quantified using digital panoramic radiographs taken at multiple time points: before grafting, after augmentation surgery, 6 months post-healing, prior to implant placement, following implant surgery, and annually thereafter. The study found both grafting techniques to be effective and reliable. Complication rates were 35.7% in the calvarial group and 33.3% in the iliac crest group. Following augmentation, an average vertical bone gain of 8.55 mm was observed; however, grafts from the iliac crest experienced significantly greater bone loss, averaging 24.16%. Implant survival rates were comparable between the two groups [22].

Different types of bone grafts exhibit varying rates of resorption. A published meta-analysis reported average bone growth of 3.7 ± 1.2 mm for grafts in granule form and 4.5 ± 1.2 mm for bone blocks, with outcomes influenced by the graft material type—autogenous, allogeneic, xenogeneic, or alloplastic—and its form (granules versus blocks) [92]. Furthermore, according to the ITI treatment guide, volumetric graft remodeling rates for repairing individual tooth defects classified as Type II to Type IV are comparable when using freeze-dried cancellous allogeneic bone blocks versus autogenous bone blocks [26, 54].

Graft site: Vascularity and mechanical stress at the site affect integration and resorption. Successful integration of grafts used in maxilla is noted, attributed to the maxilla's superior blood supply. When it comes to developing moderately to severely inadequate alveolar ridges, intraoral autogenous bone blocks have been described as a dependable and predictable method [25].

3.6.3 Strategies for Prolonging Structural Support

Strategies to prolong graft stability include the selection of slowly resorbing materials, optimization of graft size and density, surface modification, and combination with biological adjuncts. These approaches aim to balance mechanical support with biological integration rather than guaranteeing specific clinical outcomes.

3.6.3.1 Utilizing Slowly Resorbing Materials

Composite Grafts: Combinations of materials, such as a mix of natural and synthetic substances [93].

Synthetic Grafts, Alloplasts, or Xenografts: HA material resorbs very slowly and can remain in the body for years, providing long-term structural support as new bone forms around it [3].

Using barrier membranes that contain autogenous bone and/or bone substitutes, guided bone regeneration (GBR) is another way to prolong the structural support. When compared to nonresorbable membranes, resorbable ones provide several benefits, such as being easier to manipulate, having an undemanding flap design, and reducing the danger of membrane exposure. Hence, resorbable collagen membranes have been quite popular for GBR in the past few years, especially for horizontal augmentation [29, 41]. In two-stage regeneration techniques in particular, the stability of the augmented bone is thought to be a critical success factor.

The use of xenograft such as deproteinized bovine bone (DBB) provides osteoconductivity, can resist resorption, and serves as an excellent framework for bone healing [41, 71, 73]. Because of its delayed resorption qualities, DBB may be useful for preserving the volumetric stability of the graft when used in conjunction with autogenous bone [93].

The resorption rates of bone grafts in GBR and intraoral block bone grafts (RBG) impact the treatment planning and patient morbidity. Gultekin B A (2016) and colleagues found that the GBR group experienced higher resorption rates (12.5%) compared to the RBG group, which aligns with previous research indicating resorption rates of 5% to 28% for block grafts [29]. Covering recipient sites with low turnover bone substitutes can reduce resorption, with one study showing a nearly 50% reduction using direct bone barriers. The GBR method, which combines autogenous particulate bone with low turnover graft material, may reduce resorption and enhance integration. It was observed that both methods achieved sufficient horizontal bone growth for implant stability, with GBR showing greater gains than RBG and complications were minimal [41].

3.6.3.2 *Adjusting Graft Size and Density*

Larger grafts: Increasing the size of the graft slows resorption, as it takes longer for the body to break down a larger structure [93]. Denser grafts: Dense materials, such as compact xenograft particles, degrade more slowly compared to more porous options. Moreover, the physicochemical properties of graft materials significantly impact their performance and behavior *in vivo* [94].

3.6.3.3 *Surface Coatings and Modifications*

Growth factor coatings: Coating graft materials with growth factors that slow resorption, like osteoprotegerin, can help extend their durability [78]. Bioactive coatings: Applying bioactive molecules like bone morphogenetic proteins (BMPs) can promote bone formation while regulating the breakdown of the graft [95, 96].

3.6.3.4 *Cross-Linking and Polymerization*

Cross-linking Collagen: Increasing cross-linking in collagen scaffolds can enhance resistance to degradation, prolonging their stability [97]. Polymer coatings: Coating grafts with synthetic polymers such as polylactic acid slows the resorption process for fast resorbable graft materials [98].

3.6.3.5 *Controlled Release Systems*

Encapsulation: Encasing the graft in biodegradable materials that release components over time can prevent rapid resorption. Drug-eluting grafts:

Grafts that release antiresorptive drugs, like bisphosphonates, can inhibit the activity of osteoclasts, the cells responsible for resorption, thus slowing graft degradation [99].

3.6.4 Manipulating the Local Biological Environment

Vascular control: Limiting blood supply to the graft site can slow the resorption rate, though care must be taken to avoid hindering bone growth [100]. Immune modulation: Reducing inflammation-driven resorption by controlling the immune response at the graft site can also extend graft longevity. By combining these materials and techniques, the resorption rate of bone grafts can be slowed, allowing for longer-term structural support while new bone develops. Moy *et al.* conducted a histomorphometric analysis on sinus lifts using chin bone and found that, after 6 months of healing, new bone formation accounted for 59.4 ± 18.0% of the area, while connective tissue comprised 40.5 ± 17.9%. The newly formed bone was predominantly mature lamellar bone (approximately 80%), indicating superior quality compared to bovine hydroxyapatite [101].

In a long-term study tracking 36 sinus grafts over 10 years, new bone formation progressed from 29.8 ± 2.5% at 8 months to 69.7 ± 2.6% at 1 year, reaching 86.7 ± 2.84% by the end of the study. The resorption rate of bovine hydroxyapatite grafts was estimated at 3.55% per month during the first 2 years, decreasing to 0.58% per month over the subsequent 8 years. Volume loss after 4 years was 34% for Bio-Oss and 22% for Cerabone [102]. The slower resorption of Cerabone is attributed to its larger crystallite size and higher surface area, a result of its bigger average particle size (approximately 2.7 mm) compared to Bio-Oss (about 1 mm). These subtle differences contribute to the initially higher resorption rate observed with Bio-Oss [102].

Sinus augmentation using β-tricalcium phosphate (β-TCP) resulted in 29% new bone growth after 6 months. The addition of platelet-rich plasma (PRP) enhanced β-TCP's bone regenerative capacity by 38%. The resorption rate of β-TCP varies between 32% and 43%, influenced primarily by the crystal content of the graft material [103]. Following maxillary sinus augmentation with bovine xenografts (Endobon), a recent study examined biomaterial mineral degradation and bone-to-biomaterial contact in retrieved bone biopsies. Scanning electron microscopy revealed that newly formed bone was closely adherent to the xenograft. During the resorption process at the interface, calcium ions gradually diffuse from the residual biomaterial into the newly formed bone [73].

Jensen *et al.* [73] reported that bone resorption rates vary depending on the type of graft used, with average values of 1.8 mm for autografts, 2.1

mm for demineralized allografts, 0.9 mm for alloplasts, and 0.8 mm for combinations of autograft and alloplast [28]. The histologic examinations of sinus lifts [E. Nyström] revealed that all graft materials resulted in a reduction in height. Two to three years following a sinus lift, graft materials were shown to be statistically substantially decreased by [104], while mechanical stress on dental implants preserved graft height, according to another study [93, 103, 104].

3.7 Conclusion

The durability and resilience of a bone transplant are key factors in determining its ultimate success. How, when, and what kind of new bone grows depends on the graft material and the host site's healing processes. Blood vessels are revascularized and host bone is substituted for graft material in successful regeneration, which prevent mechanical stress and volume loss. The rate at which bone grafts resorb plays a crucial role in their success for skeletal repair and regeneration. An ideal graft must strike a balance between stability and biological integration resorbing slowly enough to maintain structural support, yet quickly enough to allow natural bone remodeling. Different graft types—autografts, allografts, xenografts, synthetic materials, and composites—exhibit varying resorption profiles due to their biological origin, composition, and treatment. Advances in biomaterial engineering, including growth factor coatings, cross-linking, and controlled release systems, have enabled more precise control over resorption, enhancing both safety and effectiveness. Ultimately, the choice of graft material should be individualized, based on the patient's health, defect characteristics, and desired healing outcome. Ongoing research continues to refine these materials to better mimic natural bone behavior and improve clinical results.

AI disclosure statement: The author confirms that no artificial intelligence (AI)-generated content or AI-assisted writing tools were used in the preparation of this chapter (including summaries and the abstract). All text, analysis, and conclusions are the result of the author's original work.

References

1. Szpindor, E., Evaluation of the usefulness of autogenic bone grafts in reconstruction of the mandible. *Ann. Acad. Med. Stetin.*, 1, 41, 155–169, 1995.

2. Sener, N. and Ozger, H., Bone grafts and bone banking. *Acta Orthop. Traumatol. Turc.*, 29, 4, 335–8, 1995.
3. Goto, T., Kojima, T., Iijima, T., Yokokura, S., Kawano, H., Yamamoto, A., Matsuda, K., Resorption of synthetic porous hydroxyapatite and replacement by newly formed bone. *J. Orthop. Sci.*, 1-6, 5, 444–7, 2001.
4. Di Carlo, S., De Angelis, F., Brauner, E., Rosella, D., Papi, P., Pompa, G., Saptefrati, L., Cimpean, A.M., Ciobanu, G., Histological and immunohistochemical evaluation of mandibular bone tissue regeneration. *Int. J. Immunopathol. Pharmacol.*, 32, 2058738418798249, 2018.
5. Wong, K.K. and Piert, M., Dynamic Bone Imaging with99MTC-Labeled diphosphonates and18F-NAF: Mechanisms and Applications. *J. Nucl. Med.*, 54, 4, 590–599, 2013.
6. Kühl, S., *et al.*, Three-dimensional analysis of bone formation after maxillary sinus augmentation by means of microcomputed tomography: a pilot study. *Int. J. Oral Maxillofac. Implants*, 25, 5, 930–8, 2010.
7. Kolerman, K., Goshen, G., Joseph, N., Kozlovsky, A., Shetty, S., Tal, H., Histomorphometric analysis of maxillary sinus augmentation using an alloplast bone substitute. *J. Oral Maxillofac. Surg.*, 70, 8, 1835–1843, 2012.
8. Bansal, S., Venkataraman, N., Bansal, P., Narayan, S., Dynamics of bone graft healing around implants. *J. Int. Clin. Dent. Res. Organ.*, 7, 3, 40–52, 2015.
9. Kummoona, R., *Bone Grafting - Recent Advances with Special References to Cranio-Maxillofacial Surgery*, IntechOpen (IntechOpen Limited), London, UK, 2018, doi: 10.5772/intechopen.73956. Available: https://doi.org/10.5772/intechopen.73956.
10. Khan, S.N., Cammisa, F.P., Sandhu, H.S., Diwan, A.D., Girardi, F.P., Lane, J.M., The biology of bone grafting. *J. Am. Acad. Orthop. Surg.*, 13, 1, 77–86, 2005.
11. Stevenson., S., Biology Of Bone Grafts. *Orthop. Clin. North Am.*, 30, 4, 543–552, Oct. 1999.
12. Chamay, A. and Tschantz, P., Mechanical influences in bone remodeling. Experimental research on Wolff's law. *J. Biomech.*, 5, 2, 173–180, Mar. 1972, doi: 10.1016/0021-9290(72)90053-x. Available: https://doi.org/10.1016/0021-9290(72)90053-x.
13. Claes, L., Eckert-Hübner, K., Augat, P., The effect of mechanical stability on local vascularization and tissue differentiation in callus healing. *J. Orthop. Research,*® 20, 5, 1099–1105, 2002.
14. Schwartz, Z. and Boyan, B.D., Underlying mechanisms at the bone–biomaterial interface. *J. Cell. Biochem.*, 56, 3, 340–347, 1994.
15. Heilple, K.G., Chase, S.W., Herndon, C.H., A comparative study of the healing process following different types of bone transplantation. *Plast. Reconstr. Surg.*, 34, 1, 111, 1964.
16. Boyce, B.F. and Xing, L., Functions of RANKL/RANK/OPG in bone modeling and remodeling. *Arch. Biochem. Biophys.*, 473, 2, 139–146, 2008.

17. Lieberman, J.R. and Friedlaender, G.E. (Eds.), *Bone regeneration and repair: biology and clinical applications*, Humana Press Inc., Totowa, New Jersey, United States, 2005 Feb 17.
18. Masaki, C., Nakamoto, T., Mukaibo, T., Kondo, Y., Hosokawa, R., Strategies for alveolar ridge reconstruction and preservation for implant therapy. *J. Prosthodont. Res.*, 59, 4, 220–228, 2015.
19. Sundar, S.S., Jayesh, S.R., Hussain, S., Association of matrix metalloproteinase 1 gene promoter mutation and residual ridge resorption in edentulous patients of South Indian origin. *J. Pharm. Bioallied Sci.*, 7, 6, 652, 2015.
20. Riachi, F., Naaman, N., Tabarani, C., Aboelsaad, N., Aboushelib, M.N., Berberi, A., Salameh, Z., Influence of material properties on rate of resorption of two bone graft materials after sinus lift using radiographic assessment. *Int. J. Dent.*, 2012, 1, 737262, 2012.
21. Carinci, F., Farina, A., Zanetti, U., Vinci, R., Negrini, S., Calura, G., Laino, G., Piattelli, A., Alveolar ridge augmentation: a comparative longitudinal study between calvaria and iliac crest bone grafts. *J. Oral Implantol.*, 31, 1, 39–45, 2005 Feb 1.
22. Mertens, C., Decker, C., Seeberger, R., Hoffmann, J., Sander, A., Freier, K., Early bone resorption after vertical bone augmentation–a comparison of calvarial and iliac grafts. *Clin. Oral Implants Res.*, 24, 7, 820–5, 2013 Jul.
23. Stevenson, S.D., Li, X.Q., Martin, B., The fate of cancellous and cortical bone after transplantation of fresh and frozen tissue-antigen-matched and mismatched osteochondral allografts in dogs. *JBJS*, 73, 8, 1143–56, 1991 Sep 1.
24. Abbott, L.C., Schottstaedt, E.R., Saunders, J.B., Bost, F.C., The evaluation of cortical and cancellous bone as grafting material: A clinical and experimental study. *JBJS*, 29, 2, 381–414, 1947 Apr 1.
25. Pereira, E., Messias, A., Dias, R., Judas, F., Salvoni, A., Guerra, F., Horizontal resorption of fresh-frozen corticocancellous bone blocks in the reconstruction of the atrophic maxilla at 5 months. *Clin. Implant Dent. Relat. Res.*, 17, e444–58, 2015 Oct.
26. Lumetti, S., Galli, C., Manfredi, E., Consolo, U., Marchetti, C., Ghiacci, G., Toffoli, A., Bonanini, M., Salgarelli, A., Macaluso, G.M., Correlation between density and resorption of fresh-frozen and autogenous bone grafts. *Biomed Res. Int.*, 2014, 1, 508328, 2014.
27. Chaushu, G., Mardinger, O., Peleg, M., Ghelfan, O., Nissan, J., Analysis of complications following augmentation with cancellous block allografts. *J. Periodontol.*, 81, 12, 1759–64, 2010 Dec.
28. SS, Broggini, N., Hjørting-Hansen, E., Schenk, R., Buser, D., Bone healing and graft resorption of autograft, anorganic bovine bone and β-tricalcium phosphate. A histologic and histomorphometric study in the mandibles of minipigs. *Clin. Oral Implants Res.*, 17, 3, 237–43, 2006 Jun.
29. Gultekin, B.A., Bedeloglu, E., Kose, T.E., Mijiritsky, E., Comparison of bone resorption rates after intraoral block bone and guided bone regeneration

augmentation for the reconstruction of horizontally deficient maxillary alveolar ridges. *Biomed Res. Int.*, 2016, 1, 4987437, 2016.

30. Oklund, S.A., Prolo, D.J., Gutierrez, R.V., King, S.E., Quantitative comparisons of healing in cranial fresh autografts, frozen autografts and processed autografts, and allografts in canine skull defects. *Clin. Orthop. Relat. Res.*,® 205, 269–91, 1986 Apr 1.
31. Roberts, T.T. and Rosenbaum, A.J., Bone grafts, bone substitutes and orthobiologics: the bridge between basic science and clinical advancements in fracture healing. *Organogenesis*, 8, 4, 114–24, 2012 Oct-Dec, doi: 10.4161/org.23306. Epub 2012 Oct 1. PMID: 23247591; PMCID: PMC3562252.
32. Migliorini, F., Cuozzo, F., Torsiello, E., Spiezia, F., Oliva, F., Maffulli, N., Autologous Bone Grafting in Trauma and Orthopaedic Surgery: An Evidence-Based Narrative Review. *J. Clin. Med.*, 10, 19, 4347, 2021 Sep 24, doi: 10.3390/jcm10194347. PMID: 34640364; PMCID: PMC8509778.
33. Zins, J.E. and Whitaker, L.A., Membranous versus endochondral bone: implications for craniofacial reconstruction. *Plast. Reconstr. Surg.*, 72, 6, 778–84, 1983 Dec 1.
34. Fourcade, C., Lesclous, P., Guiol, J., Assignment of autogenous bone grafts for reconstruction of the alveolar ridge before implant placement. *J. Oral Med. Oral Surg.*, 25, 1, 1, 2019.
35. Hardesty, R.A. and Marsh, J.L., Craniofacial onlay bone grafting: a prospective evaluation of graft morphology, orientation, and embryonic origin. *Plast. Reconstr. Surg.*, 85, 1, 5–14, 1990 Jan 1.
36. Cordaro, L., Amadè, D.S., Cordaro, M., Clinical results of alveolar ridge augmentation with mandibular block bone grafts in partially edentulous patients prior to implant placement. *Clin. Oral Implants Res.*, 13, 1, 103–11, 2002.
37. Iizuka, T., Smolka, W., Hallermann, W., Mericske-Stern, R., Extensive augmentation of the alveolar ridge using autogenous calvarial split bone grafts for dental rehabilitation. *Clin. Oral Implants Res.*, 15, 5, 607–15, 2004.
38. Smolka, W., Eggensperger, N., Carollo, V., Ozdoba, C., Iizuka, T., Changes in the volume and density of calvarial split bone grafts after alveolar ridge augmentation. *Clin. Oral Implants Res.*, 17, 2, 149–55, 2006.
39. Chiapasco, M., Lang, N.P., Bosshardt, D.D., Quality and quantity of bone following alveolar distraction osteogenesis in the human mandible. *Clin. Oral Implants Res.*, 17, 4, 394–402, 2006 Aug.
40. Wortmann, D.E., Klein-Nulend, J., van Ruijven, L.J., Schortinghuis, J., Vissink, A., Raghoebar, G.M., Incorporation of anterior iliac crest or calvarial bone grafts in reconstructed atrophied maxillae: A randomized clinical trial with histomorphometric and micro-CT analyses. *Clin. Implant Dent. Relat. Res.*, 23, 3, 492–502, 2021.
41. Chappuis, V., Cavusoglu, Y., Buser, D., von Arx, T., Lateral ridge augmentation using autogenous block grafts and guided bone regeneration: A 10-year prospective case series study. *Clin. Implant Dent. Relat. Res.*, 19, 1, 85–96, 2017.

42. Eriksen, E.F., Cellular mechanisms of bone remodeling. *Rev. Endocr. Metab. Disord.*, 11, 4, 219–27, 2010 Dec, doi: 10.1007/s11154-010-9153-1. PMID: 21188536; PMCID: PMC3028072.
43. Raisz, L.G., Physiology and pathophysiology of bone remodeling. *Clin. Chem.*, 45, 8 Pt 2, 1353–8, Aug. 1999, Available: https://pubmed.ncbi.nlm.nih.gov/10430818.
44. Einhorn, T.A. and Gerstenfeld, L.C., Fracture healing: mechanisms and interventions. *Nat. Rev. Rheumatol.*, 11, 1, 45–54, Sep. 2014, doi: 10.1038/nrrheum.2014.164. Available: https://doi.org/10.1038/nrrheum.2014.164.
45. Sela, J.J. and Bab, I.A., Healing of Bone Fracture: General Concepts, in: *Principles of Bone Regeneration*, pp. 1–8, Springer, New York, 2012.
46. Ma, Q., Miri, Z., Haugen, H.J., Moghanian, A., Loca, D., Significance of mechanical loading in bone fracture healing, bone regeneration, and vascularization. *J. Tissue Eng.*, 22, 14, 20417314231172573, 2023, doi: 10.1177/20417314231172573. PMID: 37251734; PMCID: PMC10214107.
47. Ferraz, M.P., Bone Grafts in Dental Medicine: An Overview of Autografts, Allografts and Synthetic Materials. *Materials (Basel)*, 16, 11, 4117, 2023 May 31.
48. Nather, A. and Zheng, S., Evolution of allograft transplantation, in: *Allograft Procurement, Processing and Transplantation: A Comprehensive Guide for Tissue Bank*, p. 1, 2010 Aug 30.
49. Negredo, E., Martínez, E., Cinquegrana, D., Estany, C., Clotet, B., Therapeutic management of bone demineralization in the HIV-infected population. *Aids*, 21, 6, 657–63, 2007; 30.
50. Boyce, T., Edwards, J., Scarborough, N., Allograft bone: the influence of processing on safety and performance. *Orthop. Clin.*, 30, 4, 571–81, 1999 Oct 1.
51. Macedo, L.G.S., Mazzucchelli-Cosmo, L.A., Macedo, N.L., Monteiro, A.S.F., Sendyk, W.R., Fresh-frozen human bone allograft in vertical ridge augmentation: clinical and tomographic evaluation of bone formation and resorption. *Cell Tissue Banking*, 13, 4, 577–586, 2011.
52. Orsini, G., *et al.*, Clinical and histologic evaluation of fresh frozen human bone grafts for horizontal reconstruction of maxillary alveolar ridges. *Int. J. Periodontics Restorative Dent.*, 31, 5, 535–44, 2011.
53. Aslan, E., Gultekin, A., Karabuda, C., Mortellaro, C., Olgac, V., Mijiritsky, E., Clinical, histological, and histomorphometric evaluation of demineralized freeze-dried cortical block allografts for alveolar ridge augmentation. *J. Craniofac. Surg.*, 27, 5, 1181–1186, 2016.
54. Spin-Neto, R., Stavropoulos, A., Pereira, L.A., Marcantonio Jr., E., Wenzel, A., Fate of autologous and fresh-frozen allogeneic block bone grafts used for ridge augmentation. A CBCT-based analysis. *Clin. Oral Implants Res.*, 24, 2, 167–73, 2013 Feb.
55. Blume, O., Hoffmann, L., Donkiewicz, P., Wenisch, S., Back, M., Franke, J., Schnettler, R., Barbeck, M., Treatment of severely resorbed maxilla due to

peri-implantitis by guided bone regeneration using a customized allogenic bone block: A case report. *Materials*, 10, 10, 1213, 2017 Oct 21.

56. Nissan, J., Marilena, V., Gross, O., Mardinger, O., Chaushu, G., Histomorphometric analysis following augmentation of the posterior mandible using cancellous bone-block allograft. *J. Biomed. Mater. Res. Part A*, 97, 4, 509–13, 2011 Jun 15.
57. Ciszyński, M., Dominiak, S., Dominiak, M., Gedrange, T., Hadzik, J., Allogenic Bone Graft in Dentistry: A Review of Current Trends and Developments. *Int. J. Mol. Sci.*, 24, 23, 16598, 2023 22, doi: 10.3390/ijms242316598. PMID: 38068918; PMCID: PMC10706024.
58. Qazi, Y. and Hamrah, P., Corneal Allograft Rejection: Immunopathogenesis to Therapeutics. *J. Clin. Cell. Immunol.*, 2013, Suppl 9, 006, 2013 Nov 20, doi: 10.4172/2155-9899.S9-006. PMID: 24634796; PMCID: PMC3954811.
59. Stevenson, S., The immune response to osteochondral allografts in dogs. *J. Bone Joint Surg.*, 69, 4, 573–582, 1987.
60. Friedlaender, G.E., Strong, D.M., Sell, K.W., Studies on the antigenicity of bone. II. Donor-specific anti-HLA antibodies in human recipients of freeze-dried allografts. *J. Bone Joint Surg.*, 66, 1, 107–112, 1984.
61. Reikerås, O., Sigurdsen, U.W., Shegarfi, H., Impact of freezing on immunology and incorporation of bone allograft. *J. Orthop. Res.*, 28, 9, 1215–9, 2010.
62. Urist, M.R., A chemosterilized Antigen-Extracted autodigested alloimplant for bone banks. *Arch. Surg.*, 110, 4, 416, 1975.
63. Jing, L. and Su, B., Resorption Rates of Bone Graft Materials after Crestal Maxillary Sinus Floor Elevation and Its Influencing Factors. *J. Funct. Biomater.*, 15, 5, 133, 2024.
64. Schmidt, A.H., Autologous bone graft: Is it still the gold standard? *Injury*, 52, S18–22, 2021 Jun 1.
65. Velasquez-Plata, D., Todd Scheyer, E., Mellonig, J.T., Clinical comparison of an enamel matrix derivative used alone or in combination with a bovine-derived xenograft for the treatment of periodontal osseous defects in humans. *J. Periodontol.*, 73, 4, 433–40, 2002 Apr.
66. Baas, J., Svaneby D, T.B., Elmengaard, B., Bechtold, J., Soballe, K., Coralline hydroxyapatite granules inferior to morselized allograft around uncemented porous Ti implants: unchanged fixation by addition of concentrated autologous bone marrow aspirate. *J. Biomed. Mater. Res. Part A*, 99, 1, 9–15, 2011.
67. Koerdt, S., Ristow, O., Wannhoff, A., Kübler, A.C., Reuther, T., Expression of growth factors during the healing process of alveolar ridge augmentation procedures using autogenous bone grafts in combination with GTR and an anorganic bovine bone substitute: an immunohistochemical study in the sheep. *Clin. Oral Investig.*, 18, 179–88, 2014.
68. Miron, R.J., Wei, L., Bosshardt, D.D., Buser, D., Sculean, A., Zhang, Y., Effects of enamel matrix proteins in combination with a bovine-derived natural bone mineral for the repair of bone defects. *Clin. Oral Investig.*, 18, 471–8, 2014 Mar.

69. Miron, R.J., Optimized bone grafting. *Periodontol. 2000*, 94, 1, 143–160, Aug. 2023.
70. Yang, S., Lan, L., Miron, R.J., Wei, L., Zhang, M., Zhang, Y., Variability in particle degradation of four commonly employed dental bone grafts. *Clin. Implant Dent. Relat. Res.*, 17, 5, 996–1003, 2015 Oct.
71. Busenlechner, D., Tangl, S., Arnhart, C., Redl, II., Schuh, C., Watzek, G., Gruber, R., Resorption of deproteinized bovine bone mineral in a porcine calvaria augmentation model. *Clin. Oral Implants Res.*, 23, 1, 95–9, 2012.
72. Otsuka, T., Kasai, H., Yamaguchi, K., Nishihara, T., Enamel matrix derivative promotes osteoclast cell formation by RANKL production in mouse marrow cultures. *J. Dent.*, 33, 9, 749–55, 2005.
73. Ramírez-Fernández, M.P., Calvo-Guirado, J.L., Delgado-Ruiz, R.A., Maté-Sánchez del Val, J.E., Negri, B., Peñarrocha Diago, M., RETRACTED: Ultrastructural study by backscattered electron imaging and elemental microanalysis of biomaterial-to-bone interface and mineral degradation of bovine xenografts in maxillary sinus floor elevation. *Clin. Oral Implants Res.*, 24, 6, 645–51, 2013 Jun.
74. Betz, R.R., Limitations of autograft and allograft: new synthetic solutions. *Orthopedics*, 25, 5, 2002May 2002.
75. Niu, C.-C., Tsai, T.-T., Fu, T.-S., Lai, P.-L., Chen, L.-H., Chen, W.-J., A comparison of posterolateral lumbar fusion comparing autograft, autogenous laminectomy bone with bone marrow aspirate, and calcium sulphate with bone marrow aspirate: a prospective randomized study. *Spine*, 34, 25, 2715–2719, December 1, 2009, doi: 10.1097/BRS.0b013e3181b47232.
76. Yahav, A., Kurtzman, G.M., Katzap, M., Dudek, D., Baranes, D., Bone regeneration: properties and clinical applications of biphasic calcium sulfate. *Dent. Clin.*, 64, 2, 453–72, 2020 Apr 1.
77. Ogose, A., Kondo, N., Umezu, H., Hotta, T., Kawashima, H., Tokunaga, K., Ito, T., Kudo, N., Hoshino, M., Gu, W., Endo, N., Histological assessment in grafts of highly purified beta-tricalcium phosphate (OSferion®) in human bones. *Biomaterials*, 27, 8, 1542–9, 2006 Mar 1.
78. Eliaz, N. and Metoki, N., Calcium phosphate bioceramics: a review of their history, structure, properties, coating technologies and biomedical applications. *Materials*, 10, 4, 334, 2017 24.
79. van Oirschot, B., Mikos, A.G., Liu, Q., van den Beucken, J.J., Jansen, J.A., Fast degradable calcium phosphate cement for maxillofacial bone regeneration. *Tissue Eng. Part A*, 29, 5-6, 161–71, 2023.
80. Jones, J.R., Review of bioactive glass: From Hench to hybrids. *Acta Biomater.*, 9, 1, 4457–4486, 2012.
81. Välimäki, V.-V. and Aro, H.T., Molecular basis for action of bioactive glasses as bone graft substitute. *Scand. J. Surg.*, 95, 2, 95–102, Jun. 2006.
82. Liu, W.C., Robu, I.S., Patel, R., Leu, M.C., Velez, M., Chu, T.M., The effects of 3D bioactive glass scaffolds and BMP-2 on bone formation in rat femoral

critical size defects and adjacent bones. *Biomed. Mater.*, 9, 4, 045013, 2014 Jul 25.
83. Moimas, L., Biasotto, M., Di Lenarda, R., Olivo, A., Schmid, C., Rabbit pilot study on the resorbability of three-dimensional bioactive glass fibre scaffolds. *Acta Biomater.*, 2, 2, 191–9, 2006 Mar 1.
84. El-Ghannam, A., Sultana, F., Dréau, D., Tiwari, A., Yang, I.H., AlFotawi, R., Knabe-Ducheyne, C., Novel 3D printed bioactive SiC orthopedic screw promotes bone growth associated activities by macrophages, neurons, and osteoblasts. *J. Biomed. Mater. Res. Part A*, 113, 1, e37801, 2025 Jan.
85. Alfotawi, R., Premnath, S., El-Ghannam, A., Alsafadi, M., Mahmood, A., *In vivo* analysis of porous bioactive silicon carbide scaffold for craniofacial bone augmentation. *J. Craniofac. Surg.*, 35, 2, 699–704, 2024 Mar 1.
86. Hernández, L., Gurruchaga, M., Goñi, I., Injectable acrylic bone cements for vertebroplasty based on a radiopaque hydroxyapatite. Formulation and rheological behaviour. *J. Mater. Sci. - Mater. Med.*, 20, 1, 89–97, 2008.
87. Breusch, S. and Malchau, H., *The Well-Cemented total hip arthroplasty: Theory and Practice*, Springer Medizin Verlag, Heidelberg, Germany, 2005.
88. Blašković, M., Butorac Prpić, I., Blašković, D., Rider, P., Tomas, M., Čandrlić, S., Botond Hangyasi, D., Čandrlić, M., Perić Kačarević, Z., Guided bone regeneration using a novel magnesium membrane: a literature review and a report of two cases in humans. *J. Funct. Biomater.*, 14, 6, 307, 2023 Jun 1.
89. Barrère, F., van Blitterswijk, C.A., de Groot, K., Bone regeneration: molecular and cellular interactions with calcium phosphate ceramics. *Int. J. Nanomed.*, 1, 3, 317–32, 2006 Sep 15.
90. Patel, R.A., Wilson, R.F., Patel, P.A., Palmer, R.M., The effect of smoking on bone healing. *Bone Joint Res.*, 2, 6, 102–111, 2013, doi: 10.1302/2046-3758.26.2000142.
91. Choukroun, E., Parnot, M., Surmenian, J., Gruber, R., Cohen, N., Davido, N., Simonpieri, A., Savoldelli, C., Afota, F., El Mjabber, H., Choukroun, J., Bone formation and maintenance in oral surgery: the decisive role of the immune system—a narrative review of mechanisms and solutions. *Bioengineering*, 11, 2, 191, 2024.
92. Shirai, Y., Okuda, K., Kubota, T., Wolff, L.F., Yoshie, H., The comparative effectiveness of granules or blocks of superporous hydroxyapatite for the treatment of intrabony periodontal defects. *Open J. Stomatol.*, 2, 2, 81–7, 2012 Jun 12.
93. Hatano, N., Shimizu, Y., Ooya, K., A clinical long-term radiographic evaluation of graft height changes after maxillary sinus floor augmentation with a 2: 1 autogenous bone/xenograft mixture and simultaneous placement of dental implants. *Clin. Oral Implants Res.*, 15, 3, 339–45, 2004 Jun.
94. Ramírez Fernández, M.P., Mazón, P., Gehrke, S.A., Calvo-Guirado, J.L., De Aza, P.N., Comparison of Two Xenograft Materials Used in Sinus Lift Procedures: Material Characterization and *In Vivo* Behavior. *Materials*

(Basel), 10, 6, 623, 2017 Jun 7, doi: 10.3390/ma10060623. PMID: 28772984; PMCID: PMC5553531.

95. Kim, B.J., Kwon, T.K., Baek, H.S., Hwang, D.S., Kim, C.H., Chung, I.K., Jeong, J.S., Shin, S.H., A comparative study of the effectiveness of sinus bone grafting with recombinant human bone morphogenetic protein 2–coated tricalcium phosphate and platelet-rich fibrin–mixed tricalcium phosphate in rabbits. *Oral Surg. Oral Med. Oral Pathol. Oral Radiol.*, 113, 5, 583–92, 2012 May 1.
96. Jun, S.H., Lee, E.J., Jang, T.S., *et al.*, Bone morphogenic protein-2 (BMP-2) loaded hybrid coating on porous hydroxyapatite scaffolds for bone tissue engineering. *J. Mater. Sci.: Mater. Med.*, 24, 773–782, 2013.
97. Lee, J.C., Pereira, C.T., Ren, X., Huang, W., Bischoff, D., Weisgerber, D.W., Yamaguchi, D.T., Harley, B.A., Miller, T.A., Optimizing collagen scaffolds for bone engineering: effects of cross-linking and mineral content on structural contraction and osteogenesis. *J. Craniofac. Surg.*, 26, 6, 1992–6, 2015.
98. Pertici, G., Carinci, F., Carusi, G., Dragos, E., Villa, T., Crivelli, F., Rossi, F., Casalini, T., Müller, M., Perale, G., Composite Polymer Coated Mineral Scaffolds for Bone Regeneration: From Material Characterization to Human Studies. *J. Biol. Regul. Homeost. Agents*, 29, 3, 1–3, 2015.
99. Zogakis, P.N., Teles, A.R., Zafeiris, EP., Zafeiris, C.P., Bisphosphonate-loaded bone cement: Background, clinical indications and future perspectives. *J. Musculoskelet. Neuronal Interact.*, 22, 4, 587, 2022.
100. Bohner, M., Resorbable biomaterials as bone graft substitutes. *Mater. Today*, 13, 1-2, 24–30, 2010 Jan 1.
101. Moy, P.K., Lundgren, S., Holmes, R.E., Maxillary sinus augmentation: histomorphometric analysis of graft materials for maxillary sinus floor augmentation. *J. Oral Maxillofac. Surg.*, 51, 8, 857–62, 1993 Aug 1.
102. Pereira, R.D.S., de Carvalho, M.V.N.B., Hochuli-Vieira, E., Statkievicz, C., Pereira Santos, D.L., Augusto Neto, R.T., Pinto, C.D.F.S., Bennardo, F., Mourão, C.F., Histomorphometric and Micro-CT Evaluation of Cerabone and Bio-Oss in Maxillary Sinus Lifting: A Randomized Clinical Trial. *Medicina*, 60, 11, 1834, 2024, https://doi.org/10.3390/medicina60111834.
103. Wiltfang, J., Schlegel, K.A., Schultze-Mosgau, S., Nkenke, E., Zimmermann, R., Kessler, P., Sinus floor augmentation with β-tricalciumphosphate (β-TCP): Does platelet-rich plasma promote its osseous integration and degradation? *Clin. Oral Implants Res.*, 14, 2, 213–8, 2003.
104. Nyström, E., Kahnberg, K.E., Albrektsson, T., Treatment of the severely resorbed maxillae with bone graft and titanium implants: histologic review of autopsy specimens. *Int. J. Oral Maxillofac. Implants*, 8, 2, 1993 Mar 1.

4
Mechanism of Action of Bone Grafts

Paramjit Kaur Khinda

Dental Faculty, King Saud bin Abdulaziz University of Health Sciences, Riyadh, Kingdom of Saudi Arabia

Abstract
Bone grafting, a cornerstone of reconstructive surgery, aims to restore structural integrity in compromised sites. This chapter explores the intricate processes governing bone regeneration following graft implantation, emphasizing the interplay between graft material properties and host tissue responses. The essential functions of osteoconduction, osteoinduction, and osteogenesis are explored, emphasizing how scaffold structure, biomaterial makeup, and growth factor release affect bone formation. This chapter also addresses common complications, including infection and graft resorption. By synthesizing current knowledge and highlighting emerging technologies, this chapter equips readers with a comprehensive understanding of bone graft mechanisms and their clinical implications.

***Keywords*:** Regeneration, remodeling, graft materials, progenitor cells, osteoinduction, osteoconduction, osteogenesis

4.1 Introduction

Bone grafts contribute to bone regeneration through a combination of biological and structural mechanisms that operate in a coordinated manner. Understanding these mechanisms informs clinical application, material selection, and interpretation of regenerative outcomes across different clinical scenarios. It includes many sequential but overlapping steps. Initial inflammation and clot formation: Following graft placement, a blood clot forms, releasing growth factors (e.g., PDGF) and cytokines (e.g., IL-8) that initiate healing and attract immune cells. Angiogenesis and vascularization:

Email: khindapammi@gmail.com

Randa A. Alfotawi (ed.) Oro-Facial Bone Grafts and Biomaterials, (73–88) © 2026 Scrivener Publishing LLC

New blood vessels form (angiogenesis) to supply nutrients and oxygen to the graft site, crucial for cell survival and recruitment of mesenchymal stem cells (MSCs). Cellular proliferation and differentiation: MSCs migrate to the graft and differentiate into osteoblasts, the bone-forming cells, influenced by growth factors and the graft material's properties [1]. Bone remodeling is replacing old bone to maintain bone strength and regulate the calcium and phosphate levels in the body. It is divided into four stages: cell activation, resorption, reversal, and, finally, bone formation. Bone healing is the process of healing of bone following a fracture [2]. This is a remarkable feat of biological engineering and is a complex process that orchestrates the repair of the skeletal system after fractures or injuries [3]. Far from being a simple patching job, this intricate process is the cascading result of various cellular and molecular events, all coordinated to restore the integrity and capacity of the damaged bone [4]. This process occurs through two main mechanisms: primary healing and secondary healing [2] (Table 4.1).

Ensuring successful bone regeneration after grafting is vital for the long-term stability of teeth and the potential for future dental implant placement, periodontal regeneration, and alveolar ridge augmentation. A thorough understanding of the various types of bone grafts and how they work is essential for effective clinical practice [8].

Bone grafts and substitute materials are mainly categorized in two ways: by their tissue origin or by their material composition [9, 10]. Therefore, based on these criteria, bone grafts and substitute materials used in dentistry are generally divided into five distinct categories [11] (Figure 4.1).

Table 4.1 Important terms used for the mechanism of bone grafts.

Terms	Definitions	Ref.
Bone healing	*is the body's natural response to a fracture*	[5]
Bone remodeling	*refers to the continuous maintenance and adaptation of existing bone*	[6]
Bone regeneration	*involves the growth of new bone to replace lost or damaged tissue, occurring during healing, and is also the aim of procedures such as bone grafting*	[7]

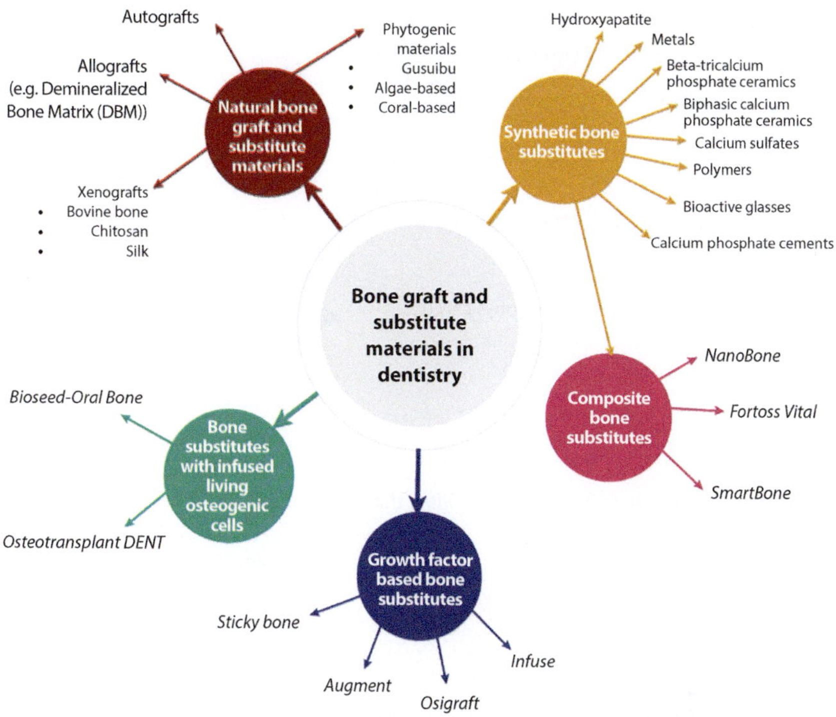

Figure 4.1 Classification of bone graft materials.

4.2 Mechanism of Action of Bone Graft Materials

The primary objective of bone grafts is to restore or replace lost bone tissue, creating an environment conducive to new bone formation and functional integration with the surrounding native bone. The mechanism by which bone grafts achieve these regenerative outcomes is multifactorial. It involves three fundamental biological processes: osteogenesis, osteoinduction, and osteoconduction as shown in Figures 4.2 and 4.3. These processes are influenced by the type of graft material used—autografts, allografts, xenografts, or alloplasts—and their inherent biological properties [12].

4.2.1 Osteogenesis

Osteogenesis refers to new bone formation mediated by viable osteogenic cells present within the graft material. This mechanism is predominantly associated with autogenous bone grafts, where transplanted cells actively participate in early bone formation at the recipient site. This process

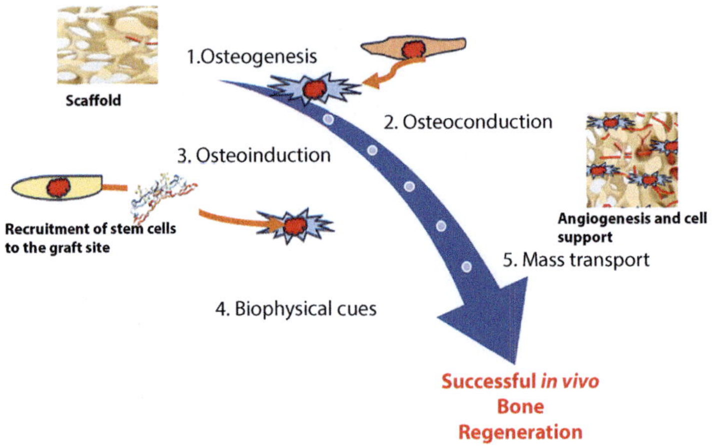

Figure 4.2 The flowchart illustrates the pillars that are required for successful bone regeneration.

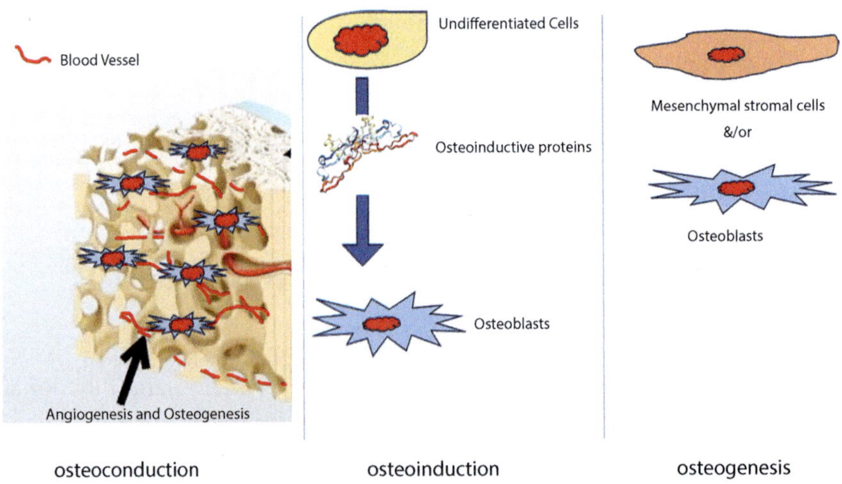

Figure 4.3 Diagram showing mechanisms of osteoconduction, osteoinduction, and osteogenesis.

depends on the survival and growth of osteoblasts and osteoprogenitor cells that are incorporated into the graft. Among the different graft materials available, only autogenous bone grafts contain living bone cells that can achieve true osteogenesis. The mechanism involves the transplantation of viable osteoblasts and osteoprogenitor cells, which then produce new bone matrix. This biological process is essential for rapid bone formation and the successful integration of the graft with the host bone [6, 13].

4.2.2 Growth Factor Signaling

Growth factors play a central role in regulating bone regeneration by modulating cell recruitment, proliferation, and differentiation. Bone morphogenetic proteins and other signaling molecules primarily act as biological modulators, influencing the regenerative cascade rather than initiating bone formation independently. Bone morphogenetic proteins (BMPs), particularly BMP-2, BMP-4, and BMP-7, play a crucial role in stimulating osteoblast differentiation. These signaling molecules bind to specific receptors on MSCs, activating intracellular pathways such as the Sma and Mad-related protein (SMAD) signaling cascade. The Smad pathway, activated by TGF-beta and BMPs, is crucial for bone regeneration as it regulates osteoblast differentiation and function. When the ligand binds to cell surface receptors, Smad proteins undergo phosphorylation, forming complexes that translocate to the nucleus to control gene expression essential for bone formation. Various Smad proteins (Smad1/5/8 for BMPs, Smad2/3 for TGF-beta) mediate distinct signals influencing osteogenic differentiation and matrix production [14]. This activation triggers the expression of osteoblast-specific genes, including *Runx2* and *osteocalcin*, which are essential for bone formation and mineralization [15].

The Wingless-related integration (Wnt) signaling pathway is essential for regulating MSC differentiation and osteoblast function. Its activation enhances osteoblastogenesis, while its inhibition suppresses bone formation. Wnt ligands bind to Frizzled receptors, initiating downstream signaling cascades that stabilize β-catenin. This stabilization subsequently influences the expression of genes vital for bone development and mineralization [16].

Fibroblast growth factors (FGFs) play a vital role in bone regeneration by stimulating MSC proliferation and differentiation. In addition to promoting osteogenesis, FGFs also enhance angiogenesis, ensuring an adequate supply of oxygen and nutrients to support tissue healing and bone formation [17].

4.2.3 Transcription Factors

Transcription factors regulate gene expression involved in osteoblastic differentiation and maturation. Key regulators such as Runx2 and Osterix coordinate the transition of mesenchymal cells toward the osteoblastic lineage, thereby supporting bone matrix production. Runt-related transcription factor 2 (Runx2) is a key regulator of osteoblast differentiation and bone formation. It regulates the expression of key osteoblast-specific genes, including *collagen type I*, *osteocalcin*, and *osteopontin*, which are vital for bone matrix synthesis and mineralization.

Osterix (Osx) is an important transcription factor required for osteoblast differentiation and bone formation. Functioning downstream of Runx2, Osx regulates the expression of key osteoblast maturation markers, ensuring proper development and mineralization of the bone matrix [18].

4.2.4 Extracellular Matrix (ECM) Synthesis

Extracellular matrix synthesis provides a structural framework that supports cellular attachment, signaling, and subsequent mineral deposition. The composition and organization of the ECM influence the quality and mechanical properties of newly formed bone. Collagen type I is the predominant structural protein in the bone matrix, essential for providing tensile strength and stability. Synthesized and secreted by osteoblasts, it forms a fibrous network that serves as a scaffold for mineral deposition, ultimately contributing to bone formation and mechanical integrity [19].

Osteocalcin, osteopontin, and bone sialoprotein are key non-collagenous proteins involved in bone mineralization and cell adhesion. Synthesized and secreted by osteoblasts, these proteins regulate matrix organization, facilitate hydroxyapatite deposition, and contribute to the structural integrity of mineralized bone tissue [20].

4.2.5 Mineralization

Mineralization involves the deposition of inorganic calcium phosphate crystals within the organic matrix, leading to progressive stiffening and maturation of bone tissue. This process occurs gradually and continues as part of long-term bone remodeling. Hydroxyapatite crystals, primarily composed of calcium and phosphate, form the mineralized component of bone, providing structural rigidity. Osteoblasts regulate the deposition of these crystals onto the collagen matrix, facilitating the mineralization process necessary for bone strength and stability. Alkaline phosphatase (ALP) is a key enzyme secreted by osteoblasts that plays a vital role in bone mineralization. It hydrolyzes phosphate esters, thereby increasing the local concentration of phosphate ions, which are essential for the nucleation and growth of hydroxyapatite crystals within the bone matrix [6].

4.2.6 Osteoinduction

Osteoinduction is the biological process by which graft materials stimulate host mesenchymal stem cells (MSCs) to differentiate into osteoblasts, promoting new bone formation [21]. This process is primarily mediated by growth factors, particularly bone morphogenetic proteins (BMPs), which are present within the graft material. Allografts and certain demineralized bone matrices (DBMs) exhibit osteoinductive properties, enhancing bone regeneration. The mechanism involves BMPs and other growth factors diffusing into surrounding tissues, where they bind to MSC receptors and activate intracellular signaling pathways that drive osteoblast differentiation. These newly formed osteoblasts then synthesize bone matrix, facilitating graft integration and bone repair [15, 22].

Bone and surrounding tissues contain both differentiated cells, such as osteoblasts, osteoclasts, and osteocytes, alongside a population of undifferentiated progenitor cells. These undifferentiated cells are critical in bone healing and implant integration, acting as a reservoir for osteoprogenitor cells. Under appropriate biological stimuli, these progenitor cells undergo differentiation into preosteoblasts, a key step in the process of bone induction as shown in Figure 4.4. This transformation is driven by inductive agents that regulate cellular commitment to the osteogenic lineage. The fundamental principles of bone induction, established through classical studies, have provided valuable insights into skeletal regeneration across different anatomical sites [23].

Modern research on osteoinduction traces back to Urist's experiments in the 1960s, when demineralized bone was identified as an osteoinductive agent. Subsequently, Urist et al. isolated bone morphogenetic proteins (BMPs), a subset of the transforming growth factor-beta (TGF-β) superfamily, as key regulators of bone formation [24]. Among the 15 known BMPs, BMP-2 and BMP-7 have demonstrated significant osteoinductive potential. Ongoing research continues to explore the role of BMPs in skeletal regeneration, as they

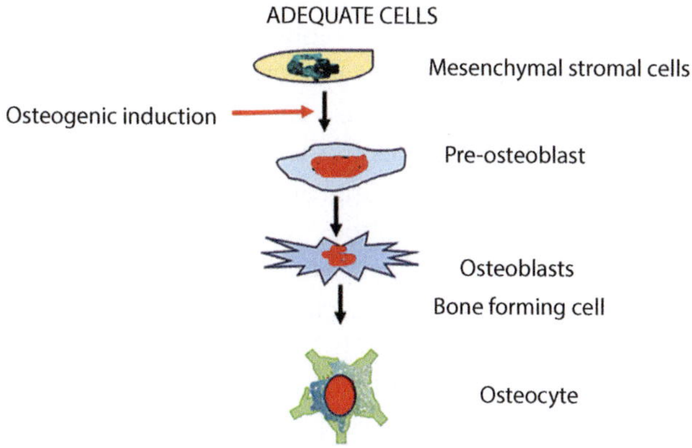

Figure 4.4 During injury, bone repair involves both differentiated and undifferentiated cells. However, the primary source of new bone formation comes from undifferentiated cells, which are stimulated to develop into preosteoblasts [23].

are endogenously released during trauma and bone remodeling. Additionally, physical stimuli such as mechanical stress and electrical signals have been implicated in modulating bone induction processes.

4.2.7 Osteoconduction

Osteoconduction is the process by which a graft material serves as a structural scaffold, facilitating the ingrowth of host bone tissue. The graft provides a framework that directs the migration of osteoblasts and supports the deposition of new bone matrix [25]. This property is observed in all types of bone grafts, including allografts, xenografts, and alloplasts. The mechanism involves the porous structure of the graft material, which enables the infiltration of blood vessels, osteoblasts, and osteoprogenitor cells from the surrounding host bone. As bone formation progresses, new bone is deposited onto the graft's surface, gradually integrating and replacing the material. The architectural characteristics of the graft play a crucial role in ensuring successful osteoconduction [26, 27].

4.3 Structural Characteristics for Osteoconduction

Structural features such as pore size, interconnectivity, surface roughness, and three-dimensional architecture influence osteoconductive performance. Porosity contributes to vascular ingrowth and cell migration but does not act as the sole determinant of regenerative capacity.

1. *Porosity:* Porosity is important for osteoconduction as it allows for the ingrowth of blood vessels and bone cells, facilitating nutrient and oxygen transport. However, excessive porosity can compromise the mechanical strength of the scaffold [28, 29]. Pores in the range of 100–500 μm are considered ideal for bone ingrowth [30]. Interconnectivity of pores ensures a continuous network for cell migration and tissue formation throughout the scaffold [31]. Well-connected pores promote vascularization, which is vital for sustaining bone tissue growth and integration [32]. By controlled pore size and interconnectivity, bone formation can be guided in a desired pattern [33].
2. *Surface roughness:* Rough surfaces enhance cell adhesion and proliferation, improving osteointegration [34].

3. *Biodegradability:* Controlled degradation allows for gradual replacement of the graft with natural bone [35]. The rate of degradation significantly impacts osteoconduction. If the graft degrades too quickly, it may lose structural support before new bone can form, whereas slow degradation may hinder bone growth [29]. As the material breaks down, the porosity of the scaffold may change, which, in turn, can influence vascularization and the transport of nutrients and oxygen, all critical factors in osteoconduction [30].

4.4 Ideal Requirements for Bone Grafts and Substitutes

An ideal bone graft material is conceptualized as one that balances biological compatibility, mechanical stability, controlled resorption, and ease of clinical handling. In practice, no single material fulfills all ideal criteria, necessitating material selection tailored to specific clinical objectives.

1. Osteoconductivity: The material must serve as a scaffold for new bone formation, facilitating the attachment, migration, and proliferation of osteoblasts, which are essential for bone matrix deposition.
2. Osteoinductivity: It should promote the differentiation of stem cells into osteoblasts, thereby initiating and accelerating the bone formation process [36].
3. Biocompatibility: The graft should be non-immunogenic and well tolerated by the host tissue, minimizing the risk of inflammatory reactions or rejection [37].
4. Porosity and interconnectivity: An interconnected porous structure is essential to support vascular infiltration, nutrient exchange, and the migration of bone-forming cells, enhancing regenerative potential [38].
5. Resorbability: The material should undergo controlled degradation, allowing for its gradual replacement by native bone without necessitating surgical removal [38].
6. Structural integrity: It must maintain mechanical stability during the early healing phase, providing necessary support to the surrounding tissues and ensuring graft success.

4.5 Factors Influencing Graft Integration and Success

Graft integration is influenced by a combination of biological, mechanical, and patient-specific factors. Adequate mechanical stability supports vascularization and bone formation but does not guarantee successful integration in isolation.

4.5.1 Biological Factors

1. Host immune response: A strong inflammatory response can hinder graft integration and lead to rejection [39].
2. Vascularization: Adequate blood supply is crucial for nutrient delivery and waste removal, supporting graft survival [40].

4.5.2 Mechanical Factors

1. Load-bearing capacity: The graft must withstand physiological stresses without fracturing or dislodging [41].
2. Stress shielding: Excessive stress shielding can lead to bone resorption and graft failure [42].

4.5.3 Patient-Specific Factors

1. Age and health status: Age-related changes in bone metabolism and overall health can influence healing and graft success [43].
2. Smoking and alcohol consumption: These habits can negatively impact bone healing and increase the risk of complications [44].

4.6 Advantages and Disadvantages of Bone Grafting

Bone grafting offers well-documented regenerative benefits but is also associated with limitations that vary according to graft type, surgical technique, and patient factors. Predictability of outcomes depends on appropriate case selection and biological compatibility rather than material choice alone.

Advantages

1. Enhanced bone healing: Bone grafts provide a scaffold for new bone growth, significantly improving the healing process for fractures and defects [13].

2. Support for implants: Crucial for patients with insufficient jawbone structure, ensuring a stable foundation for dental implants.
3. Restoration of functionality: Bone grafts can restore strength and functionality of areas affected by trauma, disease, or congenital defects, improving quality of life [45].

Disadvantages

1. Risk of infection: There is a risk of infection at the graft or donor site [46].
2. Immune rejection: Especially with allografts (donor bone) and xenografts (animal bone), though modern processing reduces this risk [47].
3. Donor site morbidity: When autografts are utilized, that is, bone taken from the patient's own body, there is added pain and recovery time at the donor site [48].

4.7 Emerging Technologies and Advanced Grafting Materials in Bone Regeneration

Emerging technologies, including bioengineered scaffolds and biologically enhanced materials, aim to improve regenerative performance by mimicking natural bone biology. Current evidence supports their potential, while long-term clinical validation remains ongoing.

1. 3D printing: Allows for the fabrication of patient-specific scaffolds with complex geometries and controlled porosity [30].
2. Nanotechnology: Utilizing nanoparticles in scaffolds can enhance cell–material interactions and promote bone regeneration [49].
3. Biodegradable polymers: These polymers degrade gradually, providing a temporary support structure while allowing for tissue ingrowth and remodeling [50].
4. Stem cell therapy: Combining scaffolds with stem cells can enhance bone regeneration by providing a source of bone-forming cells [51].
5. Gene therapy: Genetically modifying cells or delivering genes to the site of injury can stimulate bone formation and improve healing outcomes [52].

6. Biomimetic materials: Materials designed to mimic the natural extracellular matrix can provide a more physiologically relevant environment for bone regeneration [53].
7. Antimicrobial coatings: Incorporating antimicrobial agents into scaffolds can prevent infection, a major complication in bone regeneration [54].
8. Drug delivery systems: Integrating drug delivery capabilities into scaffolds allows for controlled release of growth factors and other therapeutic agents to enhance bone repair [55].
9. Personalized medicine: Tailoring graft materials and treatment strategies to individual patient needs based on genetic and other factors [56].

4.8 Clinical Outcomes and Complications

Clinical outcomes of bone graft materials are largely dependent on successful integration, evidenced by radiographic union and functional restoration. Complications, however, can significantly impact these outcomes. Infection, a major concern, can lead to graft failure and necessitate further surgical intervention [46]. Non-union, or delayed union, is another complication, often associated with patient-specific factors like smoking or poor nutrition [57]. Graft resorption, particularly with certain synthetic materials, can lead to volume loss and compromise long-term stability [13]. Donor site morbidity, especially with autografts, can cause pain and functional limitations [48]. Immunological reactions, although rare, can occur with allografts [47]. Ultimately, careful patient selection, meticulous surgical technique, and appropriate graft material selection are crucial for minimizing complications and achieving optimal clinical outcomes [58].

4.9 Future Directions in Bone Graft Mechanisms

The increasing limitations of autogenous bone harvesting, coupled with the potential immunogenic and disease transmission risks associated with allogeneic grafts, are driving a significant move towards the use of synthetic bone substitutes. Consequently, research and development are highly dedicated to engineering biocompatible, mechanically robust, and clinically efficient bone replacement materials. These advanced biomaterials aim to optimize osteoconductivity and osteoinductivity, promoting predictable bone regeneration at defect sites. Furthermore, the synergistic integration of bone replacement grafts with guided tissue regeneration (GTR) techniques is being increasingly explored to enhance periodontal and osseous repair outcomes. Future advancements aim to prioritize the development of standardized, reproducible, and clinically validated bone substitutes to ensure predictable and safe clinical outcomes, facilitating their wider application in oral and maxillofacial reconstructive therapy [59].

AI disclosure statement: The author acknowledges the use of AI-based tools for minor language editing or grammatical correction. However, all intellectual contributions, analyses, and conclusions presented in this chapter are entirely the author's own.

References

1. Abu Alfar, TM.S., Alaida, W.S., Hammudah, H.A., Mohamado, L.L., Gaw, R.R., Al-Salamah, L., Alasmari, B.A., Alotaibi, R.M., Almutairi, M.A., Exploring the Potential of Phytogenic Materials for Bone Regeneration: A Narrative Review of Current Advances and Future Directions. *Cureus*, 2, 15, 11, e48175, 2023. doi: 10.7759/cureus.48175. PMID: 38046714; PMCID: PMC10693310.
2. ElHawary, H., Baradaran, A., Abi-Rafeh, J., Vorstenbosch, J., Xu, L., Efanov, J.I., Bone Healing and Inflammation: Principles of Fracture and Repair. *Semin. Plast. Surg.*, 35, 3, 198–203, 2021, doi: 10.1055/s-0041-1732334. Epub 2021 Sep10. PMID: 34526868; PMCID: PMC8432998.
3. Bigham-Sadegh, A. and Oryan, A., Basic concepts regarding fracture healing and the current options and future directions in managing bone fractures. *Int. Wound J.*, 12, 3, 238–47, 2015.
4. Papachristou, D.J., Georgopoulos, S., Giannoudis, P.V., Panagiotopoulos, E., Insights into the Cellular and Molecular Mechanisms That Govern the Fracture-Healing Process: A Narrative Review. *J. Clin. Med.*, 10, 16, 3554, 2021;12, doi: 10.3390/jcm10163554. PMID: 34441849; PMCID: PMC8397080.
5. Sheen, J.R., Mabrouk, A., Garla, V.V., Fracture Healing Overview. [Updated 2023 Apr 8], in: *StatPearls* [Internet], StatPearls Publishing, Treasure Island (FL), 2025 Jan, Available from: https://www.ncbi.nlm.nih.gov/books/NBK551678/.
6. Dimitriou, R., Tsiridis, E., Giannoudis, P.V., Current concepts of molecular aspects of bone healing. *Injury*, 42, S2, S2–S10, 2011.
7. Rowe, P., Koller, A., Sharma, S., Physiology, Bone Remodeling. [Updated 2023 Mar 17], in: *StatPearls* [Internet], StatPearls Publishing, Treasure Island (FL), 2025 Jan, Available from: https://www.ncbi.nlm.nih.gov/books/NBK499863/.
8. Sculean, A., Gruber, R., Bosshardt, D.D., Becker, J., Bone regeneration and periodontal tissue repair in human periodontal defects. *J. Clin. Periodontol.*, 42, Suppl. 16, S86–S107, 2015.

9. Kumar, P., Fathima, G., Vinitha, B., Bone grafts in dentistry. *J. Pharm. Bioallied Sci.*, 5, 125–127, 2013, doi: 10.4103/0975-7406.113312.
10. Kolk, A., Handschel, J., Drescher, W., Rothamel, D., Kloss, F., Blessmann, M., Heiland, M., Wolff, K.-D., Smeets, R., Current trends and future perspectives of bone substitute materials—From space holders to innovative biomaterials. *J. Craniomaxillofac. Surg.*, 40, 706–718, 2012, doi: 10.1016/j.jcms.2012.01.002.
11. Zhao, R., Yang, R., Cooper, P.R., Khurshid, Z., Shavandi, A., Ratnayake, J., Bone Grafts and Substitutes in Dentistry: A Review of Current Trends and Developments. *Molecules*, 26, 10, 3007, 2021 18, doi: 10.3390/molecules26103007. PMID: 34070157; PMCID: PMC8158510.
12. Roberts, T.T. and Rosenbaum, A.J., Bone grafts, bone substitutes and orthobiologics: the bridge between basic science and clinical advancements in fracture healing. *Organogenesis*, 8, 4, 114–24, 2012, doi: 10.4161/org.23306. Epub 2012 Oct 1. PMID: 23247591; PMCID: PMC3562252.
13. Giannoudis, P.V., Einhorn, T.A., Marsh, D., Pape, H.C., Fracture healing: a current perspective of clinical problems and research directions. *J. Bone Joint Surg. (British)*, 89, 9, 1146–1156, 2007.
14. Zou, M., Chen, Z.H., Teng, Y., Liu, P., Jia, Z.K., Zhang, C., Yuan, F.L., The Smad Dependent TGF-β and BMP Signaling Pathway in Bone Remodeling and Therapies. *Front. Mol. Biosci.*, 8, 593310, 2021.
15. Wozney, J.M., Rosen, V., Celeste, A.J., Mitsock, L.M., Whitters, M.J., Kriz, R.W., Wang, E.A., Novel regulators of bone formation: molecular clones and activities. *Science*, 242, 4885, 1528–1534, 1988.
16. Logan, C.Y. and Nusse, R., The Wnt signaling pathway in development and disease. *Annu. Rev. Cell Dev. Biol.*, 20, 781–810, 2004.
17. Ornitz, D.M. and Itoh, N., The fibroblast growth factor signaling pathway: a key regulator of skeletal development and homeostasis. *Dev. Dyn.*, 244, 3, 215–229, 2015.
18. Komori, T., Regulation of proliferation, differentiation and functions of osteoblasts by Runx2. *J. Cell. Biochem.*, 94, 6, 1113–1120, 2005.
19. Prockop, D.J. and Kivirikko, K.I., Collagens: molecular biology, diseases, and potentials for therapy. *Annu. Rev. Biochem.*, 64, 1, 403–434, 1995.
20. Young, M.F., Kerr, J.M., Ibaraki, K., Heegaard, A.M., Robey, P.G., Structure, expression, and regulation of SPARC/osteonectin. *Clin. Orthop. Relat. Res.*, 282, 276–294, 1992.
21. Ferraz, M.P., Bone grafts in dental medicine: an overview of autografts, allografts and synthetic materials. *Materials*, 31, 16, 11, 4117, 2023.
22. Oryan, A., Alidadi, S., Moshiri, A., Maffulli, N., Bone regenerative medicine: classic options to innovative approaches. *J. Tissue Eng. Regener. Med.*, 11, 8, 2212–2236, 2017.
23. Albrektsson, T. and Johansson, C., Osteoinduction, osteoconduction and osseointegration. *Eur. Spine J.*, 10, Suppl 2, S96–101, 2001, doi: 10.1007/s005860100282. PMID: 11716023; PMCID: PMC3611551.
24. Urist, M.R., Bone: formation by autoinduction. *Science*, 150, 893–899, 1965.

25. Yuan, H., Fernandes, H., Habibovic, P., de Boer, J., Barradas, A.M.C., de Ruiter, A., Walsh, W.R., van Blitterswijk, C.A., de Bruijn, J.D., Osteoinductive ceramics as a synthetic alternative to autologous bone grafting. *Proc. Natl. Acad. Sci. U.S.A.*, 107, 31, 13614–13619, 2010, https://doi.org/10.1073/pnas.1003600107.
26. Geurs, N.C. and Reddy, M.S., Periodontal regenerative therapy. *Dent. Clin. North Am.*, 45, 1, 187–211, 2001.
27. Habibovic, P. and Yuan, H., Bone graft substitutes: where do we stand? *J. Tissue Eng. Regen. Med.*, 1, 1, 17–31, 2006.
28. Karageorgiou, V. and Kaplan, D., Porosity of 3D biomaterial scaffolds and osteogenesis. *Biomaterials*, 26, 27, 5474–5491, 2005.
29. Loh, Q.L. and Choong, C., Three-dimensional scaffolds for tissue engineering applications: a review of current approaches. *Tissue Eng. Part B Rev.*, 19, 6, 485–516, 2013.
30. Hutmacher, D.W., Scaffolds in tissue engineering bone and cartilage. *Biomaterials*, 21, 24, 2529–2543, 2000.
31. Jones, J.R. and Hench, L.L., Regenerating bioactive materials. *Curr. Opin. Solid State Mater. Sci.*, 7, 4–5, 301–307, 2003.
32. Murphy, S.V. and O'Brien, F.J., Pore size dependency of cell penetration, proliferation and differentiation in collagen-glycosaminoglycan scaffolds for bone tissue engineering. *Biomaterials*, 31, 1, 263–271, 2010.
33. Williams, D.F., On the mechanisms of biocompatibility. *Biomaterials*, 29, 20, 2941–2953, 2008.
34. Boyan, B.D., Lotz, E.M., Schwartz, Z., Roughness and Hydrophilicity as Osteogenic Biomimetic Surface Properties. *Tissue Eng. Part A*, 23, 23-24, 1479–1489, 2017, doi: 10.1089/ten.TEA.2017.0048. Epub 2017 Nov 4. PMID: 28793839; PMCID: PMC5729880.
35. Rezwan, K., Chen, Q.Z., Blaker, J.J., Boccaccini, A.R., Biodegradable and bioactive porous polymer/inorganic composite scaffolds for bone tissue engineering. *Biomaterials*, 27, 18, 3413–31, 2006, doi: 10.1016/j.biomaterials.2006.01.039. Epub 2006 Feb 28. PMID: 16504284.
36. Goonoo, N. and Bhaw-Luximon, A., Regenerative medicine: Induced pluripotent stem cells and their benefits on accelerated bone tissue reconstruction using scaffolds. *J. Mater. Res.*, 33, 11, 1573–1591, 2018, doi: 10.1557/jmr.2018.132.
37. Özcan, M., Hotza, D., Fredel, M.C., Cruz, A., Volpato, C.A., Materials and manufacturing techniques for polymeric and ceramic scaffolds used in implant dentistry. *J. Compos. Sci.*, 115, 3, 78, 2021.
38. Boserup, A., Biomimetic Bone Grafts: The Ideal Bone Grafting Material and its Properties. *J. Bone Res.*, 11, 246, 2023.
39. Clavero-Teran, J. and Naval-Gias, L., Graft selection in dental implantology: a systematic review. *Med. Oral Patol. Oral Cir. Bucal*, 14, 11, E568–E573, 2009.
40. Schmitz, J.P. and Hollinger, J.O., The critical size defect in canine mandible. *J. Dent. Res.*, 65, 3, 407–412, 1986.

41. Szmukler-Moncler, S., Salama, M., Reingewirtz, Y., Chiapasco, M., Timing of implant placement following immediate extraction with guided bone regeneration: a review. *Int. J. Oral Maxillofac. Implants*, 15, 3, 2000.
42. Huiskes, R., Weinans, H., Dalstra, M., Adaptive bone-remodeling theory validated for tibial component-stem design and compared with experimental observations. *J. Biomech.*, 25, 11, 1289–1307, 1992.
43. Jensen, O.T. and Cottam, J.R., Guided bone augmentation: a clinical review. *J. Oral Implantol.*, 22, 4, 263–270, 1996.
44. Palmer, R.M., Palmer, P.J., Toms, A.P., Dental implants and smoking. *Br. Dent. J.*, 199, 6, 391–394, 2005.
45. Giannoudis, P.V., Calori, G.M., Begue, T., Schmidmaier, G., Bone substitutes: handling properties, safety and efficacy. *Injury*, 42, Suppl 2, S3–S6, 2011.
46. Cierny, G. and Mader, J.T., Acute and chronic osteomyelitis. *Clin. Orthop. Relat. Res.*, 414, 7–37, 2003.
47. Tomford, W.W., Transmission of disease by transplantation of musculoskeletal allografts. *J. Bone Joint Surg. Am.*, 77, 11, 1742–1754, 1995.
48. Younger, E.M. and Chapman, M.W., 6 Morbidity at bone graft donor sites. *J. Orthop. Trauma*, 3, 3, 192–195, 1989.
49. Jain, K.K., Nanotechnology in drug delivery. *Nat. Rev. Drug Discovery*, 4, 12, 969–979, 2005.
50. Langer, R. and Vacanti, J.P., Tissue engineering. *Science*, 260, 5110, 920–926, 1993.
51. Pittenger, M.F., Mackay, A.M., Scherer, S.C., Jaiswal, R.K., Multilineage potential of adult human mesenchymal stem cells. *Science*, 284, 5411, 143–147, 1999.
52. Wagner, E. and Cotten, M., Gene therapy: approaches to human gene transfer. *Pharmacol. Rev.*, 43, 2, 145–181, 1991.
53. Ahmed, R.A.R., Atteya, M., Mahmood, A., AlHindi, A.S.M., El-Ghannam, A., Assessment of novel surgical procedures using decellularised muscle and bioactive ceramic: a histological analysis. *J. Mater. Sci.: Mater. Med.*, 32, 113, 2021.
54. Gilbert, P. and Allison, D.G., Antibacterial surface modification of biomaterials. *Biomaterials*, 21, 23, 2385–2398, 2000.
55. Langer, R., New methods of drug delivery. *Science*, 249, 4976, 1527–1533, 1990.
56. Hood, L. and Heath, J.K., Systems biology and new technologies enable predictive and preventative medicine. *Science*, 300, 5625, 619–623, 2003.
57. Einhorn, T.A., Enhancement of fracture healing. *Instr. Course Lect.*, 44, 403–415, 1995.
58. Laurencin, C.T., Nair, L.S., Nukavarapu, S.P., Tissue engineering: current concepts and challenges. *J. Cell. Biochem.*, 90, 1, 241–251, 2003.
59. Orsini, M., Orsini, G., Benlloch, D., Aranda, J.J., Lazaro, P., Sanz, M., *et al.*, Comparison of calcium sulfate and autogenous bone graft to bio absorbable membranes plus autogenous bone graft in the treatment of intrabony periodontal defects: A split mouth study. *J. Periodontol.*, 72, 296–302, 2001.

5

Osteointegration

Randa A. Alfotawi

Department of Oral and Maxillofacial Surgery, College of Dentistry, King Saud University, Riyadh, Saudi Arabia

Abstract

Dental rehabilitation and bone augmentation are used in several clinical treatments. Over the past 50 years, a variety of substitutes to natural bones have been researched, such as biomaterials that can be used to replace allogeneic or autologous bone material in the treatment of damaged and traumatized bone tissue. Material like titanium TiO_2 was shown to be superior when surface modifications were made to improve the osteointegration process. Non-toxicity, low resorption, biocompatibility, durability, early integration, non-conductivity, ease of handling and adaptability, and the ability to promote the creation of local tissues are all essential qualities of the perfect bone replacement materials. Additionally, the material needs to be manufactured, processed, and made accessible at a fair price. Many materials, including ceramics, polymers, metals and their composites, and more, are used to make bone substitutes. However, depending on the bone insufficiency, these materials can be modelled into the correct shape because of their exceptional design flexibility and biodegradability. The **biological perspectives of osteointegration**, bone-implant contact, and the impact of contact distance will all be covered in detail **in this chapter**. The gold standard material "Ti–6Al–4V" and the clinical data showing how various surface modifications affect integration will be discussed. The most recent clinical data for additional materials, such as PEEK and zirconia, will also be provided.

***Keywords*:** Titanium, PEEK, bioactive ceramics, osteointegration, BIC, implant interface, biological osseointegration, integration's dynamic

Email: ralfotawei@ksu.edu.sa

Randa A. Alfotawi (ed.) Oro-Facial Bone Grafts and Biomaterials, (89–106) © 2026 Scrivener Publishing LLC

5.1 Introduction

Osteointegration represents a fundamental biological principle underlying the long-term stability of endosseous implants used in oral and maxillofacial reconstruction. The concept describes the intimate interaction between bone tissue and implant surfaces and remains central to the predictability of implant-supported rehabilitation.

Osteointegration is the direct bone-to-implant interface, also known as bone–implant contact (BIC), which is characterized by close contact that is invisible under a microscope and extends between 4020 nm and 500 nm [1, 2]. The BIC is the ratio of the overall length of the implant profile to the linear measurement of the implant's surface that is directly in contact with the bone. This interface was previously described as a functional link between the implant material and native bone following loading with highly differentiated tissue [3, 4]. Various levels, including biological [5, 6], clinical [7], anatomical [8], histological [9], and ultra-structural [8], have been used to define osseointegration.

5.2 Biological Osseointegration

Biological osseointegration explains how the material's properties, including surface preparation, sterilization, procedures, coatings, and chemical composition, may impact the metallo-biological interface and how the healing response of the surface of the implant may impact the implant's stability over the short and long term.

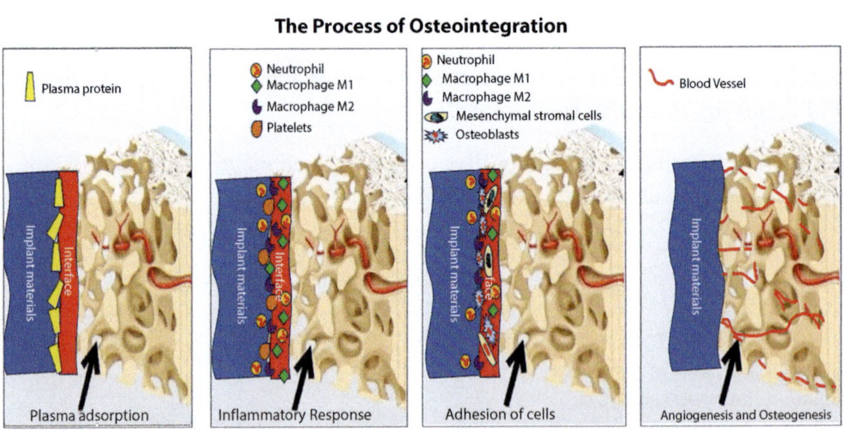

Figure 5.1 Demonstration of the stage of early osteointegration of biomaterials to native bone.

The adsorption of plasma proteins to start the osseointegration process between the bone and the implant requires a hydrophilic surface (Figure 5.1). The first interactions between platelets and blood cells and the implant surface influence the formation of clots [9, 10]. Then, adhesion, spreading, and aggregation cause morphological changes that trigger specific biological changes at the cell level (phospholipid hydrolysis, calcium release, phosphortyrosine), which ultimately result in the release of a fibrin matrix that promotes the migration and differentiation of osteogenic cells. When differentiated cells are in contact with the surface of the implant, they produce osteoid, or immature bone, which eventually develops into new trabecular bone, which mineralizes to form lamellar bone. This is followed by migration of osteoblasts and mesenchymal cells.

This integration's dynamic begins on the first day after implantation, when minerals and cells adhere to the implant's non-collagenous matrix layer, forming a calcified fibrillar layer and a weakly mineralized osteoid. According to studies, this layer, which is 0.5 mm thick and rich in proteins including osteopontin, bone sialoprotein 1, calcium, and phosphorus salts, essentially acts as a barrier between the mineralized and non-mineralized portions of the bone matrix, much like laminae limitans [7, 11].

It has been established that autocrine and paracrine growth factors regulate pre-osteoblast differentiation and proliferation. Primary callus is the thickening of the periosteal layer caused by an increase in pre-osteoblasts and osteoblast populations [12]. After four weeks of calcification, the callus is replaced by endochondral bone. The amount of time needed for callus formation is accelerated by the distance between the implant materials and the host's natural bone [13].

The development of extracellular matrix (ECM) is a necessary condition for osseointegration onto the implant interface. For instance, following titanium preparation, a nonstoichiometric layer of TiO_2 and Ti_2O_3 is oxidized on the surface of pure titanium >99%. This negatively charged oxidized layer promotes the development of extracellular matrix (ECM) and in turn promotes cell adhesion and proliferation [14–18]. Collagen fiber was detected by transmission electron microscopy (TEM) analysis at a distance of 20–25 nm from the oxidized layer [8]. Additional ECM analysis revealed the presence of additional chondroitinase and hyaluronidase-sensitive material layers [8]. The Haversian system was discovered to be 20 nm away from the oxide surface, and the bone was laid parallel to it in terms of the nature of bone attachment in pure titanium metal [19].

On the other hand, bone remodeling occurs 25–50 days after calcification of the extracellular matrix (ECM) and increases the levels of alkaline phosphatase, acidic glycosaminoglycan, and glycogen in titanium alloy (Ti-6A1-4V) implants [20].

5.2.1 Osteogenesis and the Contact Distance

Bone formation at the implant surface may occur through contact osteogenesis, where bone grows directly onto the implant, or distance osteogenesis, where bone advances from the surrounding host bed toward the implant surface. Reduced contact distance facilitates earlier bone–implant interaction but does not solely determine the quality of osseointegration. Around a titanium implant, contact osteogenesis takes place at a distance of 20–50 nm. This layer consists of a tiny mineralized area, flat osteoblast-like cells, and calcified collagen fibrils [11]. The freshly formed bone was positioned on the surface of the old bone that had been reabsorbed after osteoclastic activity. Early peri-implant osteogenesis may be encouraged by the osteoblast's reaction to the implant surface, which is believed to act as a biomimetic scaffold. Throughout this process, cement lines or a lamina of weakly mineralized osteoid denoted the point at which bone reabsorption was finished and bone formation began [11].

Cement lines and lamina limitans are secreted by osteoblasts on the implant surface a few days after implantation, and collagen matrix subsequently begins to deposit on the surface. After calcification, osteocytes and osteoblasts clustered in bone [11].

Under a microscope, the collagen fibers are arranged randomly to reestablish continuity as the woven bone first begins to develop on the

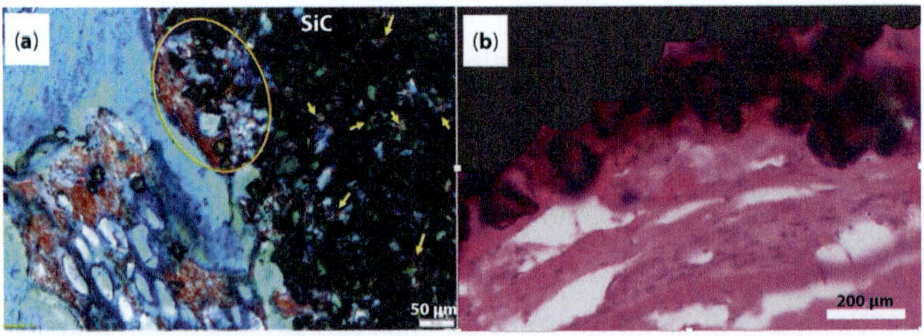

Figure 5.2 Phototomicrograph showing osteointegration of biomaterials and native bone. (a) Osteopontin immune histochemistry staining for woven bone development through the graft material's whole thickness. Direct bone contact and the graft surface interface are seen in the beginning. Differentiated osteoblasts are visible in the cells' dark brown staining. The arrows show that bone is growing inside the SiC implant's pores. Scale bar: 50 μm. (b) H&E staining at higher magnification for area of interface showed that osteoprogenitor cells and differentiated osteoblasts were found to adhere to the surface of SiC.

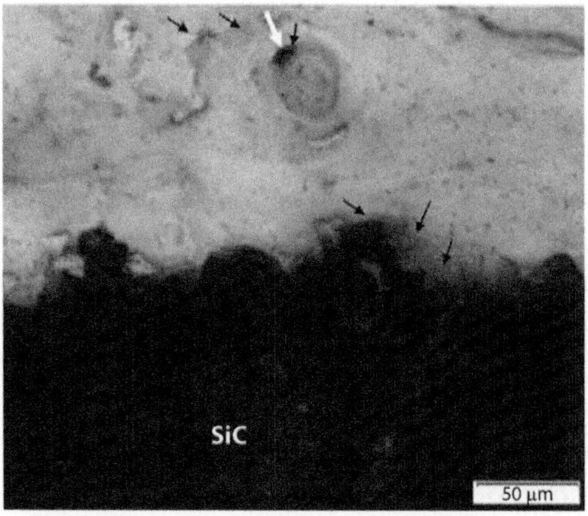

Figure 5.3 The whole thickness of the biomaterial graft, which integrates with native bone, is stained with S100 antibody immune histochemistry in this photomicrograph to demonstrate woven bone growth. It shows the interface surface and direct bone contact. The newly created tissue's innervation is indicated by the cells' dark brown staining. In *de novo* bone, a little nerve bundle (white arrow) is visibly connected to freshly formed blood vessels. Scale bar: 50 μm.

implant's surface. The interface first fills the space with a mixture of trabecular and woven bone. This bone growth, also known as biological fixation, may occur 10–14 days following surgery [21, 22]. The initial mechanical stability is typically followed by this biological fixing.

The woven bone is then mineralized and remodeled to form the lamellar bone. Histological evaluation of bone with bioactive materials or Ti implants is presented in Figure 5.2 and Figure 5.3.

5.2.2 The Effect of Loading Implant and Distance on Osseointegration

Mechanical loading influences osseointegration in a load-dependent and time-dependent manner. Controlled functional loading may support bone remodeling and maturation, whereas excessive or premature loading can disrupt early bone formation. Early loading protocols may be successful under carefully controlled conditions but should not be generalized across all clinical scenarios. Following implant loading, the frequency and masticatory pressures will be transferred to the bone–implant contact, influencing the mineralization and bone remodeling processes, respectively [2]. *In vitro* tests on osteoblastic cells exposed to cyclic strain revealed increased DNA synthesis, cell division, orientation, and elongation [23]. The amount of micromotion that may occur after loading may either improve or impair biological integration at micro-motion of 30 μm or greater than 150 μm, respectively.

The biological integration of the graft materials was found to be compromised or inhibited by micro-motions bigger than 150 μm, whereas micro-motions up to 30 μm in the elastic interface were found to be associated with osseointegration [24–26]. After arthroplasty was assessed using radiostereometric analysis, a clinical investigation was conducted to evaluate the integration. Partial and full weight-bearing following total hip replacement with uncemented implant materials was documented [27]. The patients who were instructed for full weight-bearing were evaluated, and they found no adverse effects on the movements of the stem or penetration of the femoral head [27].

Studies on the impact of the distance between bone and graft indicate that optimal integration requires the existence of an acceptable distance between bone and implant. If there is more than 500 μm between the implant material and the native bone, the quality of the newly formed bone may degrade. On the other hand, resorption would result from a tight or small gap [28]. According to studies, having the ideal amount of space is crucial for producing higher-quality peri-implant bone that supports the implant's biological fixation [10, 21, 29]. Bone remodeling occurs around the implant and extends up to 1 mm from the implant surface. The process of bone remodeling on osseointegrated implants has been assessed by looking for marrow gaps or medullary that contain lymphatic/blood vessels, mesenchymal cells, osteoblasts, and osteoclasts next to the implant surface. New osteons encircle the implant as the peri-implant bone remodels, and the presence of osteoid indicates that an active osteogenesis process is being carried out with their lamella [11, 19].

5.3 Materials Known to Osteointegrate

Several materials have demonstrated the capacity to support osseointegration through favorable biological interaction with bone tissue. The extent and quality of osseointegration depend on surface chemistry, topography, and mechanical compatibility rather than material composition alone.

5.3.1 Titanium (Ti)

Titanium (Ti) is the gold standard for osseointegration. Although other alternative materials have been presented recently, titanium is still the most popular and original material for dental implants. This can be attributed to their mechanical properties, ability to undergo osteointegration, bio-inertness, and bio-compatibility [14].

Commercially accessible Ti are graded from 1 to 4, with the purity varying according to the amount of interstitial components like carbon, oxygen, and iron. On the other hand, Grade 5 (Ti–6Al–4V), which is primarily utilized because of its fatigue and mechanical qualities, has 4% vanadium and 6% aluminum. Typically, dental implants are composed of a blend of grade 4 and grade 5 titanium. To accomplish osteointegration, the entire surface of the dental implant is oxidized, creating a coating of TiO_2. Upon preparation of the implant bed, insertion, and contact with bone, the TiO_2 layer thickens and integrates phosphorus ions and calcium from the bone matrix. This suggests a very dynamic structure at the interface between TiO_2 and bone. Future specifics have already been explained in Section 5.2.2.

5.3.1.1 Surface Modification to Enhance Osteointegration

One of the six key parameters influencing the stability of the bone-to-implant interface is the implant's surface characteristics [30]. Various surface topographies (macro–micro–nano roughness) have an impact on the interface's dynamics [31]. A rougher surface improves the contact between the bone and the implant, which in turn improves the biomechanical interlocking between the two [32]. However, when nano-surface roughness or topography was formed, it was observed that the surface topography also exerts a biological mechanism [33].

They discovered increased cell migration, proliferation, differentiation, surface matrix protein adsorption, and ultimately osteointegration [33].

Additionally, it has been demonstrated that the method employed to create surface roughness may have an impact on the chemical makeup of dental implant surfaces, raising questions about which factor—surface roughness or chemical composition—may influence bone osteointegration [34].

Also, by the creation of an ionized surface within the layer, the TiO_2 uses ions like magnesium, calcium, or nitrogen [36, 37]. Surface modification was introduced to improve implants' bioactivity, either by adding inorganic (calcium phosphate) or organic (peptide, proteins, enzymes, and drugs) phases to TiO_2 [34, 35]. This can also be achieved by employing ions such as magnesium, calcium, or nitrogen to create an ionized surface inside the TiO_2 layer [36, 37].

5.3.1.2 Implant Modification

The term "machined" or "turned" refers to the smooth, polished implants that were manufactured by machines 30 years ago. These days, they serve

Table 5.1 Various methods used for implant surface modification have been introduced to enhance clinical performance.

Methods	Techniques	Mechanism	Advantage	Material used	Remark
Subtractive methods	Grit blasting	Blasting the implant with hard materials, stable particles under high-pressure air flow	Simple Provides surface roughness Mechanical fixation	The material used for blasting needs to be sturdy. (e.g., Al_2O_2, ceramic, calcium phosphate, TiO_2)	
	Acid etching	Submerging Ti implants for a number of minutes in a solution of strong HCl and H_2SO_4 that has been heated above 100°C	Micro pits range 0.5–2 μm	Nitric acid, sulfuric acid, hydrochloric acid, hydrofluoric acid	
	Combinations Blasting +acid etch	Blasting the implant with hard materials then submerging Ti implants for a number of minutes in a solution of strong HCl	Mechanical fixation with roughness, chemical etching add micro pits and nano surface topography, which provide biological effect	The blasting material should be stable (e.g., Al_2O_2, ceramic, calcium phosphate, TiO_2) Nitric acid, sulfuric acid, hydrochloric acid, hydrofluoric acid	

(Continued)

Table 5.1 Various methods used for implant surface modification have been introduced to enhance clinical performance. (*Continued*)

Methods	Techniques	Mechanism	Advantage	Material used	Remark
Additive methods	Plasma spraying	Injecting Ti powder into plasma torch at high temperature; this Ti particles are projected on the surface	Produce, condense, and fuse together, rough film surface where they reach 10 μm	Hydroxyapatite (HA)\ it may require sand blasting before plasma spray	The spray surface can reach mm and may cause delamination of calcium phosphate coat particles [38]
	Others	Pulsed laser deposition, sputtering coating/sol-gel deposition, discrete crystalline deposition onto dual-acid etched surface, ion-beam assisted deposition, electrostatic spray deposition Biomimetic deposition	Produce thin film coat <5 μm	Bisphosphonates, calcium phosphate, Type I, II collagen, chondroitin sulfate, RGD peptide, growth factors (BMP, EGF, GH, TGF-β1, TGFF-β2, PDGF, PRGF, IGF-1, IGF-2, NGF) [34, 35]	Biomimetic deposition allows calcium phosphate deposition by submerging in simulated bodily fluid under physiological condition [39]
Subtractive/ additive methods	Anodization	Electrochemical anodized Ti surface by galvanostatic anodization or potentiostatic of Ti in concentrated acids at high voltage (200 A/m^2)	The oxide layer on Ti reach to 1000 nm and produces micro to nano pores on Ti surface [40, 41]	Requires temperature, electrolyte composition, proper current density, and concentration of acids	Complex procedure

PDGF (platelet-derived growth factor), NGF (nerve growth factor), BMP (bone morphogenic protein), TGF-β2 (transforming growth factor-β-2), IGF-2 (insulin-like growth factor 2), PRGF (plasma rich in growth factors), TGF-β1 (transforming growth factor-β-1), GH (growth hormone), EGF (epidermal growth factor), IGF-1 (insulin-like growth factor 1) as control implants in studies. Various methods have been introduced to enhance clinical performance (see Table 5.1).

5.3.1.3 *Effect of Surface Modification on Osteointegration*

5.3.1.3.1 *In Vivo* Evidence

Numerous *in vivo* investigations have offered credible proof at the histology level by measuring osseointegration using BIC and at the clinical level by employing the reverse torque test [42, 43]. The reverse torque test is described as the crucial torque threshold at which the destruction of bone–implant contact occurs or the higher force needed to eliminate implants.

A systematic review study by Shalabi *et al.* [44] that looked at the connection between surface roughness and bone healing discovered a positive correlation between BIC, surface roughness, and the implant reverse torque test. A study that compared the relationship between BIC and the surface roughness of several implants—smooth, moderate, and rough surfaces—found that the moderately rough surface had the highest BIC [31, 45].

5.3.1.3.2 The Clinical Evidence

In a human clinical investigation, histological samples from patients were examined to compare the effects of smooth machined and rough dual-etched implant surfaces. In the maxilla, threaded Ti mini-implants with two rough sides and one machined side were inserted. They were removed along with the surrounding bone after 6 months. According to the BIC assessment, there was a significant difference at $p<0.05$, and the dual etched side was found to have a higher value [46].

In the mandible and maxilla, a different study evaluated the BIC of TiO_2-blasted dental implants and contrasted them with machined implants. A histomorphometric assessment was performed on the blasted implant. For both the mandible and maxilla, high BIC was noted for blasted implants [47]. Additional research compared the surfaces of implants treated with grit blasting, etching, and anodic oxidation to those with machined surfaces. Better outcomes with improved osseointegration for implants with rough surfaces have been documented [47–51].

5.3.1.3.3 The Variables that may Contribute to Implant Failure

Factors that could cause implant failure, like enhanced bony sites, short implants, low bone density, and early loading, were evaluated in comparison to various implant surface treatments. After 3 years of loading, Khang *et al.* presented the results of evaluating 432 dual acid-etched implants in a controlled trial and comparing them to machined implants. According to the study, the success rates for machined implants and dual acid-etched were 84.8% and 96.8%, respectively. The author concluded that the failure occurs in poor bone quality sites [52]. After 4 years of loading, eight clinical investigations totaling over 4500 implants were examined in a systematic review. They concluded that the reported success rate for the modified dual acid etch was 98.1% in poor bone and 98.4% in good bone. In contrast, the machine-surfaced implants that were placed in high-quality bone had a survival rate of 93.9%, whereas those placed in low-quality bone had a survival rate of 88.2% [53]. In the same vein, a systematic review examined the implants in areas with low bone density following loading. According to the study's findings, a rough surface implant had a 97.1% survival rate compared to a survival rate of 91.6% of a machined implant [54].

Immediate implant loading is the second factor that could lead to implant failure. Twenty-two TiO_2-blasted implants were used in split-mouth studies in comparison to machined implants, and they were immediately loaded after a day. According to reports, the success rates for machined and blasted implants were 90.9% and 95%, respectively [55]. The improved surface alterations significantly shortened the time required for osseointegration. Everyone agreed that the loading period should be shortened from 3–6 months to 6–8 weeks [56–58].

On the other hand, implant length is taken into account when evaluating and assessing implants. Research revealed that short implants with a rough surface area had a higher success rate than machined implants when using sophisticated implant surface treatments [59]. The cumulative survival rate (CSR) of the short-machined implants was examined in a systematic review. The research findings revealed that for rough-surfaced implants, a higher CSR of 99.1% was recorded at an average follow-up of 3.2 years [60].

Bone grafted implants presented another area of study in comparing the rate of success of machined implants vs. those with a roughened surface. The rate of success of machined and rough surface implants inserted into grafted bone up to 5 years has been examined in a retrospective study. Comparing those inserted into native bone, the study found no statistically significant difference. However, throughout a 10-year follow-up period, the survival percentage for machined implants implanted in enlarged maxilla dropped dramatically from 81.2% to 75.1% [61]. Similarly, Del Fabbro *et al.* investigated implant survival in rats after sinus augmentation in a systematic review. For the same follow-up period, the author found that the mean survival rate for rough surface implants was up to 96.7%, but the mean survival rate for machined surface implants was 86.3% [62].

5.3.2 Yttria-Stabilized Tetragonal Zirconia Polycrystals (Y-TZPs)

Y-TZP has improved mechanical qualities, less inflammatory responses around the implant, and color and opacity resembling natural teeth. Zirconia implants have recently been commercially available as coating materials or as full or partial zirconia dental implants. *In vitro* tests revealed zirconia to be bioinert, antimicrobial, and highly cytocompatible [63–65]. Despite being bioinert, zirconia permits cell motility and plasma protein adsorption on its surface.

According to clinical studies, the rate of success of zirconia dental implants varies. Comparing zirconia implants to Ti implants, Blaschke *et al.* observed positive clinical outcomes in terms of soft tissue response [66].

In a 2007 study, Oliva *et al.* evaluated 100 zirconia implants; the overall success rate was 98%. With less than 5 mm of residual bone, there are some limitations [67]. After 2 years of loading, zirconia implants showed no signs of periodontitis or gingivitis, were stable, and showed no signs of marginal bone resorption, according to the results of another study [68]. However, some research has indicated that when zirconia implants are utilized in clinical settings, there is a slight loss of bone [69].

Since then, surface modification has been used to improve the osseointegration and biological behavior. A number of physiochemical techniques have been presented and evaluated for various coating materials. Dopamine, magnesium, silica, and graphene are a few examples of bioactive compounds found in coating materials [70]. According to a recent critical assessment and update on zirconia implants, the single-piece implant is robust, and the literature's evidence supports its comparison to Ti implants [71].

5.3.3 Polyetheretherketone (PEEK)

PEEK is a synthetic thermoplastic polymer that finds extensive use in dentistry as well as in cranial and maxillofacial implants due to its exceptional qualities [72, 73]. PEEK is bioinert, has a tooth-colored appearance, absorbs stress, resists fractures, has a low elastic modulus when compared to human bone, and is resistant to heat and chemicals [74]. However, because of its hydrophobicity and bio-inertness, the material cannot be employed without surface modification. PEEK's low surface energy hindered the osseointegration process by preventing plasma protein adsorption and, consequently, the development of extracellular matrix. PEEK surface modification is used to improve its wettability, antibacterial properties, and bioactivity [75].

Although a number of surface modification techniques have been proposed and even tried, there is a lack of long-term comprehensive assessment of osseointegration in systematic reviews that examine the evidence of PEEK implant osseointegration.

5.4 Conclusion

With a remarkable long-term survival record of over 92%, titanium-based dental implants remain a well-established management option. To overcome the difficulties that clinicians have in their day-to-day work with currently available materials such as Ti–6Al–4V, Y-TZP, and PEEK, a great deal of work has been done at the level of *in vitro* and *in vivo* evaluation for a large variety of biomaterials. Even so, implants made of zirconia and PEEK are showing great promise. However, there is not any strong evidence that it performs better than the titanium implant that is sold commercially in terms of long-term integration.

AI disclosure statement: The author confirms that no artificial intelligence (AI)-generated content or AI-assisted writing tools were used in the preparation of this chapter (including summaries and the abstract). All text, analysis, and conclusions are the result of the author's original work.

References

1. Albrektsson, T. and Johansson, C., Osteoinduction, osteoconduction and osseointegration. *Eur. Spine J.*, 10, S96–S101, 2001, DOI 10.1007/s005860100282.
2. Stanford, C.M. and Keller, J.C., The Concept of Osseointegration and Bone Matrix Expression. *Crit. Rev. Oral Biol. Med.*, 2, 1, 83–101, 1991.
3. Brånemark, P.I., Vital microscopy of bone marrow in rabbit. *Scand. J. Clin. Lab. Invest.*, 11, Suppl.38, 1–82, 1959.
4. Brånemark, P.I., Osseointegration and its experimental studies. *J. Prosthet. Dent.*, 50, 399–410, 1983.
5. Stanford, C.M., Keller, J.C., Solursh, M., Bone cell expression on titanium surfaces is altered by sterilization treatments. *J. Dent. Res.*, 73, 1061–71, 1994.
6. Swart, K.M., Keller, J.C., Wightman, J.P., Draughn, R.A., Stanford, C.M., Michaels, C.M., Short-term plasma-cleaning treatments enhance *in vitro* osteoblast attachment to titanium. *J. Oral Implantol.*, 18, 130–7, 1992.
7. Adell, R., Lekholm, U., Rockler, B., Brånemark, P.I., A 15-year study of osseointegrated implants in the treatment of the edentulous jaw. *Int. J. Oral Surg.*, 10, 387–416, 1981.

8. Linder, L., Albrektsson, T., Brånemark, P.I., Hansson, H.A., Ivarsson, B., Jönsson, U., Lundström, I., Electron microscopic analysis of the bone-titanium interface. *Acta Orthop. Scand.*, 54, 45–52, 1983.
9. Davies, J.E., Mechanisms of endosseous integration. *Int. J. Prosthodont.*, 11, 391–401, 1998.
10. Berglundh, T., Abrahamsson, I., Lang, N.P., Lindhe, J., De novo alveolar bone formation adjacent to endosseous implants. *Clin. Oral Implants Res.*, 14, 251–62, 2003.
11. Murai, K., Takeshita, F., Ayukawa, Y., Kiyoshima, T., Suetsugu, T., Tanaka, T., Light and electron microscopic studies of bone-titanium interface in the tibiae of young and mature rats. *J. Biomed. Mater. Res.*, 30, 523–33, 1996.
12. Simmons, D.J., Fracture healing perspectives. *Clin. Orthop. Relat. Res.*, 200, 100, 1985.
13. Hart, H.H., Wu, J.-J., Chao, E.Y.S., Kelly, P.J., External skeletal fixation of canine tibial osteotomies. *J. Bone Joint Surg.*, 67A, 598, 1985.
14. Kasemo, B., Biocompatibility of titanium implants:surface science aspects. *J. Prosthet. Dent.*, 49, 832, 1983.
15. Parr, G.R., Titanium: the mystery metal of implant dentistry. *J. Prosthet. Dent.*, 54, 399, 1983.
16. Lausmaa, J., Accelerated oxide growth on titanium implants during autoclaving caused by Fl contamination. *Biomaterials*, 5, 23, 1985.
17. Meenaghan, M.A., Tissue response to surface treated tantalum implants. *J. Biomed. Mater. Res.*, 13, 631, 1979.
18. Baier, R.E., Conditioning surfaces to suit the biomedical environment: recent progress. *J. Biomech. Eng.*, 104, 257, 1982.
19. Hansson, H.-A., Albrektsson, T., Branemark, P.I., Structural aspects of the interface between tissue and titanium implants. *J. Prosthet. Dent.*, 50, 108, 1982.
20. Ketenjian, A.Y. and Arsenis, C., Morphological and biochemical studies during differentiation and calcification of fracture callus cartilage. *Clin. Orthop.*, 107, 266, 1975.
21. Franchi, M., Fini, M., Martini, D., Orsini, E., Leonardi, L., Ruggeri, A., Giavaresi, G., Ottani, V., Biological fixation of endosseous implants. *Micron*, 36, 665–71, 2005.
22. Probst, A. and Spiegel, H.U., Cellular mechanisms of bone repair. *J. Invest. Surg.*, 10, 77–86, 1997.
23. Buckley, M.J., Banes, A.J., Levin, L.G., Sumpio, B.E., Sato, M., Jordan, R., Gilbert, J., Link, G.W., Tay, R.T.S., Osteoblasts increase the rate of division and align in response to cyclic, mechanical tension *in vitro*. *Bone Miner.*, 4, 225, 1988.
24. Cameron, H.U., Pilliar, R.M., MacNab, I., The effect of movement on the bonding of porous metal to bone. *J. Biomed. Mater. Res.*, 7, 301–11, 1973.

25. Maniatopoulos, C., Pilliar, R.M., Smith, D.C., Threaded versus porous-surfaced designs for implant stabilization in bone-endodontic implant model. *J. Biomed. Mater. Res.*, 20, 1309–33, 1986.
26. Soballe, K., Hansen, E.S., Brockstedt-Rasmussen, H., JØrgensen, P.H., Bünger, C., Tissue ingrowth into titanium and hydroxyapatite-coated implants during stable and unstable mechanical conditions. *J. Orthop. Res.*, 10, 285–99, 1992.
27. Thien, T.M., Ahnfelt, L., Eriksson, M., Strömberg, C., Kärrholm, J., Immediate weight bearing after uncemented total hip arthroplasty with an anteverted stem: a prospective randomized comparison using radiostereometry. *Acta Orthop.*, 78, 730–8, 2007.
28. Futami, T., Fujii, N., Ohnishi, H., Taguchi, N., Kusakari, H., Ohshima, H., Maeda, T., Tissue response to titanium implants in the rat maxilla: ultrastructural and histochemical observations of the bone-titanium interface. *J. Periodontol.*, 71, 287–98, 2000.
29. Sandborn, P.M., Cook, S.D., Spires, W.P., Kester, M.A., Tissue response to porous-coated implants lacking initial bone apposition. *J. Arthroplasty*, 3, 337–46, 1988.
30. Albrektsson, T., Brånemark, P.I., Hansson, H.A., Lindström, J., Osseointegrated titanium implants: requirements for ensuring a long-lasting, direct bone-to-implant anchorage in man. *Acta Orthop. Scand.*, 1981.
31. Wennerberg, A. and Albrektsson, T., Effects of titanium surface topography on bone integration: a systematic review. *Clin. Oral Implants Res.*, 20, 172–84, 2009.
32. Mendonça, G., Mendonça, D.B., Aragao, F.J., Cooper, L.F., Advancing dental implant surface technology–from micron-to nanotopography. *Biomaterials*, 29, 28, 3822–35, 2008.
33. Junker, R., Dimakis, A., Thoneick, M., Jansen, J.A., Effects of implant surface coatings and composition on bone integration: a systematic review. *Clin. Oral Implants Res.*, 20, 185–206, 2009.
34. Hansson, S. and Norton, M., The relation between surface roughness and interfacial shear strength for bone-anchored implants. A mathematical model. *J. Biomech.*, 32, 8, 829–36, 1999Aug1.
35. de Jonge, L.T., Leeuwenburgh, S.C., Wolke, J.G., Jansen, J.A., Organic–inorganic surface modifications for titanium implant surfaces. *Pharm. Res.*, 25, 2357–69, 2008.
36. Annunziata, M., Guida, L., Perillo, L., Aversa, R., Passaro, I., Oliva, A., Biological response of human bone marrow stromal cells to sandblasted titanium nitride-coated implant surfaces. *J. Mater. Sci.: Mater. Med.*, 19, 3585–91, 2008.
37. Annunziata, M., Oliva, A., Basile, M.A., Giordano, M., Mazzola, N., Rizzo, A., Lanza, A., Guida, L., The effects of titanium nitride-coating on the topographic and biological features of TPS implant surfaces. *J. Dent.*, 39, 11, 720–8, 2011 Nov 1.

38. Wheeler, S.L., Eight-year clinical retrospective study of titanium plasma-sprayed and hydroxyapatite-coated cylinder implants. *Int. J. Oral Maxillofac. Implants*, 11, 3, 1996.
39. Kokubo, T., Kushitani, H., Sakka, S., Kitsugi, T., Yamamuro, T., Solutions able to reproduce *in vivo* surface-structure changes in bioactive glass-ceramic A-W3. *J. Biomed. Mater. Res.*, 24, 6, 721–34, 1990.
40. Sul, Y.T., Johansson, C., Wennerberg, A., Cho, L.R., Chang, B.S., Albrektsson, T., Optimum Surface Properties of Oxidized Implants for Reinforcement of Osseointeg ration: Surface Chemistry, Oxide Thickness, Porosity, Roughness, and Crystal Structure. *Int. J. Oral Maxillofac. Implants*, 20, 3, 2005 May 1.
41. El-wassefy, N.A., Hammouda, I.M., Habib, A.N., El-awady, G.Y., Marzook, H.A., Assessment of anodized titanium implants bioactivity. *Clin. Oral Implants Res.*, 25, 2, e1–9, 2014 Feb.
42. Roberts, W.E., Smith, R.K., Zilberman, Y., Mozsary, P.G., Smith, R.S., Osseous adaptation to continuous loading of rigid endosseous implants. *Am. J. Orthod.*, 86, 2, 95–111, 1984 Aug 1.
43. Johansson, C. and Albrektsson, T., Integration of Screw Implants in the Rabbit: A 1-yr Follow-up of Removal Torque of Titanium Implants. *Int. J. Oral Maxillofac. Implants*, 2, 2, 1987.
44. Shalabi, M.M., Gortemaker, A., Hof, M.V., Jansen, J.A., Creugers, N.H., Implant surface roughness and bone healing: a systematic review. *J. Dent. Res.*, 85, 6, 496–500, 2006.
45. Lang, N.P. and Jepsen, S., Implant surfaces and design (Working Group 4). *Clin. Oral Implants Res.*, 20, 228–31, 2009.
46. Lazzara, R.J., Testori, T., Trisi, P., Porter, S.S., Weinstein, R.L., A human histologic analysis of osseotite and machined surfaces using implants with 2 opposing surfaces. *Int. J. Periodontics Restorative Dent.*, 19, 2, 1999.
47. Ivanoff, C.J., Widmark, G., Johansson, C., Wennerberg, A., Histologic evaluation of bone response to oxidized and turned titanium micro-implants in human jawbone. *Int. J. Oral Maxillofac. Implants*, 18, 3, 2003.
48. Grassi, S., Piattelli, A., De Figueiredo, L.C., Feres, M., De Melo, L., Iezzi, G., Alba Jr., R.C., Shibli, J.A., Histologic evaluation of early human bone response to different implant surfaces. *J. Periodontol.*, 77, 10, 1736–43, 2006.
49. Grassi, S., Piattelli, A., Ferrari, D.S., Figueiredo, L.C., Feres, M., Iezzi, G., Shibli, J.A., Histologic evaluation of human bone integration on machined and sandblasted acid-etched titanium surfaces in type IV bone. *J. Oral Implantol.*, 33, 1, 8–12, 2007.
50. Shibli, J.A., Grassi, S., Cristina de Figueiredo, L., Feres, M., Marcantonio, E., Iezzi, G., Piattelli, A., Influence of implant surface topography on early osseointegration: a histological study in human jaws. *J. Biomed. Mater. Res. Part B: Appl. Biomater.: An Official Journal Society Biomaterials, Japanese Society Biomaterials, Australian Society Biomaterials Korean Society Biomaterials*, 80, 2, 377–85, 2007.

51. Trisi, P., Lazzara, R., Rebaudi, A., Rao, W., Testori, T., Porter, S.S., Bone-implant contact on machined and dual acid-etched surfaces after 2 months of healing in the human maxilla. *J. Periodontol.*, 74, 7, 945–56, 2003.
52. Khang, W., Feldman, S., Hawley, C.E., Gunsolley, J., A multi-center study comparing dual acid-etched and machined-surfaced implants in various bone qualities. *J. Periodontol.*, 72, 10, 1384–90, 2001.
53. Goiato, M.C., Dos Santos, D.M., Santiago, J.J., Moreno, A., Pellizzer, E.P., Longevity of dental implants in type IV bone: a systematic review. *Int. J. Oral Maxillofac. Surg.*, 143, 9, 1108–16, 2014.
54. Stach, R.M. and Kohles, S.S., A meta-analysis examining the clinical survivability of machined-surfaced and osseotite implants in poor-quality bone. *Implant Dent.*, 12, 1, 87–96, 2003.
55. Schincaglia, G.P., Marzola, R., Scapoli, C., Scotti, R., Immediate loading of dental implants supporting fixed partial dentures in the posterior mandible: a randomized controlled split-mouth study–machined versus titanium oxide implant surface. *Int. J. Oral Maxillofac. Implants*, 22, 1, 2007.
56. Cochran, D.L., Morton, D., Weber, H.P., Consensus statements and recommended clinical procedures regarding loading protocols for endosseous dental implants. *Int. J. Oral Maxillofac. Implants*, 19, 7, 2004.
57. Weber, H.P., Morton, D., Gallucci, G.O., Roccuzzo, M., Cordaro, L., Grütter, L., Consensus statements and recommended clinical procedures regarding loading protocols. *Int. J. Oral Maxillofac. Implants*, 24, 2, 2009.
58. Gallucci, G.O., Benic, G.I., Eckert, S.E., Papaspyridakos, P., Schimmel, M., Schrott, A., Weber, H.P., Consensus statements and clinical recommendations for implant loading protocols. *Int. J. Oral Maxillofac. Implants*, 29, 2, 2014.
59. Al Hashedi, A.A., Taiyeb, A., Yunus, N., Short dental implants: an emerging concept in implant treatment. *Quintessence Int.*, 45, 6, 16, 2014.
60. Annibali, S., Cristalli, M.P., Dell'Aquila, D., Bignozzi, I., La Monaca, G., Pilloni, A., Short Dental Implants: A Systematic Review. *J. Dent. Res.*, 91, 1, 25–32, 2011, doi: 10.1177/0022034511425675.
61. Lambert, F.E., Weber, H.P., Susarla, S.M., Belser, U.C., Gallucci, G.O., Descriptive analysis of implant and prosthodontic survival rates with fixed implant-supported rehabilitations in the edentulous maxilla. *J. Periodontol.*, 80, 8, 1220–30, 2009.
62. Del Fabbro, M., Rosano, G., Taschieri, S., Implant survival rates after maxillary sinus augmentation. *Eur. J. Oral Sci.*, 116, 6, 497–506, 2008.
63. Scarano, A., Piattelli, M., Caputi, S., Favero, G.A., Piattelli, A., Bacterial adhesion on commercially pure titanium and zirconium oxide disks: an *in vivo* human study. *J. Periodontol.*, 75, 292–296, 2004.
64. Yin, L., Nakanishi, Y., Alao, A., Song, X., A review of engineered zirconia surfaces in biomedical applications. *Procedia CIRP*, 65, 284–290, 2017.

65. Blaschke, C. and Volz, U., Soft and hard tissue response to zirconium dioxide dental implants–a clinical study in man. *Neuroendocrinol. Lett.*, 27, 1, 69–72, 2006.
66. Oliva, J., Oliva, X., Oliva, J.D., One-year follow-up of first consecutive 100 zirconia dental implants in humans: a comparison of 2 different rough surfaces. *Int. J. Oral Maxillofac. Implants*, 22, 3, 2007.
67. Pirker, W. and Kocher, A., Immediate, non-submerged, root-analogue zirconia implant in single tooth replacement. *Int. J. Oral Maxillofac. Surg.*, 37, 3, 293–5, 2008 Mar 1.
68. Kohal, R.J., Schwindling, F.S., Bächle, M., Spies, B.C., Peri-implant bone response to retrieved human zirconia oral implants after a 4-year loading period: a histologic and histomorphometric evaluation of 22 cases. *J. Biomed. Mater. Res. - Part B Appl. Biomater.*, 104, 1622–1631, 2016.
69. Mouran, C.G., Pereir, R., Buciumeanu, M., Carvalho, O., Bartolomeu, F., Nascimo, R., Silva, F.S., Effect of laser surface texturing on primary stability and surface properties of zirconia implants. *Ceram. Int.*, 0–1, 2017.
70. Wiedemann, T., Clinical guideline for zirconia dental implants: a comprehensive and critical review and update. *J. Clin. Med. Res.*, 5, 1–7, 2024.
71. Bi, X., Li, M., Zhang, Y., *et al.*, Polyetheretherketone (PEEK) as a potential material for the repair of maxillofacial defect compared with E-poly(tetrafluoroethylene) (E-PTFE) and silicone. *ACS Biomater. Sci. Eng.*, 9, 4328–4340, 2023, doi: 10.1021/acsbiomaterials.2c00744.
72. Zhang, J., Su, Y., Rao, X., *et al.*, Additively manufactured polyether ether ketone (PEEK) skull implant as an alternative to titanium mesh in cranioplasty. *Int. J. Bioprinting*, 9, 634, 2023, doi: 10.18063/ijb.v9i1.634.
73. Moharil, S., Reche, A., Durge, K., Polyetheretherketone (PEEK) as a Biomaterial: An Overview. *Cureus*, 15, 8, e44307, 2023, doi: 10.7759/cureus.44307. PMID: 37779776; PMCID: PMC10536400.
74. Dondani, J.R., Iyer, J., Tran, S.D., Surface treatments of PEEK for osseointegration to bone. *Biomolecules*, 13, 3, 464, 2023.
75. Alotaibi, N.M., Naudi, K.B., Conway, D.I., Ayoub, A.F., The current state of peek implant osseointegration and future perspectives: A systematic review. *Eur. Cells Mater.*, 40, 1–20, 2020.

6

Autogenous Bone Graft

Yaser AlNatheer* **and Sameh A. Seif**

Oral and Maxillofacial Surgery Department, Dental Faculty, King Saud University, Riyadh, Saudi Arabia

Abstract

Autogenous bone grafting remains the gold standard in craniofacial reconstruction, particularly in oral and maxillofacial surgery, due to its unmatched biological properties—osteogenesis, osteoinduction, and osteoconduction. This chapter provides a comprehensive overview of autogenous bone grafts, highlighting their historical evolution, biological foundation, and clinical applications. We examine the major types of free bone grafts—cortical, cancellous, and corticocancellous—detailing their biological behavior, mechanical characteristics, and preferred donor sites, including intraoral (mandibular symphysis, ramus) and extraoral sources (iliac crest, tibia, calvarium). Special emphasis is placed on the increasingly utilized particulate cancellous bone marrow grafts (PCBM), which offer enhanced osteogenic potential and ease of harvesting, particularly in alveolar cleft and implant-related reconstructions. The chapter also reviews the rationale and evidence supporting the use of composite bone grafts, integrating autogenous bone with allografts or synthetic substitutes to improve graft volume, reduce resorption, and minimize donor site morbidity. Clinical outcomes from recent trials demonstrate promising implant success rates and reduced complications when composite grafting is employed. Despite its high success rates, autogenous grafting is not without limitations, including donor site morbidity, graft resorption, and potential infection. Careful surgical planning, appropriate material selection, and patient-centered decision-making are vital to optimize outcomes. This chapter synthesizes current evidence and practical insights to guide clinicians in selecting and utilizing autogenous bone grafts effectively in maxillofacial reconstruction.

**Corresponding author*: y.alnatheer@gmail.com

Randa A. Alfotawi (ed.) Oro-Facial Bone Grafts and Biomaterials, (107–124) © 2026 Scrivener Publishing LLC

Keywords: Autogenous bone grafts, osteogenesis, corticocancellous grafts, particulate cancellous bone marrow (PCBM), composite bone grafts, donor site morbidity

6.1 Introduction

Craniofacial defects can significantly affect a person's quality of life, whether caused by pathology, trauma, or genetic predispositions [1]. For decades, oral and maxillofacial surgeons have played a vital role in restoring function and appearance through hard and soft tissue reconstruction in the maxillofacial region. Bony reconstruction restores compromised bone volume, which is crucial for successfully rehabilitating missing teeth with dental implants. This procedure corrects jawbone deficits, ensuring sufficient implant support and promoting oral health [2].

Historically, the use of bone grafts and tissue transplantation has been known since the prehistorical era, when evidence was found in the skeletal remains [3]. However, the first reported successful clinical application of autogenous bone graft was in 1821 by von Walter, who performed a bone transplant for mandibular reconstruction [4]. Since then, scientists have carried out many investigations and breakthroughs to establish the foundation of the biology of bone grafts we know today [5].

Although there are many well-studied bone substitutes to this day, autogenous bone grafts remain the gold standard in bone grafting due to their excellent compatibility with the body and essential biological properties [6]. Autogenous bone grafting is a surgical procedure involving transferring bone tissue harvested from a donor site within the same patient's body to repair a bone defect, address a nonunion, or promote fusion in arthrodesis. These grafts facilitate bone healing by providing a scaffold for new bone growth (osteoconductive) and stimulating the formation of new bone through growth factors (osteoinductive). Additionally, it contains viable osteogenic cells, which are crucial for bone regeneration and pose no risk of disease transmission [7].

In the orofacial region, autogenous bone grafts can be utilized in many clinical applications: alveolar ridge augmentation, sinus lift procedure, cleft alveolus and palate reconstruction (Figure 6.1); mandibular and maxillary reconstruction (post-trauma or pathology) (Figure 6.2); periodontal defect repair (guided bone regeneration—GBR); and congenital and acquired craniofacial defects [8–11].

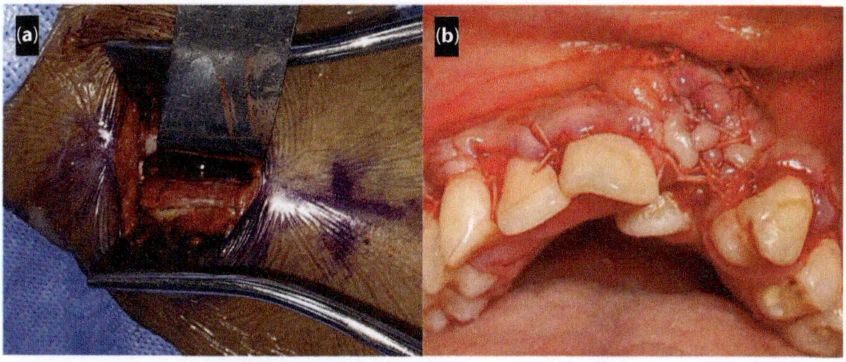

Figure 6.1 Bone graft harvested from the same patient to reconstruct their cleft alveolus. (a) Anterior iliac (donor site). (b) Reconstructed alveolus (recipient site).

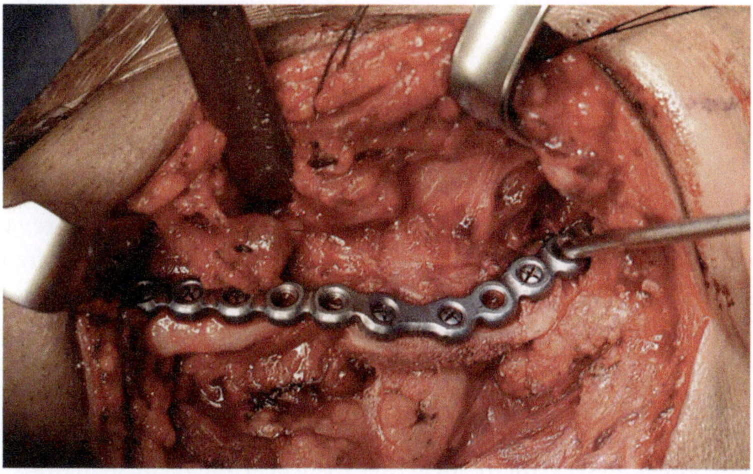

Figure 6.2 Resected mandible due to benign pathology, reconstructed with autogenous corticocancellous ilium strip.

6.2 Free Bone Graft

Generally, autogenous bone grafts can be classified based on their blood supply as free bone (no intrinsic blood supply, relies on revascularization) and vascularized bone grafts or microvascular bone graft (maintains original blood supply *via* artery and vein). Free bone grafts refer to grafts harvested from the patient's own body and transplanted to a recipient site

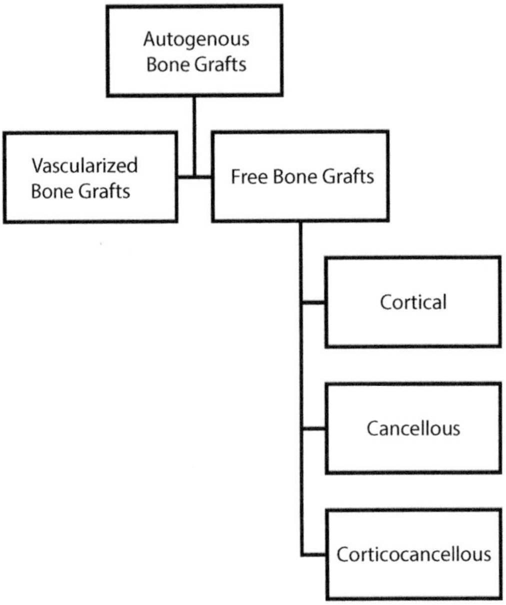

Figure 6.3 Autogenous bone grafts classification based on blood supply.

without maintaining their original blood supply, depending on revascularization from the recipient site [6]. Free autogenous bone grafts are subclassified into cortical, cancellous, and corticocancellous bone (Figure 6.3).

Cortical grafts are obtained from the dense outer layer of the donor bone. They are available in both particulate and block forms. Biologically, they act mainly as osteoconductive scaffolds with minimum osteoinductive and osteogenic properties [12]. The increased structural support of cortical grafts makes them ideal for load-bearing reconstructions and onlay augmentation for structural bony defects [13]. However, compared to cancellous grafts, cortical grafts require more time for revascularization and integration due to their smaller surface and porous area, as well as decreased cellular contents [14].

Cancellous grafts are particulate bone grafts characterized by a three-dimensional scaffold and a porous structure. They are harvested from the softer trabecular bone [15]. Biologically, they are osteogenic as they contain stem cells and osteocytes, osteoconductive as their three-dimensional structure acts as a scaffold, and osteoinductive due to their content of growth factors [16]. Although cancellous bone grafts show insufficient initial structural support, they can begin to provide adequate structural support as bone is formed. Additionally, due to their rich cellular contents, cancellous bone grafts revascularize faster than cortical bone grafts [6].

Corticocancellous grafts are bone grafts containing both cortical and cancellous bone. Combining the two provides the mechanical strength of cortical bone and the osteogenic and osteoinductive properties of cancellous bone, making them a versatile option in reconstructive surgery. Additionally, a mixture of cortical and cancellous bone could result in less bone resorption and higher bone density than traditional sole cancellous

Table 6.1 Free bone graft donor sites for orofacial reconstruction.

Category	Donor site	Characteristics	Common applications
Intraoral	Mandibular symphysis (chin)	Corticocancellous, moderate volume (1.5 to 3.0 cm^3)	Alveolar ridge augmentation, small defect repairs
	Ramus	Primarily cortical, strong structure	Alveolar ridge grafting, implant site preparation
	Maxillary tuberosity	Soft cancellous bone, easily harvested	Small defect filling, sinus lift procedures
	Palatal bone	Thin cortical bone	Minor grafting, cleft repair
Extraoral	Iliac crest	High volume, corticocancellous, rich in marrow	Large mandibular/ maxillary reconstructions, oncologic defects
	Calvarium (cranial bone)	Primarily cortical, strong, low resorption	Craniofacial reconstruction, contour augmentation
	Tibia	Cancellous, moderate volume	Small to medium bone defects, periodontal applications
	Rib	Corticocancellous, elastic	Mandibular and nasal reconstructions, TMJ grafting

bone grafts. In contrast to sole cancellous bone grafts, corticocancellous bone grafts could preserve a more significant bone volume with comparable bone density and prevent excessive bone resorption [17, 18].

Free bone grafts utilized in orofacial reconstruction can be harvested from extra- or intraoral donor sites, each with its unique characteristics (Table 6.1). Intraorally, they can be harvested from mandibular symphysis, ramus, palatal bone, and maxillary tuberosity. Extraorally, the iliac crest, tibia, ribs, and calvarium are all optional donor sites [13, 19, 20].

6.2.1 Techniques

6.2.1.1 The Mandibular Symphysis

The mandibular symphysis (chin) is a reliable intraoral donor site for corticocancellous bone grafts, offering good access, moderate graft volume, and favorable healing. The surgical technique includes a horizontal vestibular incision made approximately 5 mm below the mucogingival junction, extending from canine to canine. A full-thickness mucoperiosteal flap is then carefully reflected to expose the anterior surface of the mandible, with particular attention to avoid injury to the mental nerve and adjacent muscular attachments (Figure 6.4).

6.2.1.2 Ramal Bone Grafts

For the harvesting of ramal bone grafts, various incision techniques may be employed. In edentulous patients, a crestal incision is typically made and extended posteriorly to the ascending ramus at the level of the occlusal plane. In patients with natural teeth, an intrasulcular incision is preferred, also extended posteriorly to the ascending ramus. Once the incision is made, a full-thickness mucoperiosteal flap is elevated along the lateral surface of the mandible, thereby exposing the lateral aspect of the mandibular ramus. A rectangular cortical bone block, typically up to 4 mm in thickness, 3.5 cm in anteroposterior length, and 1 cm in height (superoinferiorly), can be harvested. The medial osteotomy cut is placed lateral to the posterior teeth and approximately 4 to 6 mm medial to the external oblique ridge.

6.2.1.3 Ilium Bone Grafts

The ilium is widely recognized as the most preferred donor site for harvesting autogenous bone grafts. Grafts may be obtained from either the

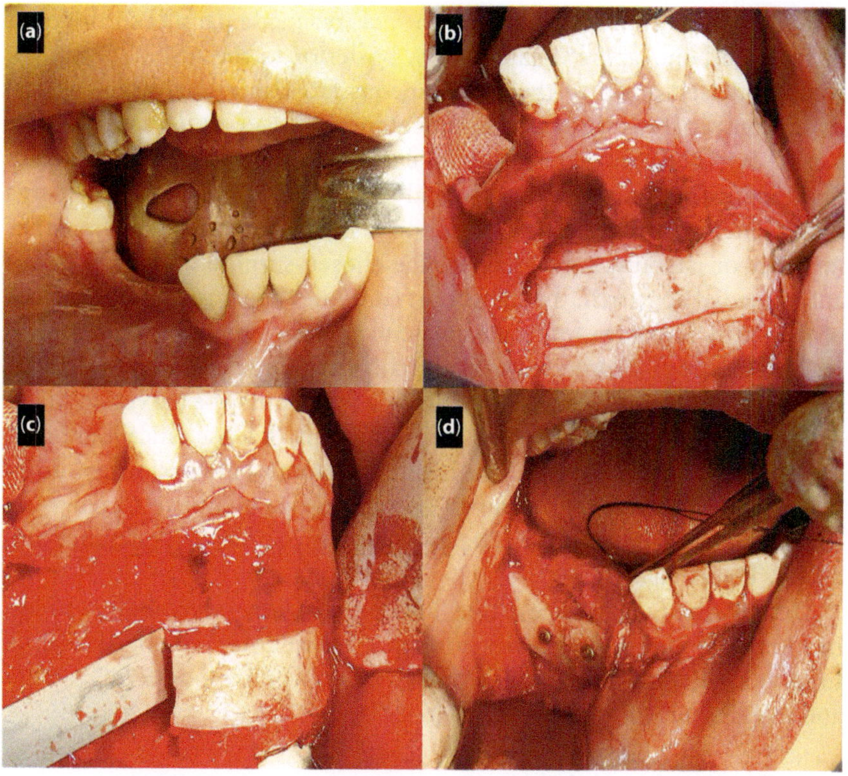

Figure 6.4 Intraoperative sequence of mandibular symphysis (chin) bone graft harvesting. (a) Preoperative view showing alveolar defect. (b) Horizontal vestibular incision and reflection of a full-thickness mucoperiosteal flap exposing the symphyseal bone. (c) Osteotomy cuts are made within safe anatomical margins, followed by elevation of a corticocancellous block graft. (d) Donor site closure after graft harvesting, showing placement of fixation screws and flap repositioning.

anterior or posterior portions of the ilium, depending on the clinical requirement and surgeon preference. This site offers the greatest absolute volume of cancellous bone and possesses the highest cancellous-to-cortical bone ratio among commonly used donor locations. When approaching the anterior iliac crest, particular care must be taken to avoid injury to surrounding neurovascular structures. Specifically, surgeons must be cautious of the lateral cutaneous branch of the subcostal nerve (T12) and the lateral cutaneous branch of the iliohypogastric nerve (L1). Additionally, the lateral femoral cutaneous nerve, located anterior and medial to the anterior superior iliac spine (ASIS), necessitates gentle superior and medial traction of the overlying skin to allow incision placement away from this nerve. The procedure begins with an incision made parallel to the crest of the iliac bone, approximately 2 cm posterior to the ASIS. The skin is sharply incised down to the subcutaneous fat. Using electrocautery, the dissection proceeds through the subcutaneous tissue to the fascia covering the fascia lata and external oblique muscles. Next, a precise incision is made along the iliac crest down to and through the periosteum. Once this layer is incised, subperiosteal dissection is initiated and carried out either medially or laterally, depending on the chosen surgical approach. In the anteromedial approach, the dissection continues along the medial surface of the ilium. In contrast, the anterolateral approach involves stripping the periosteum from the lateral surface, facilitating better access for graft harvesting. Following exposure of the ilium, the graft may be harvested in the form of a corticocancellous block, a cortical graft, or loose cancellous bone. The intended graft size is outlined, and osteotomies are performed using saws, osteotomes, or surgical burs. Cancellous bone may be retrieved using curettes, gouges, or trephines, depending on the surgeon's preference and access (Figure 6.5).

Despite their advantages, free bone grafts have several drawbacks, including donor site morbidity, limited graft volume, prolonged healing time, and potential resorption, which can compromise long-term stability and integration with the host bone [6, 21].

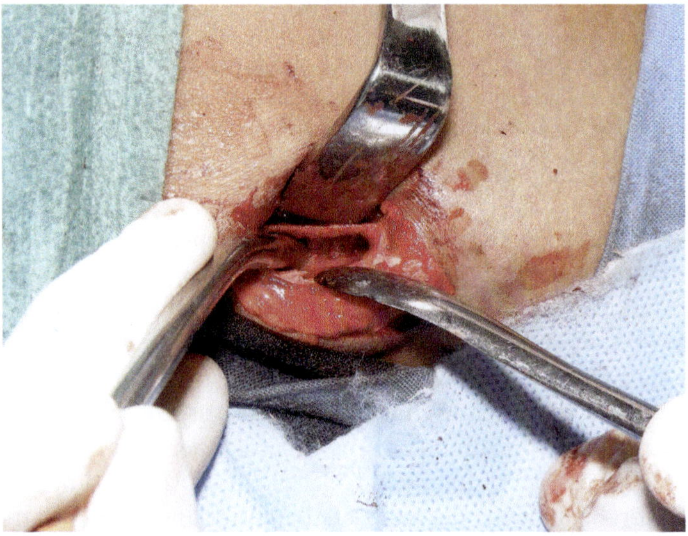

Figure 6.5 Intraoperative view of anterior iliac crest bone graft harvesting, showing retrieval of cancellous bone using curettes, following corticocancellous block harvesting.

6.3 Particulate Cancellous Bone Marrow Grafts (PCBMs)

Recently, particulate cancellous bone marrow grafts (PCBMs) in orofacial defects have been employed in many clinical scenarios [22–25]. PCBM grafts are autogenous bone grafts composed of small fragments of cancellous bone harvested along with bone marrow, typically from highly vascularized medullary bone such as the iliac crest. These grafts are rich in osteogenic cells, growth factors, and hematopoietic elements, providing osteogenic, osteoinductive, and osteoconductive properties essential for bone regeneration [26]. PCBM grafts demonstrate superior efficacy to block cortical or corticocancellous grafts because it is relatively easy to harvest, reduce the operative time, contain a more significant number of osteogenic precursor cells, and more readily incorporate into the alveolus with the capacity for postoperative remodeling [17].

In clinical applications, PCBM grafts have been effectively used to reconstruct orofacial defects. For instance, Giordano *et al.* reported the successful reconstruction of mandibular defects using PCBM grafts within a metallic mesh crib, demonstrating the grafts' capacity to restore function and stability to mandibular structures [27]. Another study by Ames *et al.* showed the use of PCBM in reconstructing alveolar clefts by analyzing more than 40 cases, and they concluded that the use of these grafts offers a dynamic and biologically viable approach that currently appears to be the preferred technique for rehabilitating patients with alveolar clefts [28]. Additionally, a study by Yusa *et al.* evaluated the use of PCBM in implant prosthetic rehabilitation, assessing the survival rates of the implants [22]. The illustration highlights the main features and clinical applications of PCBM grafts in orofacial reconstruction (Figure 6.6).

PCBM grafts are typically harvested using curettage, trephine drills, or bone gouges to collect small cancellous bone particles along with bone marrow aspirate. The technique is designed to preserve the viable osteogenic cells present in the marrow and trabecular matrix [29, 30]. The common sites for harvesting PCBM grafts are the anterior and posterior iliac crest, tibia, proximal humerus, and intraorally. Table 6.2 highlights their main characteristics and clinical applications (Table 6.2).

Although PCBM grafts have many favorable features, they present certain drawbacks:

- **Donor site morbidity:** Harvesting PCBM typically involves an additional surgical procedure, often from the iliac crest,

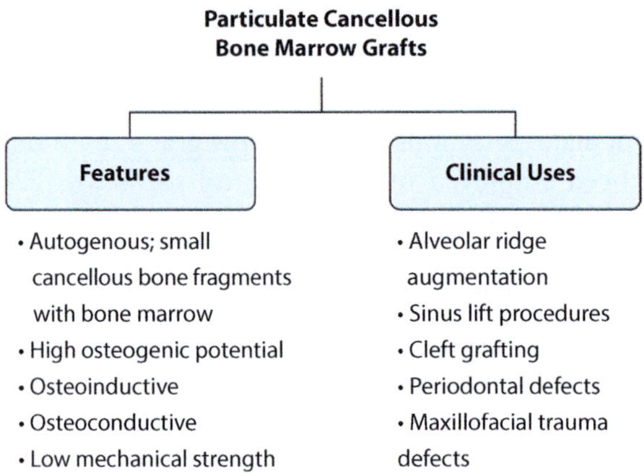

Figure 6.6 Overview of particulate cancellous bone marrow grafts.

Table 6.2 Common donor sites and their characteristics for PCBM grafts.

Donor site	Characteristics	Common applications
Anterior iliac crest	Most common; abundant cancellous bone and marrow	Jaw reconstruction, sinus lift, cleft repair
Posterior iliac crest	Higher bone volume, more invasive	Larger reconstructions, spinal surgeries
Tibia	Less morbidity; moderate cancellous bone	Small to moderate oral defects
Proximal humerus	Occasionally used	Orthopedic and trauma-related reconstructions
Intraoral sites	Ramus, symphysis, and maxillary tuberosity (limited marrow)	Small volume grafts for localized defects

which can lead to complications such as pain, infection, excessive bleeding, inflammation, and scarring at the donor site [31].

- **Limited mechanical strength:** PCBM grafts lack the structural integrity required for load-bearing applications, necessitating supplementary support, such as titanium mesh, to maintain the desired shape and stability during the healing process [32].
- **High resorption rates:** Due to their trabecular nature, PCBM grafts may experience significant resorption over time, potentially compromising the long-term stability of the reconstruction [33].
- **Volume limitations:** The amount of cancellous bone available for harvesting is finite, which may be insufficient for extensive reconstructions. This limits the applicability of PCBM grafts in large defect repairs [21].

6.4 Evidence of Using Composite Bone Grafts

The limited availability of autologous bone grafts and the depletion of cancellous bone at common donor sites have underscored the need for alternative grafting materials that offer comparable biological and regenerative properties. Nevertheless, since no existing bone substitute fully replicates the biological properties of autologous bone grafts, clinicians have adopted the concept of composite grafting as a strategy to overcome this limitation [34]. Composite grafts combine the advantageous properties of different grafting materials and have been successfully utilized in clinical settings for craniofacial reconstruction [35]. Composite bone grafts are engineered by combining autogenous bone with other materials such as allografts, xenografts, or synthetic substitutes. This combination aims to leverage the osteogenic properties of autogenous bone alongside the structural support, resorption rate, and volume provided by additional materials.

The rationale for using composite bone grafts is to overcome the individual limitations of single-source graft materials by combining their complementary properties through enhancing volume stability, improving biological performance, and reducing surgical burden and morbidity. Autogenous bone, while biologically superior due to its osteogenic, osteoinductive, and osteoconductive properties, is limited in quantity and often undergoes rapid resorption post-transplantation; by integrating it with slow-resorbing materials such as xenografts, allografts, or synthetic scaffolds (e.g., hydroxyapatite, β-TCP), the graft maintains its volume and shape over time, especially in large or non-contained defects [36]. In terms of improving biological performance, composite grafts aim to retain the osteogenic capacity of autogenous bone (stem cells and growth factors), increase scaffold stability and porosity through osteoconductive materials, facilitate cell migration and vascular ingrowth, and reduce donor site morbidity by minimizing the amount of autogenous bone required [37]. In reducing surgical burden and morbidity, using composites allows clinicians to harvest smaller volumes of autogenous bone and to avoid additional surgeries or complications associated with extensive graft harvesting (e.g., iliac crest morbidity) [38].

Composite grafts have demonstrated successful applications in craniofacial reconstruction and implant dentistry. Galindo-Moreno *et al.*'s clinical trial [39] assessed the effectiveness of a composite graft combining autogenous cortical bone, inorganic bovine bone, and platelet-rich plasma (PRP) for maxillary sinus augmentation. Their results demonstrated that this composite graft can be successfully used for sinus augmentation procedures. Another randomized clinical trial by Thuaksuban *et al.* [40] compared autogenous bone grafting alone to a composite graft of autogenous bone and deproteinized bovine bone for alveolar cleft repair. The study found that both techniques resulted in comparable bone remodeling and canine eruption outcomes. Yet, the composite graft significantly reduced patient morbidity, hospital stay, and the amount of autogenous bone required. A similar recent study by Shen *et al.* [36] explored the efficacy of combining BMP2-loaded calcium phosphate cement with autogenous bone for alveolar cleft reconstruction [36]. The findings indicated that this composite grafting strategy significantly enhanced bone regeneration and defect healing, offering a promising approach to reduce donor site morbidity while maintaining high clinical success rates. A prospective study by Maiorana *et al.* [41] investigated the impact of covering autogenous onlay block grafts with deproteinized bovine bone (Bio-Oss) to mitigate graft resorption [41]. The findings indicated that Bio-Oss coverage effectively reduced resorption of the autogenous grafts, leveraging its osteoconductive properties to compensate for natural bone remodeling processes. In terms of the use of composite grafts with dental implants, a review by Goyal *et al.* [42] emphasizes composite bone grafts—particularly those combining autogenous bone with xenografts [42]. The authors utilized deproteinized bovine bone (DBB) accompanied with autogenous bone for sinus augmentation, ridge preservation, and large defect reconstructions. The tested composite graft group has achieved high implant success rates exceeding 90–95%, depending on the case and graft composition.

6.5 Success Rate vs Complications

Autogenous bone grafts are widely regarded as the gold standard in bone regeneration due to their osteogenic, osteoinductive, and osteoconductive properties. Despite their biological advantages, their use entails inherent limitations and potential complications. Evaluating the clinical success rates alongside associated risks is essential for evidence-based surgical planning.

Clinical studies consistently report high success rates for autogenous bone grafts in both maxillofacial and orthopedic applications. In alveolar ridge augmentation, reported success rates range from 85% to 95%, with favorable long-term outcomes for implant placement. Vertical ridge augmentation procedures have demonstrated average vertical bone gains of 4–6 mm, with implant survival rates exceeding 90% over a 5-year period. Similarly, iliac crest grafts have shown integration rates surpassing 90% in cleft alveolus repair [43]. A meta-analysis by Moraschini *et al.* [44] evaluated the long-term outcomes of dental implants placed in areas reconstructed with extraoral autogenous bone grafts [44]. Their findings demonstrated high implant survival rates and minimal marginal bone loss over time, supporting the efficacy of extraoral autogenous grafts in complex maxillofacial reconstructions.

Despite their clinical effectiveness, autogenous bone grafts are associated with a range of complications, both at the donor and recipient sites:

6.5.1 Donor Site Morbidity

Harvesting autogenous bone, particularly from extraoral sites like the iliac crest, can result in considerable postoperative morbidity. Reported complications include

- Pain and discomfort
- Infection or hematoma formation
- Gait disturbance (especially with iliac crest harvesting)
- Cosmetic issues such as scarring or deformity
- Nerve disturbances

Studies have shown donor site morbidity in up to 20–30% of iliac crest graft cases [21]. A prospective cohort study by Heimes *et al.* [45] compared morbidity-related outcomes between autologous and allogeneic bone grafts for alveolar ridge augmentation, focusing on patient-reported experience [45]. While both graft types yielded high satisfaction rates, autologous grafts were associated with significantly greater swelling, nerve disturbances, and discomfort from a second surgical site. Conversely, allogeneic grafts caused less postoperative morbidity and were preferred by patients in terms of comfort, highlighting the importance of shared decision-making when selecting grafting materials.

6.5.2 Graft Site Complications

Complications at the graft site may include:

- Graft resorption: Particularly prevalent in cortical grafts lacking adequate fixation or vascularization, leading to partial or complete loss of the grafted material.
- Graft exposure: The most common complication in oral regenerative procedures is when the barrier membrane or block graft becomes exposed, increasing the risk of infection and compromising the graft's success.
- Infection: Postoperative infections can occur, necessitating interventions ranging from antibiotic therapy to graft removal, depending on severity.
- Delayed healing or soft tissue dehiscence [46].

These complications underscore the importance of meticulous surgical technique, proper patient selection, and postoperative care to enhance graft success rates.

6.6 Conclusion

While autogenous bone grafts remain the most reliable material for bone regeneration, the associated risks necessitate careful patient selection and surgical planning. In many cases, particularly those involving large defects or patients with systemic risk factors, composite or synthetic graft alternatives may be considered.

AI disclosure statement: The author acknowledges the use of AI-based tools for minor language editing or grammatical correction. However, all intellectual contributions, analyses, and conclusions presented in this chapter are entirely the author's own.

References

1. Hurley, C.M., McConn Walsh, R., Shine, N.P., O'Neill, J.P., Martin, F., O'Sullivan, J.B., Current Trends in Craniofacial Reconstruction. *Surgeon*, *21*, 3, e118–e125, 2023, https://doi.org/10.1016/j.surge.2022.04.004.
2. Doonquah, L., Holmes, P.-J., Ranganathan, L.K., Robertson, H., Bone Grafting for Implant Surgery. *Oral Maxillofac. Surg. Clin.*, *33*, 2, 211–229, 2021, https://doi.org/10.1016/j.coms.2021.01.006.
3. Hernigou, P., Bone Transplantation and Tissue Engineering, Part I. Mythology, Miracles and Fantasy: From Chimera to the Miracle of the Black Leg of Saints Cosmas and Damian and the Cock of John Hunter. *Int. Orthop. (SICOT)*, *38*, 12, 2631–2638, 2014, https://doi.org/10.1007/s00264-014-2511-y.
4. Von Walter, P.H., Wiedereinheilung Der Bei Der Trapanation Ausgebohrten Knochenscheibe. *J. Chir. Augen Heilk.*, *2*, 571, 1821.
5. Schlickewei, W. and Schlickewei, C., The Use of Bone Substitutes in the Treatment of Bone Defects – the Clinical View and History. *Macromol. Symp.*, *253*, 1, 10–23, 2007, https://doi.org/10.1002/masy.200750702.
6. Schmidt, A.H., Autologous Bone Graft: Is It Still the Gold Standard? *Injury*, *52*, S18–S22, 2021, https://doi.org/10.1016/j.injury.2021.01.043.
7. Fillingham, Y. and Jacobs, J., Bone Grafts and Their Substitutes. *Bone Joint J.*, *98-B*, 1 Suppl A, 6–9, 2016, https://doi.org/10.1302/0301-620X.98B.36350.
8. Sakkas, A., Wilde, F., Heufelder, M., Winter, K., Schramm, A., Autogenous Bone Grafts in Oral Implantology—Is It Still a "Gold Standard"? A Consecutive Review of 279 Patients with 456 Clinical Procedures. *Int. J. Implant Dent.*, *3*, 1, 23, 2017, https://doi.org/10.1186/s40729-017-0084-4.
9. Valentini, V., Cassoni, A., Marianetti, T.M., Romano, F., Terenzi, V., Iannetti, G., Reconstruction of Craniofacial Bony Defects Using Autogenous Bone Grafts: A Retrospective Study on 233 Patients. *J. Craniofacial Surg.*, *18*, 4, 953–958, 2007.
10. Zhang, J., Li, S., He, H., Han, L., Zhang, S., Yang, L., Han, W., Wang, X., Gao, J., Zhao, J., Shi, W., Wu, Z., Wang, H., Zhang, Z., Zhang, L., Chen, W., Zhu, Q., Sun, T., Tang, P., Zhang, Y., Clinical Guidelines for Indications, Techniques, and Complications of Autogenous Bone Grafting. *Chin. Med. J.*, *137*, 01, 5–7, 2024, https://doi.org/10.1097/CM9.0000000000002691.
11. Starch-Jensen, T., Deluiz, D., Vitenson, J., Bruun, N.H., Tinoco, E.M.B., Maxillary Sinus Floor Augmentation with Autogenous Bone Graft Compared with a Composite Grafting Material or Bone Substitute Alone: A Systematic Review and Meta-Analysis Assessing Volumetric Stability of the Grafting Material. *J. Oral Maxillofac. Res.*, *12*, 1, e1, 2021.
12. Manson, P.N., Facial Bone Healing and Bone Grafts: A Review of Clinical Physiology. *Clin. Plast. Surg.*, *21*, 3, 331–348, 1994.
13. Misch, C.M., Maxillary Autogenous Bone Grafting. *Dent. Clin.*, *55*, 4, 697–713, 2011.

14. Burchardt, H., The Biology of Bone Graft Repair. *Clin. Orthop. Relat. Res.,*® *174*, 28–34, 1983.
15. Roden Jr., R.D., Principles of Bone Grafting. *Oral Maxillofac. Surg. Clin. North Am.*, *22*, 3, 295–300, 2010.
16. Heiple, K.G., Goldberg, V.M., Powell, A.E., Bos, G.D., Zika, J.M., Biology of Cancellous Bone Grafts. *Orthop. Clin. North Am.*, *18*, 2, 179–185, 1987.
17. Ma, L., Yali, H., Guijun, L., Dong, F., Effectiveness of Corticocancellous Bone Graft in Cleft Lip and Palate Patients: A Systematic Review. *J. Stomatol. Oral Maxillofac. Surg.*, *122*, 1, 33–38, 2021, https://doi.org/10.1016/j.jormas.2020.04.012.
18. Robinson, P.G., Abrams, G.D., Sherman, S.L., Safran, M.R., Murray, I.R., Autologous Bone Grafting. *Oper. Tech. Sports Med.*, *28*, 4, 150780, 2020.
19. Gianluca, I. and Valente, N.A., Intraoral and Extraoral Autologous Bone Block Graft Techniques: A Review of the Recent Literature. *Int. J. Contemp. Dent. Med. Rev.*, *2016*, 2016.
20. Kainulainen, V.T., Sandor, G.K., Caminiti, M.F., Clokie, C.M., Oikarinen, K.S., Extraoral Bone Harvesting Sites for Oral and Maxillofacial Surgery. *Suom. Hammaslaakarilehti*, 10–11, 2002.
21. Younger, E.M. and Chapman, M.W., Morbidity at Bone Graft Donor Sites. *J. Orthop. Trauma*, *3*, 3, 192–195, 1989.
22. Yusa, K., Ishikawa, S., Suzuki, N., Kunii, S., Okuyama, N., Hemmi, T., Iino, M., Clinical Evaluation of Bone Quality of Particulate Cancellous Bone and Marrow, and Implant Prosthetic Rehabilitation. *J. Stomatol. Oral Maxillofac. Surg.*, *125*, 5, Supplement 1, 101862, 2024, https://doi.org/10.1016/j.jormas.2024.101862.
23. Iino, M., Fukuda, M., Nagai, H., Hamada, Y., Yamada, H., Nakaoka, K., Mori, Y., Chikazu, D., Saijo, H., Seto, I., Ohkubo, K., Takato, T., Evaluation of 15 Mandibular Reconstructions with Dumbach Titan Mesh-System and Particulate Cancellous Bone and Marrow Harvested from Bilateral Posterior Ilia. *Oral Surg. Oral Med. Oral Pathol. Oral Radiol. Endod.*, *107*, 4, e1–e8, 2009, https://doi.org/10.1016/j.tripleo.2008.12.018.
24. Takato, T., Mori, Y., Fujihara, Y., Asawa, Y., Nishizawa, S., Kanazawa, S., Ogasawara, T., Saijo, H., Abe, T., Abe, M., Suenaga, H., Kanno, Y., Sugiyama, M., Hoshi, K., Preclinical and Clinical Research on Bone and Cartilage Regenerative Medicine in Oral and Maxillofacial Region. *Oral Sci. Int.*, *11*, 2, 45–51, 2014, https://doi.org/10.1016/S1348-8643(14)00008-1.
25. Ferretti, C., Muthray, E., Rikhotso, E., Reyneke, J., Ripamonti, U., Reconstruction of 56 Mandibular Defects with Autologous Compressed Particulate Corticocancellous Bone Grafts. *Br. J. Oral Maxillofac. Surg.*, *54*, 3, 322–326, 2016.
26. Atasoy, A. and Kose, G.T., Biology of Cancellous Bone Graft Materials and Their Usage for Bone Regeneration. *JSM Biotechnol. Biomed. Eng.*, 2016.

27. Giordano, A., Brady, D., Foster, C., Adams, G., Particulate Cancellous Marrow Crib Graft Reconstruction of Mandibular Defects. *Laryngoscope, 90*, 12, 2027–2036, 1980, https://doi.org/10.1288/00005537-198012000-00014.
28. Ames, J.R., Ryan, D.E., Maki, K.A., The Autogenous Particulate Cancellous Bone Marrow Graft in Alveolar Clefts: A Report of Forty-One Cases. *Oral Surg. Oral Med. Oral Pathol., 51*, 6, 588–591, 1981, https://doi.org/10.1016/S0030-4220(81)80005-9.
29. Isoda, Y., Imamura, E., Ueno, D., Akaike, T., Hamada, Y., Use of a Trephine Bur and Curette for Minimally Invasive Harvesting of Particulate Cancellous Bone and Marrow from the Iliac Crest: A Case of Alveolar Ridge Reconstruction. *Int. J. Implant Dent., 2*, 1, 1, 2016, https://doi.org/10.1186/s40729-015-0033-z.
30. Cakar, A., Egerci, O.F., Dogruoz, F., Tasatan, E., Ozturk, S., Sindel, M., Kose, O., Comparison of Curettage vs. Trephination Technique for Harvesting Anterior Iliac Crest Bone Graft: A Cadaveric Study. *Chin. J. Traumatol., 28*, 2, 151–156, 2025, https://doi.org/10.1016/j.cjtee.2023.10.007.
31. Zhao, R., Yang, R., Cooper, P.R., Khurshid, Z., Shavandi, A., Ratnayake, J., Bone Grafts and Substitutes in Dentistry: A Review of Current Trends and Developments. *Molecules, 26*, 10, 3007, 2021, https://doi.org/10.3390/molecules26103007.
32. Yagihara, K., Okabe, S., Ishii, J., Amagasa, T., Yamashiro, M., Yamaguchi, S., Yokoya, S., Yamazaki, T., Kinoshita, Y., Mandibular Reconstruction Using a Poly(l-Lactide) Mesh Combined with Autogenous Particulate Cancellous Bone and Marrow: A Prospective Clinical Study. *Int. J. Oral Maxillofac. Surg., 42*, 8, 962–969, 2013, https://doi.org/10.1016/j.ijom.2013.03.010.
33. Shabaan, A.A., Salahuddin, A., Aboulmagd, I., Ragab, R., Salah, K.A., Rashid, A., Ayad, H.M., el Aty Ahmed, W.A., Refahee, S.M., Alveolar Cleft Reconstruction Using Bone Marrow Aspirate Concentrate and Iliac Cancellous Bone: A 12-Month Randomized Clinical Study. *Clin. Oral Investig., 27*, 11, 6667–6675, 2023, https://doi.org/10.1007/s00784-023-05276-9.
34. Hakimi, M., Grassmann, J.-P., Betsch, M., Schneppendahl, J., Gehrmann, S., Hakimi, A.-R., Kröpil, P., Sager, M., Herten, M., Wild, M., Windolf, J., Jungbluth, P., The Composite of Bone Marrow Concentrate and PRP as an Alternative to Autologous Bone Grafting. *PLoS One, 9*, 6, e100143, 2014, https://doi.org/10.1371/journal.pone.0100143.
35. Khan, S.N., Tomin, E., Lane, J.M., Clinical applications of bone graft substitutes. *Orthop. Clin. North Am., 31*, 3, 389–398, 2000, https://doi.org/10.1016/S0030-5898(05)70158-9.
36. Shen, H., Li, L., Zhang, C., Chen, Y., Yu, H., Si, J., Shen, G., The Strategy of Composite Grafting with BMP2-Loaded Calcium Phosphate Cements and Autogenous Bone for Alveolar Cleft Reconstruction. *Front. Physiol., 13*, 1023772, 2022.
37. Troeltzsch, M., Troeltzsch, M., Kauffmann, P., Gruber, R., Brockmeyer, P., Moser, N., Rau, A., Schliephake, H., Clinical Efficacy of Grafting Materials

in Alveolar Ridge Augmentation: A Systematic Review. *J. Craniomaxillofac. Surg.*, *44*, 10, 1618–1629, 2016, https://doi.org/10.1016/j.jcms.2016.07.028.

38. Tessier, P., Kawamoto, H., Posnick, J., Raulo, Y., Tulasne, J.F., Wolfe, S.A., Complications of Harvesting Autogenous Bone Grafts: A Group Experience of 20,000 Cases. *Plast. Reconstr. Surg.*, *116*, 5 Suppl, 72S–73S, 2005, https://doi.org/10.1097/01.prs.0000173841.59063.7e.
39. Galindo-Moreno, P., Ávila, G., Fernández-Barbero, J.E., Aguilar, M., Sánchez-Fernández, E., Cutando, A., Wang, H.-L., Evaluation of Sinus Floor Elevation Using a Composite Bone Graft Mixture. *Clin. Oral Implants Res.*, *18*, 3, 376–382, 2007, https://doi.org/10.1111/j.1600-0501.2007.01337.x.
40. Thuaksuban, N., Nuntanaranont, T., Pripatnanont, P., A Comparison of Autogenous Bone Graft Combined with Deproteinized Bovine Bone and Autogenous Bone Graft Alone for Treatment of Alveolar Cleft. *Int. J. Oral Maxillofac. Surg.*, *39*, 12, 1175–1180, 2010, https://doi.org/10.1016/j.ijom.2010.07.008.
41. Maiorana, C., Beretta, M., Salina, S., Santoro, F., Reduction of Autogenous Bone Graft Resorption by Means of Bio-Oss Coverage: A Prospective Study. *Int. J. Periodontics Restorative Dent.*, *25*, 1, 2005.
42. Goyal, S., Masood, M., Le, C., Rajendran, Y., Nanjapa, S., Vaderhobli, R., Comparative Bone Graft Evaluation for Dental Implant Success: An Evidence-Based Review. *J. Long-Term Eff. Med. Implants*, *31*, 3, 2021.
43. Chiapasco, M., Casentini, P., Zaniboni, M., Bone Augmentation Procedures in Implant Dentistry. *Int. J. Oral Maxillofac. Implants*, *24 Suppl*, 237–259, 2009.
44. Moraschini, V., Louro, R.S., Son, A., Calasans-Maia, M.D., Sartoretto, S.C., Shibli, J.A., Long-Term Survival and Success Rate of Dental Implants Placed in Reconstructed Areas with Extraoral Autogenous Bone Grafts: A Systematic Review and Meta-Analysis. *Clin. Implant Dent. Relat. Res.*, *26*, 3, 469–481, 2024, https://doi.org/10.1111/cid.13319.
45. Heimes, D., Pabst, A., Becker, P., Hartmann, A., Kloss, F., Tunkel, J., Smeets, R., Kämmerer, P.W., Comparison of Morbidity-related Parameters between Autologous and Allogeneic Bone Grafts for Alveolar Ridge Augmentation from Patients' Perspective—A Questionnaire-based Cohort Study. *Clin. Implant Dent. Relat. Res.*, *26*, 1, 170–182, 2024.
46. Sanz-Sánchez, I., Sanz-Martín, I., Ortiz-Vigón, A., Molina, A., Sanz, M., Complications in Bone-Grafting Procedures: Classification and Management. *Periodontol. 2000*, *88*, 1, 86–102, 2022, https://doi.org/10.1111/prd.12413.

7

Allografts in Oral and Maxillofacial Reconstruction

Sree Lalita Kotha[1]*, Shams Altwaim[1] and Antonio Palma[2]

[1]Department of Basic Dental Sciences, College of Dentistry, Princess Nourah bint Abdulrahman University, Riyadh, Saudi Arabia
[2]Department of Surgery, King Abdullah bin Abdulaziz University Hospital, Riyadh, Saudi Arabia

Abstract

Allografts have emerged as a reliable alternative to autografts in contemporary oral and maxillofacial surgery for reconstruction of critical sized defects, offering structural stability and biologic compatibility. Derived from human donors of the same species, these materials undergo stringent processing and sterilization to eliminate immunogenic components while preserving the extracellular matrix architecture. They overcome the limitations of autografts like donor site morbidity and limited availability. This chapter comprehensively reviews allografts derived from bone, cartilage, nerve, epithelium, and other connective tissues, focusing on their clinical applications and outcomes. Allogeneic bone grafts support osteoconduction and, in some forms such as demineralized bone matrix (DBM), exhibit osteoinductive potential, making them effective in procedures including sinus floor elevation, guided bone regeneration, alveolar cleft grafting, orthognathic defects, and reconstruction after trauma or tumor resection. Osteochondral grafts having cartilage with subchondral bone are used to restore TMJ, nasal, and auricular structures. Cellular cartilage from nasal septum or auricle is used in rhinoplasty and facial contouring. Acellular dermal matrix from human dermis supports soft tissue regeneration after trauma or surgery. Amniotic membrane, rich in growth factors, is an effective dressing for burns, traumatic, and chronic wounds. Fascia lata, known for tensile strength, aids in facial reanimation and orbital or nasal reconstruction. Processed nerve allografts enable trigeminal or facial nerve repair over short gaps. Extracellular matrix (ECM) derived through decellularization of tissue or cultured cells preserves native matrix and bioactivity, showing promise in regeneration and 3D bioprinting.

**Corresponding author*: sreelalitacelur@gmail.com

Randa A. Alfotawi (ed.) Oro-Facial Bone Grafts and Biomaterials, (125–148) © 2026 Scrivener Publishing LLC

Additionally, the chapter addresses donor screening protocols and ethical aspects associated with tissue banking. Finally, it concludes with insights into future directions, including tissue-engineered allografts, growth factor-enriched matrices, and personalized graft design. This resource serves as a comprehensive guide for oral and maxillofacial surgeons, periodontists, and implantologists seeking to optimize grafting outcomes through the judicious use of allograft materials in reconstructive and regenerative procedures.

***Keywords*:** Allogeneic, extracellular matrix, implantologists, cartilage, bone, connective tissues, donors, demineralized bone matrix

7.1 Introduction

Human body is made up of living cells and extracellular materials that are organized in the form of tissues, organs, and systems. Oral and maxillofacial region is a complex area comprising tissues like skin muscles, nerves, blood vessels, bone, cartilage, tendons, ligaments, fat, and teeth. Injury caused to any of these tissues due to trauma, infections, degenerative disease, congenital deformities, tumor resection, and teeth loss may result in a defect. Based on the size, these defects are either sub-critical, which can be repaired by itself, or critical, which do not heal spontaneously, due to the limited healing capabilities of injured tissues. Moreover, the defects could be simple or composite, involving multiple tissue types, leading to structural, functional, and cosmetic repercussions. Many of these defects can be managed by primary closure; however, flaps and grafts from own body or other sources are required for the others. Autologous cortico-cancellous grafts and vascularized or free flaps remain as the gold standard for definitive reconstruction of critical-sized defects. Along with the advantages of low immunogenicity and fewer complications, autografts are associated with disadvantages of donor site morbidity and limited availability. To overcome the drawbacks, other options like allografts, allotransplants, xenografts, and biomaterials are widely being considered currently. To enhance the healing abilities, alternative modalities like hyperbaric oxygen therapy to promote fibroblast activity and angiogenesis, bisphosphonates to inhibit osteoclast mediated bone resorption, antioxidants to reduce inflammation and support collagen synthesis, pentoxifylline to improve microcirculation, platelet-rich plasma to deliver growth factors, and bone morphogenetic proteins (BMPs) to induce osteogenic differentiation of mesenchymal stem cells are considered. This chapter focuses on allografts, which are a viable alternative to autografts. Allografts are the grafts obtained from individuals of the same species, but with a different genetic makeup.

7.2 History

Tooth transplantation from other individuals has been reported since the time of ancient Egyptian mummies. In 1700s, it was a practice to perform live tooth transplants from rich to poor, particularly in France and England. As medicine and dentistry advanced, this was no longer practiced due to ethical and immunologic reasons. The credit of first successful bone allografting goes to a Scottish surgeon, Sir William MacEwen, who repaired a humeral defect with a transplanted tibial shaft in 1878. The successful remodeling of the allograft and functional recovery led to further exploration of graft viability, incorporation, and transplant immunology. However, there have been major concerns of availability and safety of allografts for more than a century. In 1965, Marshall R. Urist, an orthopedic surgeon, discovered BMPs and introduced the concept of osteoinduction with demineralized bone matrix [1]. Soft tissue allografts are used as a biological dressing, while bone grafts with a more complex action are used for bone regeneration. With the developments in donor screening, tissue banking, processing, and sterilization techniques, the safety and efficacy of allografts have been greatly enhanced leading to its wide use. Despite this evolution, the integration of allograft with the host bone, its remodeling potential, and combination with BMPs are still being studied [2, 3].

7.3 Processing and Sterilization Techniques

Processing of allografts aims to reduce disease transmission, minimize immunogenicity, and preserve structural and biological integrity. Common techniques include freeze-drying, gamma irradiation, and chemical processing, each of which may influence graft incorporation and resorption behaviour. After thorough donor screening like medical history evaluation, serological testing, and infectious disease screening, allografts obtained from live or cadaveric donors are subjected to meticulous processing by physical and biochemical means, followed by terminal sterilization to

- Decrease the risk of disease transfer without losing biologic healing potential
- Increase the availability of growth factors (by demineralization)
- Decrease the immunogenic reaction (by decellularization)
- Shape bone grafts and improve usability
- Enhance the shelf life

7.3.1 Decreasing the Risk of Disease Transfer

Rigorous donor screening, sterilization, and tissue handling protocols have substantially reduced the risk of disease transmission associated with allograft use. Tissue bioburden of allografts can be reduced by debridement, physical lavage, centrifugation, ultrasonic cleaning, low irradiation prior to chemical processing, and chemo modification with mild (detergents, alcohol, antibiotics) and aggressive (hydrogen peroxide/H_2O_2) chemicals. Contamination and immunogenicity of the graft are lowered by cleaning processes that eliminate microbes, bone marrow elements, lipids, and low-molecular-weight proteins. Aggressive chemicals are used to disinfect bone but not to treat soft tissues. After the bioburden is reduced, the graft sample is tested for sterility or subjected to terminal sterilization, most commonly by gamma irradiation. Irradiation of allografts at low temperatures and dose approximating 25 kGy are shown to have better clinical outcomes. Subjecting the final package to plasma H_2O_2, ethylene oxide, carbon dioxide in supercritical fluid form (SCO_2), and electron beam irradiation are other terminal sterilization methods with their own risks and benefits [4].

7.3.2 Increasing the Availability of Growth Factors (Demineralization)

Bone matrix comprises 60% inorganic component–crystalline hydroxyapatite [$Ca_{10}(PO_4)_6(OH)_2$], 10% water, and 30% organic component (collagenous and non-collagenous proteins) [5]. Careful controlled demineralization of allograft cortical bone with dilute hydrochloric acid results in the release of growth factors like BMPs belonging to transforming growth factor b (TGF-b), insulin-like growth factors (IGFs), fibroblast growth factors (FGFs), and vascular endothelial growth factors (VEGFs). BMP-2 is the most clinically potent and can stimulate mesenchymal stem cells to differentiate into osteoblasts, thus aiding in osteoinduction. This process is like the natural osteoclastic action during bone remodeling. IGF also promotes osteoblast proliferation and matrix formation, FGF enhances collagen production and stimulates angiogenesis, and VEGF is crucial for angiogenesis. Hypodemineralization would trap the growth factors in the bone matrix, making them unavailable to signal osteoinduction and hyperdemineralization would deplete the growth factors. Thus, optimally demineralized bone matrix (DBM) is both osteoinductive and osteoconductive, acting as a scaffold for host cell migration. Cellular bone allografts consisting of osteogenic cells adherent to native bone or derived from adipose or amniotic tissue is a recent development [4]. David M. Alfi and his associates successfully reconstructed a 6.5-cm-long segmental defect of mandible with cellular bone graft possessing autograft properties (VF-CBA; LifeNet Health®, Virginia Beach, VA) [6].

7.3.3 Decreasing the Immunogenic Reaction (Decellularization)

Decellularization techniques aim to remove antigenic cellular components while preserving the extracellular matrix. This process reduces host immune response and supports graft integration. Physical methods (including freeze-thawing, SCO_2 treatment), chemical treatment (with acetic acid, peracetic acid, hydrochloric acid, calcium hydroxide, sodium hydroxide, detergents), and enzymatic methods (using nucleases and proteases) can remove the cellular and bone marrow elements from allografts, thereby reducing the immunogenicity [7]. Meticulous care must be taken in the selection and duration of chemical treatment, as the mechanical strength of the graft is adversely affected if collagen is removed in this process [4].

7.3.4 Enhancing the Shelf Life

To increase the longevity of allografts, they are subjected to either freezing, freeze-drying, cryopreservation with liquid nitrogen, or treating with preservatives like ethanol and glycerol. Frozen grafts are fully hydrated but require monitored storage freezer and thawing before use. Freeze-dried allografts can be stored at ambient temperature but have altered biomechanical properties and need to be adequately rehydrated prior to use. Glycerol-based preservation (GBP) keeps the allograft fully hydrated at ambient temperature, maintains the biomechanical properties, and cuts down the cost associated with freezing and freeze-drying. Glycerol preserved demineralized bone grafts and dermis have been used in medicine for more than two decades. Refrigeration is another preservation method for fresh allografts, but with a limited shelf life [4, 8, 9].

7.4 Types of Allografts

The first level of description of a graft is dependent on its origin; accordingly, they are categorized as autograft (obtained from the same individual),

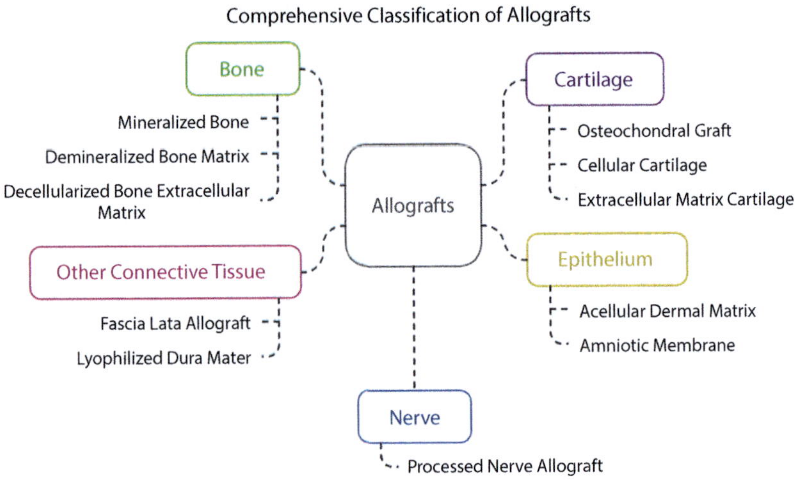

Figure 7.1 Classification of allografts.

allograft (obtained from a genetically different individual of the same species), xenograft (obtained from a member of different species), and isograft (obtained from a monozygotic twin). The second level of description is postulated on the tissue type from which the graft is obtained. Based on this schema, allografts are further classified as bone-derived, cartilage-derived, epithelium-derived, nerve-derived, and other connective tissue-derived to replace the respective critical tissue deficits (Figure 7.1).

7.4.1 Bone Grafts

Bone grafts are available as cortical, cancellous, and cortico-cancellous forms, in various shapes and sizes. Although literature provides multiple classifications of allogenic bone grafts, practically, they can be categorized as mineralized bone, demineralized bone matrix, and decellularized extracellular bone matrix.

When a bone graft is placed in a host bed, a series of biological processes take place leading to bone regeneration and graft incorporation, which are as follows:

- Osteogenesis—synthesis of new bone by cells of the graft
- Osteoinduction—synthesis of new bone by inductive action of growth factors (BMPs)

- Osteoconduction—acting as a friendly environment for bone growth by allowing ingrowth of capillaries and osteoprogenitor cells from the recipient bed
- Creeping substitution—resorption of graft by osteoclasts and formation of new bone by osteoblasts

Osteoconduction is a property of all bony allografts. Osteoinduction is seen only in demineralized and decellularized bone matrix, which is derived by processing methods preserving the BMPs. Osteogenesis is not a characteristic of allografts (seen only in autografts) (Table 7.1).

The incorporation of a bone graft is like the healing of a fractured bone. The initial response is the formation of hematoma and recruitment of platelets and inflammatory cells, and release of growth factors and cytokines. This is followed by inflammation and clearance of cell debris by macrophages and monocytes, fibroblastic infiltration, and initiation of angiogenesis, leading to an initial connection of graft with the host tissue. The graft acts as an osteoconductive scaffold, allowing the host blood vessels to penetrate through the Haversian and Volkmann canals. Monocytes and macrophages differentiate into osteoclasts, which resorb necrotic bone, and demineralize graft matrix, resulting in the release of growth factors. These growth factors in turn drives osteoinduction by differentiation of MSCs into osteoprogenitor cells. Graft remodeling begins with osteoclastic and osteoblastic action, along with maturation of matrix and mineralization.

Table 7.1 Properties of allogenic bone grafts.

Type of bone allograft	Mechanical properties	Osteogenesis	Osteoinduction	Osteoconduction	Resorption time frame
Mineralized, cortical	+++	-	-	++	+++
Mineralized, cancellous	+	-	-	+	++
Demineralized bone matrix	+/-*	-	++	+	+
Decellularized extracellular bone matrix	++	+/-**	++	++	++

*Depends on the range of demineralization and cortical/cancellous type
**Depends on the presence of mesenchymal stem cells

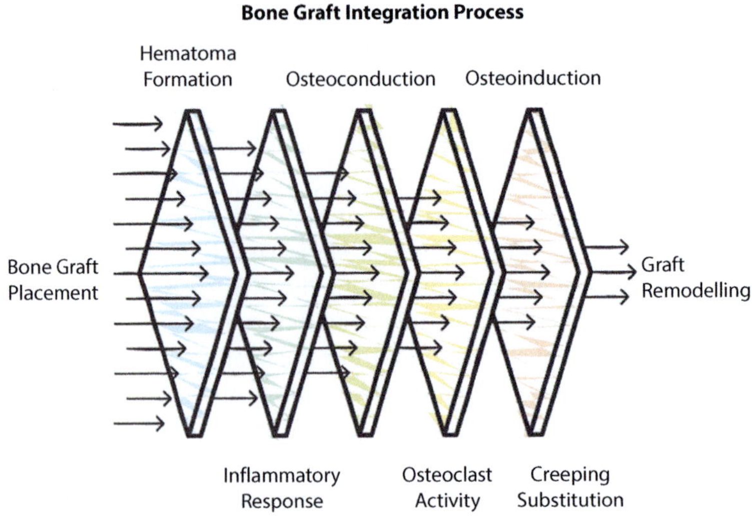

Figure 7.2 Incorporation of bone graft.

Full remodeling of graft continues for several weeks to months, under functional loads according to Wolff's law [10] (Figure 7.2).

A biological balance between the graft and host bed is needed for successful graft incorporation, and allografts may remain as a mixture of graft and host bone for many years. Cancellous bone graft incorporates faster due to higher porosity and greater surface area that is in contact with the host bone. To improve the available surface area of the cortical bone, researchers have perforated the graft, which showed better bone in growth compared to non-perforated grafts. Theoretically, if a graft has the same geometry and mechanical properties as that of the host bone, it may function immediately. If the properties of the graft are inferior to the host, either additional material must be used or the augmented graft must be stabilized by internal fixation until remodeling occurs so that it can take up functional loads. A clean, infection-free, well-vascularized recipient bed is important. Finally, immobilization of the graft, with greater host bone–graft contact, and complete tension-free soft tissue coverage is necessary for successful graft incorporation. Also, the graft must be protected from full loads until it is remodeled [11].

Clinical Applications

- Periodontal regeneration
- Socket preservation after tooth extraction

- Augmentation of atrophic alveolar ridge
- Sinus floor elevation
- Alveolar cleft grafting
- Filling of cystic enucleation defects
- Filling of bony gaps during orthognathic surgery
- Reconstruction of defects following trauma
- Reconstruction of defects due to tumor resection

7.4.1.1 *Mineralized Bone Allograft*

Although fresh allogenic bone block is the basic form of mineralized bone allografts, it is rarely used due to the high risk of disease transmission and immunogenetic potential. The other forms are fresh-frozen bone and freeze-dried grafts, which are currently obtained as cortical, cancellous, or combined forms. Cortical bone is available in the form of whole bone segment, blocks, and pieces; cancellous bone in the form of chips, wedges, pegs, and powder; and cortico-cancellous bone as blocks and particles. The structural strength of frozen bone far exceeds that of freeze-dried bone, as it is less processed. However, freeze-dried bone has reduced immunogenicity as it is lyophilized, where water is removed from the tissues, thereby destroying the osteogenic cells. The osteoblast surface harbors the major histocompatibility complex (MHC) antigens, which are responsible for graft recognition and provoking either a humoral or T-cell response [11, 12]. Cancellous bone has a faster incorporation into the host bone as it is less dense, leading to enhanced revascularization of large intertrabecular spaces. Cortico-cancellous bone has advantages of bone types, with the cortical component providing mechanical strength and the cancellous component ensuring precise fit [7] (Figure 7.3).

A recent systematic review showed fresh-frozen allogeneic bone blocks in the form of cortical, cancellous, and cortico-cancellous types as a reliable option for augmentation of atrophic maxilla before implant placement. The grafts underwent minimal resorption and had a low failure rate, and their clinical performance was comparable to autografts [13, 14]. Similar results were obtained with cancellous freeze-dried bone blocks too; however, it was recommended to avoid overcontouring of allografts in contrast to autologous bone harvested from iliac crest [15, 16].

7.4.1.2 *Demineralized Bone Matrix (DBM)*

As the name suggests, DBM is an acid extracted organic extracellular bone matrix consisting of collagen (mostly type I) and non-collagenous

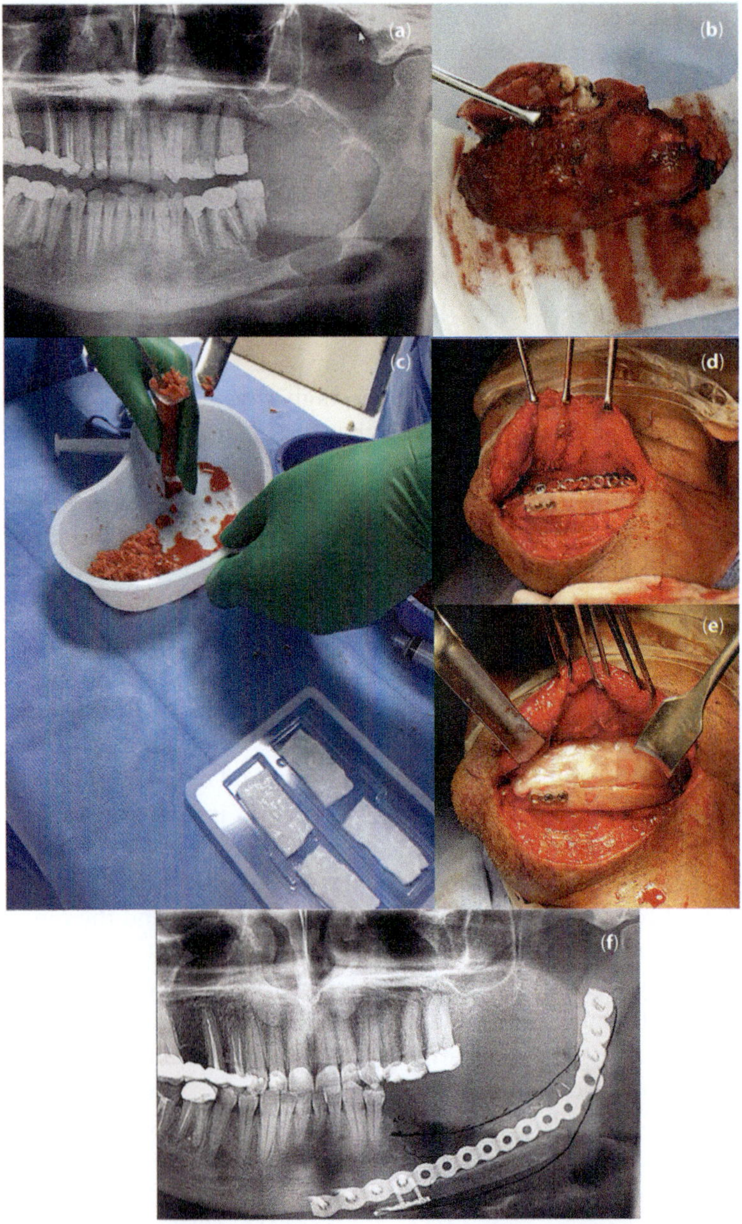

Figure 7.3 Ameloblastoma of left body and ramus of mandible, (a) Pre-operative OPG. (b) Segmental resection. (c) Compression of autogenous bone harvested from posterior iliac crest, and BMP infused on collagen sponges. (d) Allogenic rib as a bone container for autograft stabilized by reconstruction plate. (e) Application of BMP. f. 4-month post-operative OPG.

proteins, small amounts of calcium and phosphates, and trace cell debris [17]. Careful bone decalcification exposes the growth factors to aid in osteoinduction. Recent studies have shown that in addition to BMPs, other non-collagenous proteins like bone sialoproteins, osteopontin, osteocalcin, and proteoglycans also aid in bone regeneration [18]. Since DBM has poor mechanical properties, some commercial formulations included mixing with traditional allografts. Also, the original DBM was less cohesive and difficult to handle; hence, it had to be mixed with hardening agents like glycerol, hyaluronic acid, starch, or saline. However, these additions exert a deleterious effect on osteoinduction as the DBM per unit volume of graft is reduced. As DBM lacks structural rigidity, it is mainly used as fillers for defects with walls and contraindicated in areas where high compressive forces would be exerted. When used for cranial and facial contour defects, they tend to resorb. DBM is available in the form of blocks, putty, particles, and powder and can be stored at ambient temperature as they are freeze-dried [7]. DBM has been successfully used for defects of naso-maxillary clefts, cysts and tumors, Lefort I osteotomies, periodontal regeneration, socket preservation, sinus augmentation, and peri-implant defects (Figures 7.4, 7.5, and 7.6). To date, most impactful implant results are obtained when DBM is used in conjunction with autografts. Since there is a lot of variation in the processing and composition of commercially available DBM, the osteoinductive ability cannot be generalized [17].

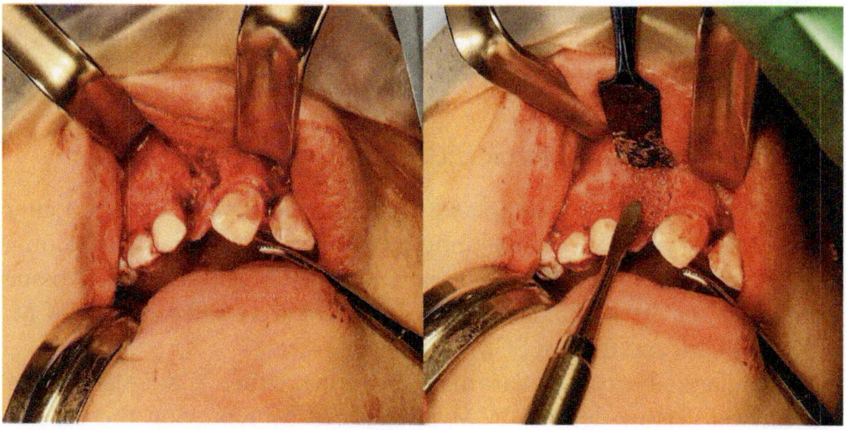

(a) (b)

Figure 7.4 Alveolar bone grafting in cleft palate case. (a) Bone defect after closure of nasal and palatal layer. (b) Allogeneic demineralized cancellous bone sponge placed in the bony defect.

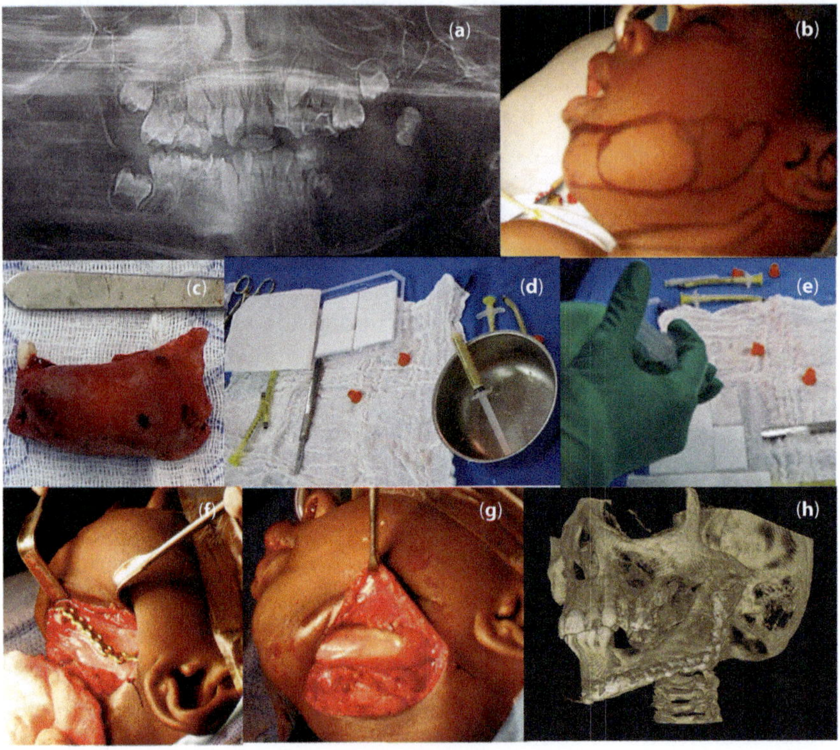

Figure 7.5 Ghost cell tumor of left body and ramus of mandible. (a, b) Pre-operative OPG and marking. (c) Segmental resection. (d) Preparation of ExFuse™ demineralized bone matrix with cancellous bone gel. (e) Infusion of BMP onto collagen sponges. (f, g) Reconstruction of defect with DBM, BMP stabilized by reconstruction plate. (h) 2-year post-operative CBCT showing excellent bone regeneration.

7.4.1.3 Extracellular Matrix (ECM)

Extracellular matrix is a complex 3-dimensional scaffold obtained after the removal of cells and cellular antigens from a tissue while still retaining the biological cues for tissue regeneration. Depending on the native tissue from which the extracellular matrix is derived, it is classified as bone ECM, cartilage ECM, and dermal ECM.

Decellularized extracellular matrix can be either tissue-derived or cell-derived. Tissue-derived ECM is obtained by removing the cellular components responsible for immunogenicity by either physical, chemical, or enzymatic processes. The quantity of DNA in the matrix before and after the process is used as a measure of decellularization. Tissue-derived ECM

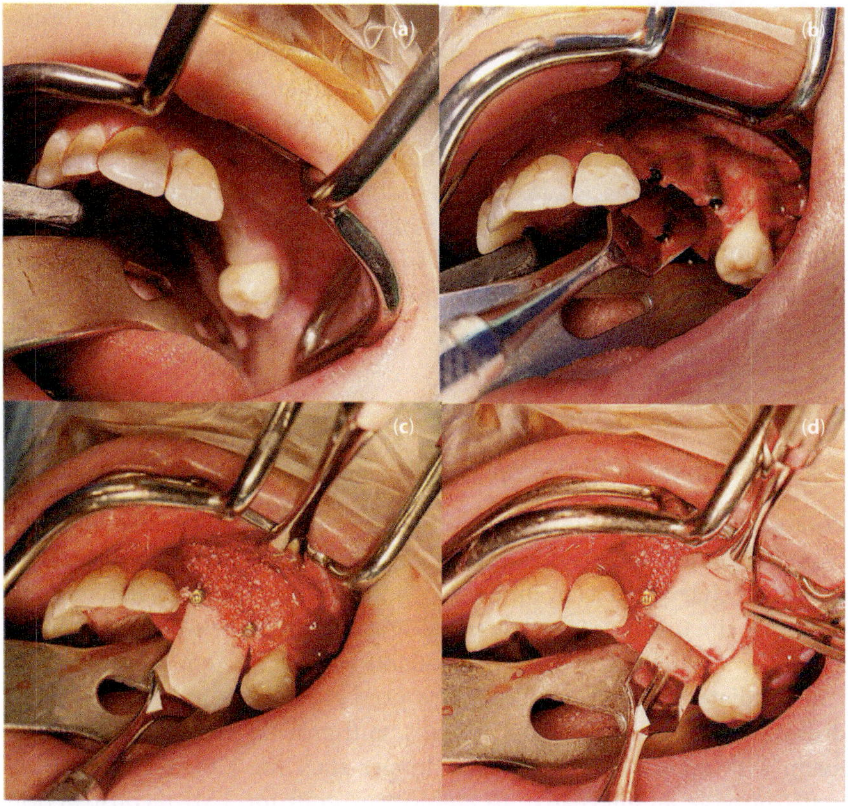

Figure 7.6 Guided bone regeneration. Allogenic demineralized bone chips and collagen membrane to cover dental implants with one-walled defects.

retains the memory specific to a particular tissue, thereby promoting the cell differentiation of a specific lineage. Cell-derived ECM is obtained by *in vitro* culturing of human cells. ECM releases growth factors, stimulates angiogenesis, controls tissue remodeling, and undergoes degradation in few months.

7.4.1.4 Decellularized Bone Extracellular Matrix (dECM)

Bone extracellular matrix consists of inorganic and organic phases. Calcium-deficient apatite, which is poorly crystalline, and trace metal ions (magnesium, zinc, strontium, copper) constitute the inorganic phase. Collagen type I, non-collagenous proteins (osteopontin, osteocalcin, proteoglycans, glycosaminoglycans) and growth factors (BMPs, transforming growth factor/TGF-b) constitute the organic phase [18].

Bone dECM, which is tissue-derived, maintains the structural architecture, resulting in favorable mechanical properties. Cell-derived bone dECM is obtained by *in vitro* culturing of mesenchymal stem cells, usually on a hydroxyapatite scaffold. It has a reduced risk of disease transmission. Recently, dECM has been used as bioink for 3D-printing [7]. Although dECM allograft has a great potential in the bone regeneration of the maxillofacial region due to their biomimetic properties, current clinical evidence is limited.

7.4.2 Cartilage Grafts

7.4.2.1 Osteochondral Graft

Osteochondral grafts due to their composite structure of cartilage with subchondral bone offer mechanical stability and functional versatility. They are usually harvested as hyaline osteochondral graft from distal femur and proximal tibia, and as costochondral grafts from 5th or 6th rib in women and 8th or 9th rib in men. They are available as fresh, frozen, cryopreserved, and irradiated forms [19]. Novel cryopreserved forms have viable chondrocytes, extracellular matrix proteins, and growth factors like the fresh form, with an added advantage of longer shelf life [20]. Osteochondral grafts provide an alternative to autologous graft for TMJ reconstruction and functional and reconstructive rhinoplasty, and to provide a helical framework of ear [21].

7.4.2.2 Cellular Cartilage

Cellular cartilage is harvested from nasal septum, auricle, and costal cartilage. The cartilaginous structure consists of collagen, elastin, and chondrocytes within the extracellular matrix. Chondrocytes have antigens and can invoke an immune reaction; however, the cartilage grafts are less immunogenic mainly due to their avascular nature [22]. It is available as fresh frozen, freeze-dried, and irradiated forms. Though allogenic cartilage is used for primary rhinoplasty, it is mainly reserved for revision rhinoplasty, cases with insufficient septal cartilage, and severe saddle nose deformities. It is an appropriate alternative for reconstruction of auricle, orbital floor, and midface contouring. Studies show comparable outcomes between allogenic cartilage grafts, both frozen and irradiated, and autografts in terms of graft infection, warping, and resorption [23, 24].

7.4.2.3 Cartilage ECM/Extracellular Matrix Cartilage Allograft (EMCA)

Cartilage ECM is composed of mainly collagen type II, non-collagenous proteins like proteoglycans and glycosaminoglycans, and hyaline cartilaginous growth factors [25]. It is a decellularized tissue-derived cartilage ECM harvested from nasal septum costal cartilage, providing mechanical integrity and an environment conducive for chondrogenesis [26]. It is available as particles, hydrogel, and paste, which can be recellularized and transformed as cell-laid matrix [7, 18]. EMCA is indicated for rhinoplasty, auricular and facial contouring, and as a soft tissue support for perinasal and periorbital regions.

7.4.3 Epithelial Grafts

7.4.3.1 Dermal ECM (Acellular Dermal Matrix)

Acellular dermal matrix is a derivative of human dermis after the removal of epidermal and dermal cells by chemical means and freeze-drying. Structural integrity and elasticity of dermal ECM are maintained by collagen type I and III (comprising 90%) and a small amount of elastin and proteoglycans. These components along with blood vessel channels aid in revascularization, cell infiltration, and tissue remodeling [27]. It is primarily used as a graft over vascularized soft tissue wounds [28]. It has versatile indications for reconstruction of soft tissue defects of oral and maxillofacial region, resulting from trauma, burns, oncologic resection, and parotidectomy [29] (Figure 7.7). Recent studies also concluded its successful use to augment soft tissues during dental implant placement and as a replacement after temporomandibular joint discectomy [28, 30, 31].

7.4.3.2 Amniotic Membrane

Human amniotic membrane obtained from the inner layer of placenta is composed of stratified epithelium and mesenchymal stromal layer, with collagen, proteoglycans, adhesive glycoproteins, and an abundance of growth factors [including epidermal growth factor (EGF), TGF-β, VEGF] [32, 33]. It is available as fresh, processed, and decellularized forms. Both structural and biological properties of amniotic membrane favorably modulate the wound microenvironment reducing fibrosis, inflammation, and infection [34–36]. In maxillofacial surgery, it has been used as a dressing

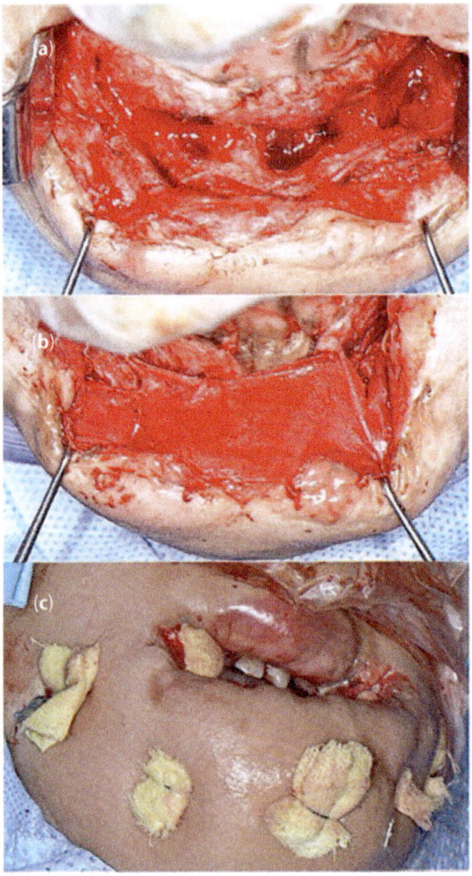

Figure 7.7 Chemical burn with constricted mucosa. (a) De-epithelialized large size mucosal defect with a lack of healthy donor site. (b) Acellular dermal matrix as an allogenic soft tissue coverage. (c) Matrix secured with bolster sutures.

for burns, traumatic and chronic wounds, and for oral mucosal and periodontal reconstruction. It has also been proved as a treatment strategy for medication-related osteonecrosis of the jaw [37, 38].

7.4.4 Other Connective Tissue Grafts

7.4.4.1 Fascia Lata Allograft

Allogeneic fascia lata is dense, fibrous, collagen-rich connective tissue harvested from the iliotibial tract of the lateral thigh. After harvesting, it is subjected to decellularization, sterilization, lyophilization, or cryopreservation.

Due to its tensile strength and pliability, it is used to create temporalis muscle sling for facial reanimation. Studies reported improvement in static and dynamic facial symmetry with minimal complications [39]. It has also been successfully used for orbital floor repairs, nasal dorsum and tip augmentation, oral mucosal defects, guided tissue regeneration, and gingival recession, and as a less explored option as a replacement for TMJ disc [40, 41].

7.4.4.2 Lyophilized Dura Mater

Freeze-dried allogeneic dura mater has historically been used as a collagen barrier for guided tissue regeneration of periodontal defects [42], to replace TMJ disc [43], to repair dural defects [44], and orbital floor fractures [45]. It is no longer in use due to its potential to transmit prion borne diseases, notably Creutzfeldt–Jakob disease in humans [46].

7.4.5 Nerve Grafts

7.4.5.1 Processed Nerve Allograft

In case of peripheral nerve injuries, adequate functional recovery is obtained by tension-free coaptation of residual nerve stumps at the epineurium level. Processed nerve allografts are a comparable alternative to autografts, where primary closure of transected nerves is not possible. These are human cadaveric peripheral nerves, which are processed to remove the cellular and antigenic components, while retaining the native extracellular matrix, endoneurial microstructure, and basal lamina to guide axonal growth. In the maxillofacial region, they are used to reconstruct defects of trigeminal and facial nerves. Due to the lack of viable Schwann cells, processed nerve allografts are highly effective for sensory and motor recovery of short gap distances (<2 cm) [47–50].

7.5 Advantages of Allografts

The biggest advantage of allografts is that there is no need for a second surgical site, eliminating donor site morbidity and reducing the surgical time. They are available in ample quantities from tissue banks, in various forms and sizes to suit different patient needs.

7.6 Limitations and Concerns

Limitations include variable biological activity, slower incorporation compared with autogenous grafts, and residual concerns regarding immunogenicity and disease transmission, despite modern processing standards. Despite their widespread clinical use, allografts present several significant limitations that impact their safety and efficacy. A major concern is the risk of disease transmission, including HIV, hepatitis B/C, and prion diseases, even with rigorous donor screening and sterilization protocols [51]. Ethical sourcing is a critical consideration for allografts, in terms of maintaining public trust, legal compliance, and patient safety.

Another issue is immunogenicity as allografts can trigger host immune responses, leading to inflammation, delayed incorporation, or complete graft rejection [52, 53]. Although processing methods such as freezing and irradiation reduce immunogenicity, they also compromise the graft's structural integrity and biological activity [54, 55]. Since there is a greater variation in the composition and manufacture process of individual allografts, material and type specific validation of clinical performance is lacking [16]. Furthermore, limited donor availability combined with stringent storage requirements (e.g., cryopreservation) results in logistical challenges, supply shortages, and higher costs compared to synthetic alternatives.

7.7 Future Directions

The future of allografts is promising, with innovations in tissue engineering, growth factor enhancement, and stem cell therapy. Techniques such as gene-activated grafts, 3D bioprinting, and composite grafts combining allografts with biologics like platelet-rich fibrin (PRF) or BMPs are under exploration. There is a great scope for customized allografts with the combination of 3D printing and advanced imaging, thereby improving the functional and aesthetic outcomes of maxillofacial reconstruction [56].

7.8 Conclusion

Allografts have revolutionized oral and maxillofacial reconstruction by offering reliable, non-toxic, biocompatible, and bio-active grafting options. Though they are not a replacement for autografts in all cases, they provide an effective solution for many clinical scenarios with minimal risk and optimal success rates. Ongoing research and technological advances are poised to further amplify their role in the reconstructive surgeons' toolkit.

AI disclosure statement: The author acknowledges the use of AI-based tools for minor language editing or grammatical correction. However, all intellectual contributions, analyses, and conclusions presented in this chapter are entirely the author's own.

References

1. Urist, M.R. and Strates, B.S., Bone Morphogenetic Protein. *J. Dent. Res.*, 50, 6, 1392–406, 1971 Nov 1.
2. Ahmed, N., Eras, V., Pruß, A., Perka, C., Brune, J., Vu-Han, T.L., Allografts: expanding the surgeon's armamentarium. *Cell Tissue Banking*, 24, 1, 273–83, 2023 Mar 1.
3. Tomford, W.W., Bone allografts: Past, present and future. *Cell Tissue Banking*, 1, 2000.
4. Moore, M.A., Samsell, B., McLean, J., Allograft tissue safety and technology, in: *Biologics in Orthopaedic Surgery*, pp. 49–62, Philadelphia, PA, Elsevier, 2018.
5. Feng, X., Chemical and Biochemical Basis of Cell-Bone Matrix Interaction in Health and Disease. *Curr. Chem. Biol.*, 3, 2, 189–96, 2009 Apr 30.
6. Alfi, D.M., Hassan, A., East, S.M., Gianulis, E.C., Immediate Mandibular Reconstruction Using a Cellular Bone Allograft Following Tumor Resection in a Pediatric Patient. *Face*, 2, 4, 490–5, 2021 Dec 1.
7. Ciszyński, M., Dominiak, S., Dominiak, M., Gedrange, T., Hadzik, J., Allogenic Bone Graft in Dentistry: A Review of Current Trends and Developments. *Int. J. Mol. Sci.*, 24, Multidisciplinary Digital Publishing Institute (MDPI), 2023.
8. Samsell, B., Softic, D., Qin, X., McLean, J., Sohoni, P., Gonzales, K., *et al.*, Preservation of allograft bone using a glycerol solution: A compilation of original preclinical research. *Biomater. Res.*, 23, 1, 2019 Feb 13.
9. Magadum, M., K.L.M., Chitragar, D.D., Allograft sterilization and processing: impact on biomechanical strength. *Int. J. Res. Orthop.*, 10, 2, 484–9, 2024 Feb 26.
10. Salyer, K.E. and Taylor, D.P., Bone grafts in craniofacial surgery. *Clin. Plast. Surg.*, 14, 1, 27–35, 1987.
11. Goldberg, V.M. and Akhavan, S., Biology of Bone Grafts, in: *Bone Regeneration and Repair*, pp. 57–65, Humana Press, Totowa, NJ, 2005.
12. Langer, F., Czitrom, A., Pritzker, K.P., Gross, A.E., The immunogenicity of fresh and frozen allogeneic bone. *J. Bone Joint. Surg. - Ser. A*, 57, 2, 216–9, 1975.

13. Monje, A., Pikos, M.A., Chan, H.L., Suarez, F., Gargallo-Albiol, J., Hernández-Alfaro, F., *et al.*, On the feasibility of utilizing allogeneic bone blocks for atrophic maxillary augmentation. *Biomed Res. Int.*, 2014, Hindawi Publishing Corporation, 2014.
14. Kloss, F.R., Offermanns, V., Kloss-Brandstätter, A., Comparison of allogeneic and autogenous bone grafts for augmentation of alveolar ridge defects—A 12-month retrospective radiographic evaluation. *Clin. Oral Implants Res.*, 29, 11, 1163–75, 2018 Nov 1.
15. Kloss, F.R., Kämmerer, P.W., Kloss-Brandstätter, A., Risk Factors for Complications Following Staged Alveolar Ridge Augmentation and Dental Implantation: A Retrospective Evaluation of 151 Cases with Allogeneic and 70 Cases with Autogenous Bone Blocks. *J. Clin. Med.*, 12, 1, 6, 2022 Dec 20.
16. Perez, A., Pierantozzi, E., Di Felice, R., Lombardi, T., Clinical and Biological Validation of an Allogeneous Cancellous Bone Block for Alveolar Maxillary Ridge Reconstruction: A Case Series. *Dent. J. (Basel)*, 12, 2, 2024 Feb 1.
17. Gruskin, E., Doll, B.A., Futrell, F.W., Schmitz, J.P., Hollinger, J.O., Demineralized bone matrix in bone repair: History and use. *Adv. Drug Delivery Rev.*, 64, 1063–77, Elsevier B.V., 2012.
18. Mansour, A., Mezour, M.A., Badran, Z., Tamimi, F., Extracellular matrices for bone regeneration: A literature review. *Tissue Eng. Part A*, 23, 1436–51, Mary Ann Liebert Inc.; 2017.
19. Roselló-Añón, A., Mirabet Lis, V., Fariñas, O., Gelber, P., Sanchís-Alfonso, V., Fresh osteochondral graft. Indications, surgical technique and scientific evidence. *Rev. Española de Artroscopia y Cirugía Articular English Ed.*, 28, 1, 2021 Jan.
20. Geraghty, S., Kuang, J.Q., Yoo, D., LeRoux-Williams, M., Vangsness, C.T., Danilkovitch, A., A novel, cryopreserved, viable osteochondral allograft designed to augment marrow stimulation for articular cartilage repair. *J. Orthop. Surg. Res.*, 10, 1, 66, 2015 Dec 14.
21. Read-Fuller, A.M., Yates, D.M., Radwan, A., Schrodt, A.M., Finn, R.A., The Use of Allogeneic Cartilage for Grafting in Functional and Reconstructive Rhinoplasty. *J. Oral Maxillofac. Surg.*, 76, 7, 1560.e1–1560.e7, 2018 Jul 1.
22. Harutyunyan, A. and Hakobyan, G., Dorsal Augmentation Rhinoplasty by Cartilage Allograft. *J. Cosmet. Dermatol.*, 2024 Feb 1.
23. Hanna, S.A., Mattos, D., Datta, S., Reish, R.G., Outcomes of the Use of Fresh-Frozen Costal Cartilage in Rhinoplasty. *Plast. Reconstr. Surg.*, 154, 2, 324–8, 2024 Aug 9.
24. Pfaff, M.J., Bertrand, A.A., Lipman, K.J., Malapati, S.H., Kim, D.H., Rezzadeh, K.S., *et al.*, Cadaveric Costal Cartilage Grafts in Rhinoplasty and Septorhinoplasty: A Systematic Review and Meta-Analysis of Patient-Reported Functional Outcomes and Complications. *J. Craniofac. Surg.*, 32, 6, 1990–3, 2021 Sep.
25. Butler, J., Hartman, H., Dhilllon, R., Wingo, T., Vargas, L., Cole, W.W., *et al.*, Outcomes Following the Use of Extracellular Matrix Cartilage Allograft

for the Management of Osteochondral Lesions of the Talus: A Systematic Review. *Cureus*, 2024 Jun 10.

26. Lee, K.W., Chung, K., Nam, D.H., Jung, M., Kim, S.H., Kim, H.G., Decellularized allogeneic cartilage paste with human costal cartilage and crosslinked hyaluronic acid-carboxymethyl cellulose carrier augments microfracture for improved articular cartilage repair. *Acta Biomater.*, 172, 297–308, 2023 Dec.
27. Neiva, R. and Giannobile, W.V., Mucosal and gingival tissue engineering, in: *Preprosthetic and Maxillofacial Surgery*, pp. 305–26, Elsevier, 2011.
28. Patel, M.H., Kim, R.Y., Aronovich, S., Skouteris, C.A., Clinical assessment of acellular dermal matrix (AlloDerm©) as an option in the replacement of the temporomandibular joint disc: A pilot study. *J. Stomatol. Oral Maxillofac. Surg.*, 121, 5, 496–500, 2020 Nov 1.
29. Dominguez, A., Liang, Y., Abbed, T.M., Mukhatyar, V., Shimoga, S., Real-world Use of AlloDerm Acellular Dermal Matrix in Head and Neck Procedures in the United States. *Plast. Reconstr. Surg. Glob. Open*, 12, 11, e6339, 2024 Nov 26.
30. Jiang, N., Chen, H., Zhang, J., Cao, P., Wang, P., Hou, Y., *et al.*, Decellularized-disc based allograft and xenograft prosthesis for the long-term precise reconstruction of temporomandibular joint disc. *Acta Biomater.*, 159, 173–87, 2023 Mar 15.
31. Puisys, A., Vindasiute, E., Linkevciene, L., Linkevicius, T., The use of acellular dermal matrix membrane for vertical soft tissue augmentation during submerged implant placement: A case series. *Clin. Oral Implants Res.*, 26, 4, 465–70, 2015 Apr 1.
32. Davis, J.W., Skin transplantation with a review of 550 cases at the Johns Hopkins Hospital. *Johns Hopkins Med. J.*, 15, 307, 1910, References - Scientific Research Publishing [Internet]. [cited 2025 Apr 2]. Available from: https://www.scirp.org/reference/referencespapers?referenceid=1040417.
33. Mamede, A.C., Carvalho, M.J., Abrantes, A.M., Laranjo, M., Maia, C.J., Botelho, M.F., Amniotic membrane: from structure and functions to clinical applications. *Cell Tissue Res.* [Internet], 349, 2, 447–58, 2012 Aug 1 [cited 2025 Apr 2], Available from: https://pubmed.ncbi.nlm.nih.gov/22592624/.
34. Grémare, A., Jean-Gilles, S., Musqui, P., Magnan, L., Torres, Y., Fénelon, M., *et al.*, Cartography of the mechanical properties of the human amniotic membrane. *J. Mech. Behav. Biomed. Mater.* [Internet], 99, 18–26, 2019 Nov 1 [cited 2025 Apr 2], Available from: https://pubmed.ncbi.nlm.nih.gov/31325833/.
35. Insausti, C.L., Blanquer, M., Bleda, P., Iniesta, P., Majado, M.J., Castellanos, G., *et al.*, The amniotic membrane as a source of stem cells. *Histol. Histopathol.* [Internet], 25, 1, 91–8, 2010 Jan [cited 2025 Apr 2], Available from: https://pubmed.ncbi.nlm.nih.gov/19924645/.
36. Talmi, Y.P., Sigler, L., Inge, E., Finkelstein, Y., Zohar, Y., Antibacterial properties of human amniotic membranes. *Placenta* [Internet], 12, 3, 285–8,

1991 [cited 2025 Apr 2], Available from: https://pubmed.ncbi.nlm.nih.gov/1754577/.
37. Fénelon, M., Catros, S., Fricain, J.C., What is the benefit of using amniotic membrane in oral surgery? A comprehensive review of clinical studies. *Clin. Oral Investig.* [Internet], 22, 5, 1881–91, 2018 Jun 1 [cited 2025 Apr 2], Available from: https://pubmed.ncbi.nlm.nih.gov/29682688/.
38. Odet, S., Louvrier, A., Meyer, C., Nicolas, F.J., Hofman, N., Chatelain, B., *et al.*, Surgical Application of Human Amniotic Membrane and Amnion-Chorion Membrane in the Oral Cavity and Efficacy Evaluation: Corollary With Ophthalmological and Wound Healing Experiences. *Front. Bioeng. Biotechnol.* [Internet], 9, 2021 Jun 10 [cited 2025 Apr 2], Available from: https://pubmed.ncbi.nlm.nih.gov/34178969/.
39. Silan, F., Consiglio, F., Dell'Antonia, F., Montagner, G., Trojan, D., Berna, G., Cryopreserved fascia lata allograft use in surgical facial reanimation: a retrospective study of seven cases. *Maxillofac. Plast. Reconstr. Surg.*, 42, 1, 2, 2020 Dec 8.
40. Çeliköz, B., Duman, H., Selmanpakoğlu, N., Reconstruction of the orbital floor with lyophilized tensor fascia lata. *J. Oral Maxillofac. Surg.*, 55, 3, 240–4, 1997 Mar.
41. Papakosta, V., Mourouzis, C., Komis, C., Saranteas, T., Rallis, G., Solvent-dehydrated fascia lata allograft for covering intraoral defects: Our experience. *Oral Surg. Oral Med. Oral Pathol. Oral Radiol. Endod.*, 103, 4, e13–5, 2007 Apr.
42. Lobo Gajiwala, A. and Shah, A.V., Clinical Evaluation of Irradiated, Freeze-Dried Dura Mater Allograft as a Collagen-Based Barrier in Periodontal Osseous Defects. *Cell Tissue Banking*, 4, 2–4, 101–7, 2003.
43. Hartog, J.M., Slavin, A.B., Kline, S.N., Reconstruction of the temporomandibular joint with cryopreserved cartilage and freeze-dried dura: A preliminary report. *J. Oral Maxillofac. Surg.*, 48, 9, 919–25, 1990 Sep.
44. Curry, J. and Sargi, Z., Principles of Skull Base Reconstruction After Ablative Head and Neck Cancer Surgery. *Otorhinolaryngol. Clin. - Int. J.*, 2.
45. Muñoz Guerra, M.F., Pérez, J.S., Rodriguez-Campo, F.J., Gías, L.N., Reconstruction of orbital fractures with dehydrated human dura mater. *J. Oral Maxillofac. Surg.*, 58, 12, 1361–6, 2000 Dec.
46. Sato, T., Masuda, M., Utsumi, Y., Enomoto, Y., Yamada, M., Mizusawa, H., *et al.*, Dura mater related Creutzfeldt–Jakob disease in Japan: Relationship between sites of grafts and clinical features, in: *Prions*, pp. 31–40, Tokyo, Springer, Verlag, 2004.
47. Brooks, D.N., Weber, R.V., Chao, J.D., Rinker, B.D., Zoldos, J., Robichaux, M.R., *et al.*, Processed nerve allografts for peripheral nerve reconstruction: A multicenter study of utilization and outcomes in sensory, mixed, and motor nerve reconstructions. *Microsurgery*, 32, 1, 1–14, Hoboken, NJ, Wiley-Liss. 2012 Jan.

48. Matus, G., Aravena, J.P., Mariño, D., Niklander, S.E., Decellularized allografts as an alternative for reconstruction of large inferior alveolar nerve defects: a systematic review. *Med. Oral Patol. Oral Cir. Bucal Med. Oral S.L.*, 28, 183–90, 2023.
49. Moore, A.M., MacEwan, M., Santosa, K.B., Chenard, K.E., Ray, W.Z., Hunter, D.A., *et al.*, Acellular nerve allografts in peripheral nerve regeneration: A comparative study. *Muscle Nerve*, 44, 2, 221–34, 2011 Aug.
50. Yampolsky, A., Ziccardi, V., Chuang, S.K., Efficacy of Acellular Nerve Allografts in Trigeminal Nerve Reconstruction. *J. Oral Maxillofac. Surg.*, 75, 10, 2230–4, 2017 Oct 1.
51. Snydman, D., Fishman, J.A., Greenwald, M.A., Grossi, P.A., Transmission of infection with human allografts: essential considerations in donor screening. *Clin. Infect. Dis.* [Internet], 55, 5, 720–7, 2012 Sep 1 [cited 2025 Mar 29], Available from: https://pubmed.ncbi.nlm.nih.gov/22670038/.
52. Heyligers, I.C. and Klein-Nulend, J., Detection of living cells in non-processed but deep-frozen bone allografts. *Cell Tissue Banking* [Internet], 6, 1, 25–31, 2005 Mar [cited 2025 Mar 29], Available from: https://pubmed.ncbi.nlm.nih.gov/15735898/.
53. Zeevi, A., Girnita, A., Duquesnoy, R., HLA antibody analysis: sensitivity, specificity, and clinical significance in solid organ transplantation. *Immunol. Res.* [Internet], 36, 1–3, 255–64, 2006 [cited 2025 Mar 29], Available from: https://pubmed.ncbi.nlm.nih.gov/17337786/.
54. Nguyen, H., Morgan, D.A.F., Forwood, M.R., Sterilization of allograft bone: effects of gamma irradiation on allograft biology and biomechanics. *Cell Tissue Banking* [Internet], 8, 2, 93–105, 2007 Jun [cited 2025 Mar 29], Available from: https://pubmed.ncbi.nlm.nih.gov/17063262/.
55. Cornu, O., Boquet, J., Nonclercq, O., Docquier, P.L., Van Tomme, J., Delloye, C., *et al.*, Synergetic effect of freeze-drying and gamma irradiation on the mechanical properties of human cancellous bone. *Cell Tissue Banking* [Internet], 12, 4, 281–8, 2011 Nov [cited 2025 Mar 29], Available from: https://pubmed.ncbi.nlm.nih.gov/20703816/.
56. Baniameri, S., Aminianfar, H., Gharehdaghi, N., Yousefi-Koma, A., Mohaghegh, S., Nokhbatolfoghahaei, H., *et al.*, Tissue Engineering 3D-Printed Scaffold Using Allograft/Alginate/Gelatin Hydrogels Coated With Platelet-Rich Fibrin or Adipose Stromal Vascular Fraction Induces Osteogenesis *In Vitro*. *J. Cell. Physiol.*, 240, 1, 2025 Jan 19.

8

Xenografts

Manju Roby Philip

Department of Maxillofacial Surgery and Diagnostic Sciences, College of Dentistry, King Saud Bin Abdulaziz University for Health Sciences, Riyadh, Saudi Arabia

Abstract

Xenotransplantation refers to the transplantation of living cells, tissues, or organs from genetically similar individuals of one species into another species. In the context of bone grafting, the donor bone must possess a similar structure to that of human bones exhibiting osteoinduction and osteoconduction properties to meet the criteria for an ideal bone graft. Many reviews indicate that the rates of implant survival using xenografts are equal or superior to those achieved with autogenous bone. The desire to reduce patient morbidity by eliminating the need for a second surgical site, thereby decreasing the operating time and recovery duration, positions xenografts as the preferred graft material. Although bone formation ability is lower compared with autografts, heterogeneous bone graft materials possess a porous microstructure that positively influences angiogenesis and bone formation resulting in faster bone deposition than other bone graft materials. Histologic sections revealed a "bone bridging" pattern in the studies with xenografts where the xenograft residues are enveloped partly by new vital bone, which interdigitate through this mechanism. Eliminating antigens that may trigger an immune response is essential for the success of xenogenic bone grafting. Deproteinization removes their immune reactivity retaining osteoinduction and osteoconduction properties. The physicochemical properties and mechanical strength of tissue-engineered bone have been shown to meet the requirements of ideal scaffolds. Despite the mitigating factors such as risk for infection, xenografts become popular as the widely preferred biomaterial for orofacial reconstruction. Here we discuss about general properties, types, and sources of xenografts currently in use and its various applications in the orofacial region.

***Keywords*:** Xenograft, hydroxyapatite, tissue reaction, alveolar ridge preservation, peri-implant defect, critical-size defect, osteogenesis

Email: drmanjuphilip@gmail.com

Randa A. Alfotawi (ed.) Oro-Facial Bone Grafts and Biomaterials, (149–174) © 2026 Scrivener Publishing LLC

8.1 Introduction

Autologous bone grafting, being the gold standard for reconstructing complex osseous deformities, is often hindered by inadequate donor bone for grafting, morbidity of the donor site, and high resorption [1]. The success of bone engineering technique relies on the regenerative potential when the pluripotent stem cells, inductive growth factors, and a bone graft are combined to induce bone growth within the three-dimensional scaffold after implantation at the defect sites. Growth factors, such as recombinant human BMP-2, which is the only BMP known to induce osteoblastic differentiation from mesenchymal stem cells [2] and vascular endothelial growth factor (VEGF), also present significant limitations and risks associated with their doses [3]. High costs and risks such as viral transmission make allografts an imperfect substitute when compared with synthetic grafts, which are strictly osteoconductive [2]. Meanwhile, xenografts gained consensus because of their documented reliability and efficacy regarding its osteoconductive properties as scaffold to guide new bone formation [4]. Xenografts have their origin from a species, commonly like bovine or porcine origin other than human. Xenografts, which are demineralized and freeze-dried, have reported satisfactory clinical outcomes in dental surgery, but scarce validation with poor results in hip surgery was mentioned in orthopedics with 25% pseudo infections [5]. Bone xenografts reduce morbidity of donor site and operating time. As a surgical alternative to autologous bone graft, xenografts have been explored almost exclusively in implant dentistry [6]. Long-term follow-up evaluations and future research are mandated in the literature as the lack of bone loading could compromise its integration and autologous bone replacement [7].

8.2 Types and Sources

Bauermeister A and Maatz R introduced bovine bone as a calcified matrix in 1957 [8]. Xenografts can be derived from demineralized bovine, porcine, equine bone mineral, algae, and corals [9]. Madrepore and Millipore types of corals are harvested and processed to form granules primarily composed of calcium carbonate similar to the composition found in human bone with hydroxyapatite, thus playing an important role to stimulate new bone formation. The coral material can be manufactured as a non-resorbable bone substitute of hydroxyapatite through a hydrothermal process, or it can remain in its calcium carbonate state serving as a resorbable graft saturated with growth-enhancing solutions [5, 10–12]. Coral-based products currently in clinical use include Interpore and Pro-osteon (Interpore International, Inc., Irvine, CA) [9].

Xenografts used for alveolar ridge preservation (ARP) most commonly utilize deproteinized bovine bone mineral (DBBM) [10]. Bovine-derived products such as Bio-Oss (Geistlich Biomaterials, Geistlich, Switzerland), Osteograf-N (CeraMed Co., Denver, CO), Endobon (Merck Co., Darmstadt, Germany), and Freossi granules (Fredna Dental Systems, India) are some of the commercially available substitutes currently in use [10, 11]. Particulate bovine bone can form a cohesive moldable graft with the addition of protein-based regenerating gels such as Emdogaine [12, 13]. A recent study compared the effects of healing in critical-size bone defects for xenografts derived from three different sources such as bovine, ostrich, and camel [14]. The sources of bone grafts used in the study were from bovine (OCS-B, NIBEC), ostrich (Bone PLUS O, NovaTeb Holding (DOB)], and camel [Bone PLUS C, NovaTeb holding (DCB)]. Micro CT and histology results were generated to show that all three grafts proved good in repairing bone defects; camel bone grafts had better results in terms of new bone formation after 12 weeks ($p<0.05$) indicating that the final characteristics are affected to some extent by the origin and the processing of xenografts [15]. Osteoinductive properties demonstrated by equine derived bone substitutes that enhanced new bone development in resected areas of malignant tumors of the orofacial region and bimaxillary atrophy were observed in case reports [4, 6] with adequate follow-up after implant integration.

Cuttlefish is a marine invertebrate with calcium carbonate in the bone or outer shell-like structure resembling the chemical, crystalline, and morphologic characteristics of the natural bone mineral [16]. Cuttlefish serves as an economical and abundant source of bone biomaterial. Hydroxyapatite porous scaffolds were fabricated in one study from cuttlefish bone derived from *Sepia officinalis.* Fish scales, considered as biowaste materials, also present as a potential source for hydroxyapatite powder. Fish scale scaffolds replicate the crystallographic nature, morphology, and composition of native bone [17]. Another biowaste product derived from consumed cockles or mollusks is the Cockle shells. The pure antagonite polymorph form of calcium carbonate seen in these shells can be substituted by bone mineral for its applications as bone scaffolds [18, 19]. Xenografts from other sources have applications in dentistry particularly in preventing the transmission of bovine-specific disease. Porcine bone graft is an effective alternative to bovine bone graft when deproteinized. Many studies have utilized this biomaterial for clinical use in dentistry due to the similar structural and physiological characteristics to human bone. Due to their proven efficacy as a bone biomaterial, e.g., Symbios® granules of 0.25–1.0 mm (Dentsply Sirona Implants, Mölndal, Sweden), xenografts gained popularity in maxillary sinus augmentation procedures [20].

Xenografts are also available as resorbable collagen barrier membrane for guided bone regeneration. Kontour Adapt is a strong stable collagen barrier membrane manufactured from purified porcine peritoneum having shown resorption in 3 to 4 months. Resorbable collagen membranes like Cytoplast RTM are manufactured from bovine bone with high strength and flexibility and medium resorption between 4 and 6 months. They are made from Type 1 bovine bone collagen, which constitutes nearly 95% of the bone collagen, thus influencing the mineralization of bone and ultimately the bone strength [21].

8.3 Factors Affecting Selection

New bone formation seen with xenografts is affected by multiple factors such as its origin, manufacturing process, morphology, and size of particles. The angiogenesis, cell adhesion, osteogenesis, and diffusion of nutrients and drugs are affected by the surface area, porosity, and intercell connections in the pore system [22]. Selection of a xenograft for clinical use should depend on factors such as type or size of defects and the expected time of healing. The collagen derived from animal bones contains proteins that stimulate the growth of new bone tissue. If calcium is combined in the material, it can create a three-dimensional structure to assist in bone growth.

8.3.1 Type of Materials and Manufacturing

In vivo study using two xenograft materials for maxillary sinus augmentation reported that the physical and chemical characteristics differed between the two hydroxyapatite xenografts determining the behavior response for the materials when they were deproteinized at different temperatures [20]. Hydroxyapatite (HA) was the main component in both xenografts but differed strongly in its porosity, crystallinity, and calcium phosphate composition. The calcium/phosphate ratios for the xenografts were 2.31 ± 0.09 for the bovine material (BBM) with high crystallinity in X-ray diffraction studies and 2.22 ± 0.08 for the porcine material (PBM) with low crystallinity. Based on bone biopsies, the sintered xenografts demonstrated better osteoconductivity, with incomplete resorption (30.80

± 0.88% residual material). The non-sintered xenografts reported osteoinduction of 25.92 ± 1.61% with a higher resorption after 6 months of implantation [20]. Processing BBM at high temperature of 1200 °C and PBM at low temperature of 130 °C achieved successful results in ridge augmentation after sinus elevation with increased vertical dimension of ridges from baseline values adequate for implant placement.

8.3.2 The Particle Size and Morphology

The particle size reported in one study with xenografts from different sources ranged from 250 to 1000 μm. Under scanning electron microscopy with magnifications × 50 and × 10 000, the differences in particle morphology ranged from polyhedral and spindle granules to spheroid crystal and rod-like structures [15]. Also the osteoconductivity of xenografts may get enhanced if the particle size has similarity close to native bone, although the subject is controversial [23].

The surface area that aids in matrix formation also plays a crucial role in bone healing. The larger surface area facilitates the diffusion of growth factors and nutrients to form an extracellular matrix. The surface area differed in three different sources of xenografts used in same critical-sized bone defects in a study. The xenograft surface area used in this study was as follows: Bovine-OCS-B (45.109 m^2/g), Camel-DCB (23.817 m^2/g), and Ostrich-DOB (5.676 m^2g) [15]. New bone formed was at the lowest level in the ostrich DOB group.

Microporosity is another major factor determining the properties of scaffolds in terms of osteoconductivity as well as vascularization [24]. Scaffolds with optimal pore size is necessary to maintain oxygen tension and pH levels within a scaffold that closely resembles the values measured on the scaffold's exterior. These scaffolds, also known as oxygen tension-controlled matrices, are promising to support cell proliferation and mineralization both *in vitro* and *in vivo.* Research indicates that pore sizes greater than 300 μm along with sufficient interconnectivity are necessary for effective cell migration and vascular ingrowth [25]. Both diameter and interconnections between pores have influenced significantly the type and quantity of bone formation as demonstrated in various studies [22].

8.3.3 Patient Factors

The clinical parameters that affect selection include the size and anatomical site of the defect, bone quality at the recipient site, thickness of bone, blood supply, maxillary or mandibular defect due to the cortico-cancellous bone ratio, type of teeth such as incisors or molars, functional load at defect, pressure from adjacent tissues, and whether external or internal augmentation is required. Animal bone grafting biomaterials are biocompatible and pose no risk of rejection in terms of bone growth as reported in many studies. However, incorrect surgical procedures and poor patient care can result in complications like infection or graft exposure. Surgical protocols should be strictly followed while providing the patient with adequate post-operative instructions and follow-up consultation.

8.4 Biodegradation

Slower resorption rate for xenografts have been reported in many animal studies when they were used as bone grafts in critical-size bone defects [14, 26]. A study that compared the presence of residual material at 8 weeks in rabbit calvaria using two different xenograft sources and an alloplast observed that the resorption rate was slower in xenografts compared to alloplasts [26]. Also a study that compared the same effect with three different xenografts observed 53% and 37% residual material at 8 and 12 weeks, respectively, which was significantly higher than that of the bovine group. In a histomorphometric analysis comparing bovine xenografts with nano-hydroxyapatite in rodent cranial defects, after 2 months, residual material was more observed in xenografts ($p<0.03$) [27]. Erythropoietin inclusion resulting in rapid integration of spongy xenograft granules to the host bone was reported in orthopedics in an animal study [28].

8.5 Uses in Maxillofacial Surgery, Outcomes, and Success Rates

8.5.1 Sinus Floor Augmentation

The posterior edentulous maxilla poses a surgical dilemma for implantologists due to the dip in the sinus floor into the edentulous region and lack of adequate anchorage impeding successful implant placement to support the prosthesis. Lateral window approach as shown in Figure 8.1 or crestal approach is required for sinus floor augmentation to address the vertical bone atrophies in this region. If a sinus floor elevation of more than 2 mm is required, bone graft substitutes are inevitable [29]. In one study that compared biphasic calcium phosphate with xenograft particles

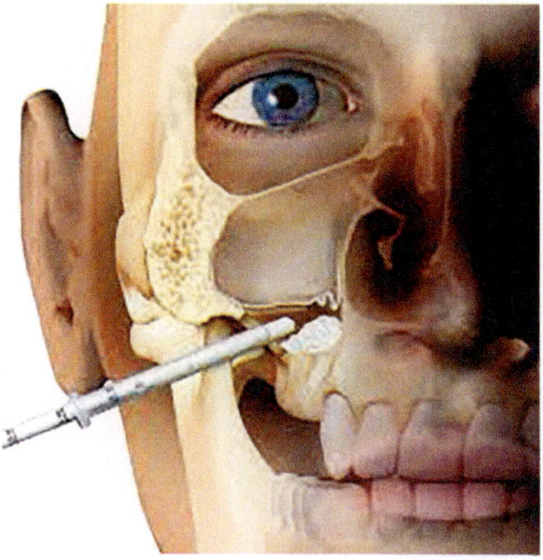

Figure 8.1 Maxillary sinus augmentation (lateral window approach) with xenograft particles.

as control, highly statistically significant sinus height gain of 7.25 ± 1.78 mm for the test group and 7.26 ± 1.47 mm for the control is achieved in both groups ($p < 0.000001$) with a statistically significant gain in width seen with xenografts [29]. The implant stability measured by resonance frequency measurement was not statistically different between the groups post-operatively at 180 days [29, 30]. In a split mouth randomized clinical trial comparing two xenografts derived from bovine and porcine bone mixed in the ratio of 80:20 with autogenous bone scraped off from the access window in the two-stage bilateral sinus augmentation, no significant difference was observed after 6 months in the bone biopsies with similar histologic, histomorphometric, immune-histochemical findings and graft resorption rates [31]. A systematic review compared the histological outcomes of bovine bone composed of particles of different sizes used for maxillary sinus elevation. The percentages of connective tissue, newly formed bone, and residual xenograft based on the granule sizes were not different. Results were similar to previous studies, but the smaller number of studies included in the review calls for more clinical evidence [32].

8.5.2 Alveolar Ridge Preservation (ARP)

ARP procedures are advocated for successful osseointegration of dental implants as the overall changes in alveolar dimensions may be minimized. In a recent Cochrane systematic review [33], five clinical trials compared

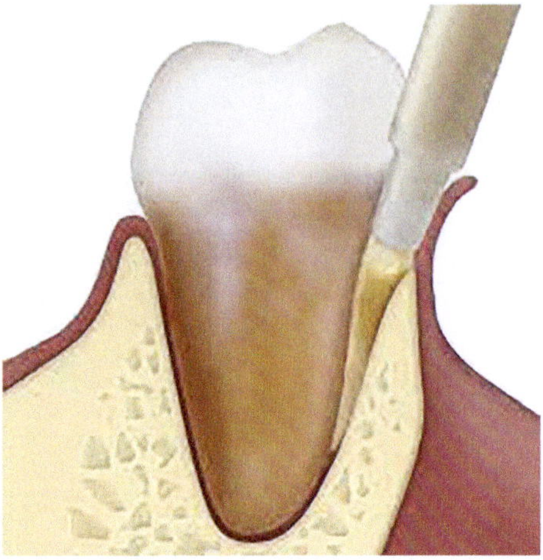

Figure 8.2 Injectable xenografts for socket preservation.

xenografts with allografts and alloplasts. But evidence was not certain regarding the need for ARP for implant placement within 6 months after extraction and reported no clinically significant differences between different graft materials with or without a membrane [33]. In a pilot clinical trial on socket preservation after minimally invasive extractions, two xenograft particles taken from commercially available bovine bone with different processing such as Bio-Oss and Cerabone in 20 adjacent extraction sockets of 10 patients were compared [34]. Mean transverse crestal ridge resorption and mean implant primary stability were in favor of treatment with Bio-Oss particles in the study. Histomorphometric analysis of sites with ARP using bovine and porcine bone particles in a clinical trial reported no significant differences in the dimensional stability and vital bone formation after 5 months [35]. All these reports underline the fact that xenogeneic-derived bovine bone materials are among the most frequently and successfully employed biomaterials for socket preservation of extraction sites. Figure 8.2 shows injectable xenografts intended for socket preservation.

8.5.3 Ridge Augmentation (Horizontal and Vertical)

For implant successful osseointegration, there are different surgical procedures such as ridge splitting done along with placement of bone grafts including both inlay and onlay bone grafts to achieve adequate width and height of ridges. The moldability of xenografts for successful use in ridge

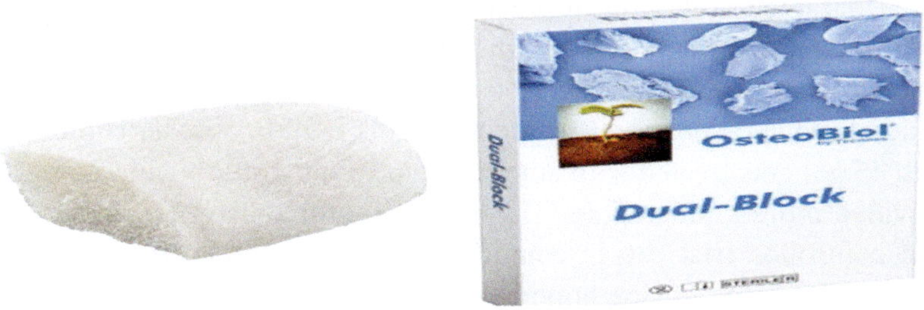

Figure 8.3 Block xenografts for ridge augmentation.

splitting to boost implant osseointegration has been enhanced with the use of simvastatin gel (SMV) as reported in a recent study [36]. They evaluated clinical and radiographic changes after 6 and 9 months in groups with the same treatment protocol using xenografts with membranes, with and without SMV in horizontal atrophy. The study observed statistically significant expansion of alveolar ridge ($p < .001$) with increased bone density and minimum marginal bone loss in the group with SMV.

Dual block xenografts as shown in Figure 8.3 are cortico-cancellous xenogeneic bone blocks with osteoconductive properties when regeneration of big volumes is required. It is rigid and collagenated promoting blood clotting and migration of reparative cells. The graft exhibits gradual resorption while new bone formation occurs.

8.5.4 Local Bone Defect Filling/Peri-Implant Defects

Bone biomaterials with or without barrier membranes demonstrated better clinical outcomes and reduction of radiographic defect depth for the treatment of well-contained intrabony defects, although success in regenerative techniques in peri-implantitis is limited in the literature. A randomized clinical pilot study evaluated on the surgical management of peri-implantitis defects in 25 patients with two different xenografts such as Endobon and Bio-Oss [37]. Results after 12 months have shown similar values for both materials with no statistical differences suggesting their successful use. The study reported a defect reduction of more than 1 mm radiographically in all patients at 12 months. In another study with 22 patients, treated with porous titanium granules (PTG) and xenografts, clinical attachment levels and radiographic defect reduction were found to be more appropriate for PTG favoring their inert nature compared with xenografts [38]. One study reported improved soft tissue and hard tissue parameters in clinical outcomes with xenografts when compared with untreated mineralized dentine grafts, although similar radiographic results in defect reduction were observed in previous studies with treated mineralized and demineralized dentin grafts [39]. In another clinical trial with 45 patients treated with autografts and xenografts, bovine xenografts provided more radiographic fill after 12 months [40]. A recent randomized controlled trial (RCT) compared autologous bone from tuberosity and deproteinized bovine bone mineral (DBBM) for buccal bone defects in the esthetic region after implant placement. Both sites did not differ with respect to ridge alterations, peri-implant clinical attachment levels, and patient-reported outcomes after 1 year suggesting its use in esthetic regions after immediate implants [41].

Orbital wall fracture defects can be reconstructed as shown in Figure 8.4 using semi-soft lamina made from 100% cortical bone of heterologous origin, which undergoes a semi-decalcification process, preserving the typical consistency and collagen content of the bone tissue from which it originates. It can be shaped with sterile instruments until the desired size is achieved, after which it must be hydrated for 3 to 5 minutes in a sterile physiological solution. Once it attains the desired plasticity, it can be adapted to the grafting site. Although these bone grafts provide structural support, they are not suitable in load-bearing situations.

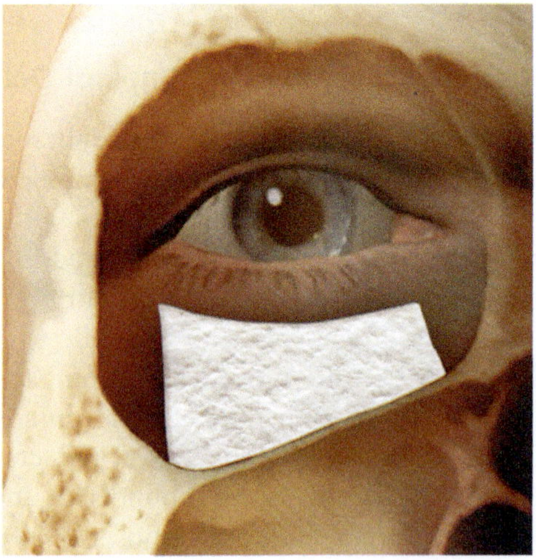

Figure 8.4 Semi-soft Lamina xenograft for orbital wall defect reconstruction.

8.5.5 Injectable Dermal Fillers/Skin Substitutes

Bovine-derived collagen fillers like Zyderm and Zyplast are available for facial augmentation and dominated the United States market for over two decades [42]. Zyplast and Zyderm are highly purified bovine collagen filler introduced in 1980s and approved by FDA for cosmetic treatment to reduce fine wrinkles and folds in the face and for lip augmentation with the treatment results lasting for 6 months. Without subsequent treatments, collagen will get absorbed into the face returning to original contours. It is primarily composed of bovine dermal collagen combined with 0.3% lignocaine. Dermal sensitivity testing required before its application precludes its use with other synthetic dermal fillers [42].

The primary indications for the use of porcine and bovine xenografts as skin substitutes include burn wounds and post-traumatic wounds. Xenografts have become mainstay in the management of wound dressings [43]. As our discussion here focuses on bone xenografts, this topic is further not mentioned.

8.5.6 Reconstruction of Critical-Size Bone Defects

The management of critical-sized bone deformities is complex as the bone regeneration capacity is compromised with factors such as post-traumatic defects, infections, and tumor resection existing. The three-dimensional matrix of a bone scaffold serves as a platform that is implanted into the defect area to provide mechanical support, vascularization, recruitment of growth factors, and nutrients that facilitate osteoconduction and osteogenesis. Researchers have utilized scaffolds derived from various animal sources such as bovine, cuttlefish, fish, and cockles to investigate their effects on bone regeneration [16, 18, 44]. Cancellous bone scaffolds (5-mm diameter × 2-mm height) from the epiphyseal bovine femur bone were fabricated in a study that was then subjected to cell lysis by demineralization and freeze–thaw cycles followed by gentle agitation treatment with chemical agents such as sodium dodecyl sulfate. *In vivo*, after seeding with mice bone marrow mesenchymal stem cells (BMSCs), it showed increased cell growth and integration on the bone scaffold was observed in scanning electron microscopy and histology [45]. In a study by Bianco *et al.*, a combination of biological and physical agents was used to fabricate decellularized bone scaffolds from bovine metacarpal and metatarsal bone. The scaffold has exhibited a mechanical strength similar to that of native bone with presence of vessels, adipose tissues, and collagen fibers [46]. Moest *et al.* [47] compared the effects of bovine and equine bone minerals with autologous bone in an experimental model with a critical-size defect on the frontal skull area of pigs. Among the xenogeneic groups, equine bone exhibited significantly higher *de novo* bone formation after 30 days. After 60 days, no statistically significant difference was observed between the bovine and equine groups; concerning the residual bone substitute, *de novo* bone formation was higher in the bovine bone group [48]. Overall, clinical studies on the repair of jaw bone defects with biomaterials are scarce, with case reports of low evidence value [48].

Hydroxyapatite porous scaffolds fabricated through the hydrothermal transformation of cuttlefish bone derived from *Sepia officinalis* were utilized in a study done by Battistella *et al.* [16]. This transformation process converted the calcium carbonate of cuttlefish bone into calcium phosphate (hydroxyapatite). The scaffold was then evaluated for osteogenesis using mouse osteoblast-like cells (MC3T3-E1) for the expression of osteogenic markers. The level of alkaline phosphatase (ALP) was elevated initially, while the expression of osteocalcin (OCN) was higher in the later stages. Mondal *et al.* prepared another natural hydroxyapatite scaffold that exhibited greater tensile and compressive strength compared to the native bone from various sources such as human, bovine, swine, and horse using fish scales from tilapia (*Oreochromis mossambicus*) [17]. *In vitro* experiment with this scaffold demonstrated similar cell viability on the fish scale-derived hydroxyapatite scaffold to that without fish scales when cultured with human osteoblast cells (MG63). When histologically tested *in vivo*, the scaffold manifested both osteoconductivity and bio-affinity in a critical-sized bone defect at the rabbit's left femur by showing cellular infiltration with new cell lining [17]. Yet another source of bio-waste products derived from mollusks and cockles, cockleshells are composed of polymorph of calcium carbonate, which can be replaced by bone tissue [18]. Bharatham *et al.* incorporated cockle shell powder (60%) with alginate (40%) to fabricate nano-biocomposite bone scaffolds. This natural scaffold presented with favorable features such as adequate pore size, moderate resorption rate, and high mechanical strength to be suitable as bone graft substitutes [18]. A biomimetic scaffold from tricalcium phosphate derived from chitosan, gelatin, and bovine ash was successfully developed using an eggshell membrane as a template in another study [19]. Gelatin, being biodegradable and biocompatible, promotes the adherence of cells with minimal immune response, while chitosan mimics the glycosaminoglycans of extracellular matrix of mineralized tissue, providing excellent cellular proliferation and osteogenesis [19, 44, 49]. Chitosan, derived from the exoskeletons of insects, cell walls of algae, and fungi, is a natural biomaterial [49].

Due to its high biocompatibility, chitosan is preferred as a scaffold by many investigators. Scaffolds from animal sources facilitate cellular growth, adhesion, and proliferation supporting function. Limitations of *in vitro* studies include a static environment for culture, frequently employed on animal bone scaffolds. Cell growth stagnation with appearance of irregular cell density can occur due to insufficient oxygen, nutrients, and the metabolic waste product accumulation within the scaffold. Establishing a bioreactor system can solve this limitation to a certain extent by providing a dynamic environment for scaffolds when cells are used for culture [50]. Additionally, the low mechanical strength of animal bone scaffolds compromises its application on load-bearing areas in critical-size defects of the maxillofacial region. As a result, incorporation of biological substances or synthetic polymers is necessary to enhance its features. Again, bone scaffolds derived from various animal sources and parts may compromise in stability and structure. The need for standardization of bone scaffolds with necessary features such as shape, porosity, and geometrical design requires consideration due to the difficulty in predicting the success rates for the microstructure of the scaffold under investigation [44].

8.6 Products: Common Trade Names and Applications

Bio-Oss® (BO) is a leading natural sterilized bone substitute available worldwide. It is derived from bovine deproteinized cancellous bone with 75% to 80% porosity. The biomaterial is available as tiny granules of 250–1000 μm sizes. This material is hydrophilic and facilitates the uptake of cells, leading to osteogenesis and osseointegration around implants that mimic the bone formation in normal extraction sites [51]. Therefore, Bio-Oss is largely being used for the treatment of defects associated with peri-implantitis achieving satisfactory results radiographically by reduction of defect size and improved clinical outcomes. Two granule sizes are available commercially (i.e., 0.25–1 and 1–2 mm) for BO, which is having a crystal size of approximately 10 nm with a calcium-deficient carbonate apatite structure. This material is highly osteoconductive with similarity in chemical and physical characteristics to human bone [52–54].

Endobon® (EB) is also derived from bovine bone with hydroxyapatite ceramic available as small granule sizes of 500–1000 μm. This material is deproteinized at high temperatures by a two-step process for safety from contamination. This two-step process begins with pyrolysis above 900°C to eliminate the protein antigen followed by ceramization above 1200°C to achieve a crystalline framework [32]. The crystallinity achieved results in minimizing resorption of graft [23]. This microstructure with pores facilitates the adsorption of osteogenic cells accelerating bone formation [20, 55]. Clinical and histologic outcomes suggest that both Endobon and BO have similar efficacy as bone grafts when used for socket preservation [56]. Many clinical trials emphasized the use of EB for the management of defects in peri-implantitis [57].

OsteoBiol® mp3 is a pre-hydrated cortico-cancellous bone mix with 10% collagen gel. This porcine bone derivative is deproteinized and composed of small granules available from 600–1000 to 1000–2000 μm in sizes, which are dispensed in ready-to-use syringes. It can be easily applied avoiding the hydration and manipulation phases. It is characterized by slow resorption with a reentry period of 5 months. A low processing temperature at 130 °C is enough to obtain this material for commercial use, which preserves the components of natural bone in its structure and composition.

Cerabone and Cerabone Plus

Osteoconductive bovine bone grafts combined with hyaluronic acid to form a sticky bone material upon hydration. It provides easy handling for delivery to the site of application without displacement. In order to prevent any disturbance to the area of healing, a barrier membrane needs to be placed to prevent ingrowth of soft tissues. Also, excess liquid should be removed from the defect site prior to application.

Gen-Os: (OsteoBiol by Tecnoss Dental, Torino-Italy)

A cortico-cancellous heterologous bone mix with granule size ranging from 250 to 2000 μm serves as a natural replicate of autologous bone with the similar matrix and pore size with highly osteoconductive properties. The porcine bone mineral is commonly used for alveolar ridge preservation, periodontal regeneration of deep infrabony pockets, and for lateral maxillary sinus lift approach. The collagen content and hydrophilic nature contribute to combine well with blood. The cortico-cancellous nature allows for the progressive resorption of graft material occurring parallel to a similar rate in bone formation providing volume stability.

Ivory Dentin Graft

This porcine tooth-derived product is available in granule form consisting of both organic and inorganic non-cellular components that exhibit physical and chemical similarities to the mineralized matrix of human bone. This graft is contraindicated, similar to other xenografts, in the presence of acute inflammation, suspected hypersensitivity, and immunologic disorders. The graft creates an excellent microenvironment for successful osteogenesis as reported in clinical studies with greater amount of new bone formation observed in alveolar bone core biopsies. This porcine origin, dentin-derived material has demonstrated clinical safety and performance as bone grafts at 4 months, when implants were placed following tooth extraction, comparable to a commercial bone-derived material [58].

8.7 Other Clinical Indications

Xenografts derived from bovine bone material as shown in Figure 8.5, are deproteinized and available as small and large particle sizes having applications in minor and major bone regeneration procedures. The pore size ensures a stable support for osteogenesis and is an FDA-approved product.

MatrixOss is a highly osteoconductive porcine particulate material with carbonate apatite structure and is biocompatible with high porosity facilitating cell adhesion. It is dispensed in jars or delivery syringes.

Osseo-Seal is a bovine bone derivative that mimics human bone in its inorganic micro- and macroporous structures. It is indicated when autogenous bone is insufficient in quantity or not indicated for use.

Bovine collagen fillers (Zyplast, Zyderm; Inamed Corporation, Santa Barbara, California):

Products include Zyderm 1, Zyderm 2, and Zyplast, which are cross-linked with glutaraldehyde to specifically strengthen the collagen fibers. These products are injectable, and a more popular lighter version is Zyderm.

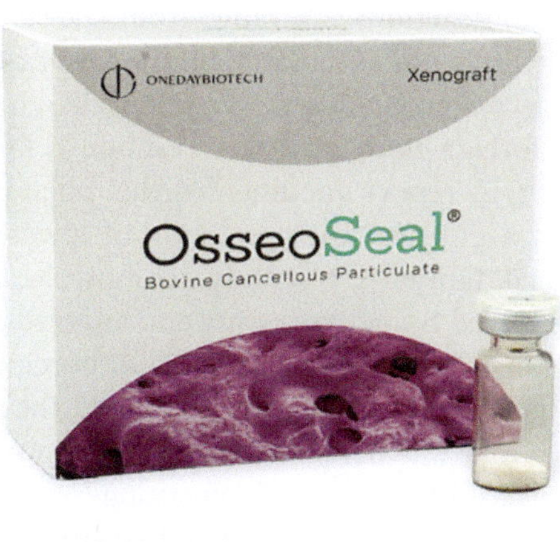

Figure 8.5 Cancellous particle xenografts.

tarSys™ (IOP Ophthalmics, Costa Mesa, California, USA) has been launched successfully as posterior lamella graft of the lower eyelid. tarSys™, a porcine derivative consisting mainly of decellularized small intestinal submucosa, acts as a scaffold upon which cellular infiltration, integration, and remodeling of host cells occur. Therefore, this material has an extracellular matrix rich in various proteins and collagens. Such xenografts have been utilized in a variety of clinical scenarios, including repair of nasal septal perforation. tarSys™ graft is unique in that it mimics the collagen and glycosaminoglycan profile of the tarsal plate, thus providing structural integrity to the eyelid. It has demonstrated favorable clinical outcomes in cases of lagophthalmos and Graves ophthalmopathy. On the other hand, foreign body reaction FBGC was reported after grafting tarSys™ that requires its removal [59].

8.8 Complications

8.8.1 Delayed Type of Hypersensitivity

Approximately 3% of the human population is known to have allergy to bovine type 1 collagen. The emergence of diseases such as mad cow disease and transmissible spongiform encephalopathies renders the use of bovine-derived products risky [21]. A study reported foreign body reaction to xenografts obtained from three different sources in critical-size defects of 8 mm created in rat calvaria at 8 and 12 weeks [14]. At 8 weeks, foreign body reaction occurred in 23 out of 28 defects, while at 12 weeks, 20 defects exhibited this reaction.

Normally, only 3–4% of tested patients exhibit positive reaction to dermal injectable fillers [42]. Reactions can range from transient erythema, tenderness, swelling, itching, and discoloration. In some cases, extrusion may occur where the injected collagen can appear on the skin as a small raised and white area. A foreign body giant cell reaction (FBGC) may develop with xenografts [59]. A report documented this phenomenon following the introduction of a graft for the correction of lower eyelid retraction using the biomaterial, tarSys™. This study demonstrated that the porcine cellular material survived tissue processing and induced antigenicity causing prolonged swelling. Therefore, skin testing for porcine hypersensitivity may be advisable before implantation. Additionally, the age of the animal from which the scaffold was derived is also a determining factor for the host graft response; scaffolds derived from younger animals tend to facilitate effective remodeling of host tissue than that from older animals [60].

Transmission of zoonotic diseases from animals to humans such as BSE (bovine spongiform encephalopathy) or PERV (porcine endogenous retroviruses) was also argumented [61].

8.8.2 Delayed Bone Regeneration

Delayed bone healing with DBBM was reported in a clinical trial that compared DBBM grafts with non-grafted sites. The DBBM sites presented with less vital bone (25% versus 44%) with similar findings reported in other studies [62]. Histologic analysis at 9–12 months also indicated slow resorption as residual DBBM particles were found [63, 64]. Although osteoconductive in nature, successful osseointegration can be compromised for placement of implants at 3–5 months post-extraction due to the slow graft resorption and replacement with new vital bone [64]. When compared with allografts, xenografts present with slower rates of resorption, increased connective tissue ingrowth, and delayed angiogenesis as reported in studies [13, 65, 66].

8.9 Xenografts—Ethics and Public Policy

Xenotransplantation is the transplantation of living cells, tissues, or organs from genetically similar individuals of one species into another species. For bone grafting, the donor bone should have a similar structure to that of human bone, exhibiting osteoinductive and osteoconductive properties, to meet the criteria of an ideal bone graft. The use of xenografts is complicated by factors such as hypersensitivity, immune rejection, late resorption, and disease transmission. Researches have documented that bones derived from one species or host can elicit an immune response in another species or host after implantation due to the presence of cellular components that act as foreign antigens forming major histocompatibility complexes (MHCs), causing graft rejection [67]. By decellularization, the cellular components are removed from the bone matrix while retaining its composition. Such a well-preserved extracellular matrix can provide structural and mechanical characteristics facilitating cellular growth and survival. Commonly, chemical, biological, and physical agents have been employed for decellularization of bone material. The chemical agents include cell lyses with detergents such as Triton X-100, sodium dodecyl sulfate, and ethylene diamine tetra-acetic acid (EDTA). The biologic measures include enzymatic digestion with nucleases, such as deoxyribonuclease or ribonucleases. Physical agents involve methods such as freezing, sonication, agitation, direct pressure, and vacuum-assisted decellularization. Demineralization of bone is another effective method used in combination with decellularization to improve the osteoinductive potential of bone scaffolds by eliminating fat residues, inorganic minerals, and impurities, while preserving the collagen matrix and bone morphogenetic proteins in the bone. By demineralization, the bioavailability of osteogenic proteins can be enhanced, thereby inducing cell differentiation and osteogenesis. Special cells that result from fusion of macrophages such as multinucleated giant cells (MNGCs) are known to induce foreign body reaction. Recent studies report the presence of MNGCs as favorable because growth factors and angiogenic factors such as VEGF are expressed around bone grafts by MNGC, which stimulate bone formation, reduce inflammation, and thereby promote healing [68, 69].

Ethical issues, including the risks versus benefits to individuals, the risks of porcine-derived infectious agents to cross into humans, animal welfare and rights, identity concerns of humans and animals, fair allocation of organs, and appropriate resource utilization, are being addressed through various strategies. One recently published effective strategy is based on virtue ethics emphasizing on the moral purpose of the research, the character of the research, as well as patient preferences [67]. According to the new approach, the needs of the recipients should be taken into consideration by the research-clinician particularly their long-term desires. Information regarding the potential benefits and consequences of therapy, such as the need for long-term medication and follow-up, should be made readily available. Moreover, the FDA-approved xenograft materials are harvested ethically and in compliance with the regulations, and the processing methods are thorough ensuring safety and efficacy to meet patient expectations.

8.10 Patient-Derived Xenograft Models

The "patient-derived xenograft" (PDX) is a relatively new concept for tumor xenograft model employing immune-deficient mice for personalized tumor chemotherapy as it is emerging as the most efficient method for the management of malignant tumors. This model retains various characteristics of primary tumor grafts, which include histologic and pathologic features, including molecular heterogeneity, and expression of gene profiles. Consequently, the PDX model combined with technologies for drug screening represents a future direction for research in tumor therapy.

Studies have reported developing PDX models for oral malignancies such as squamous cell carcinoma (OSCC) [70, 71]. The establishment of a personalized chemotherapy regimen requires a biological model that closely resembles squamous cell carcinoma retaining the stromal, molecular diversity, histologic, and micro-environmental features. The PDX model is a xenograft model where fresh tumor cells from individuals are implanted onto immune-deficient mice, depending on the growth environment [71]. Such patient-derived models when combined with specific pharmacodynamic and clinical data with gene expression profiles can enhance drug specificity, suited for personalized treatment of tumors contributing to improved clinical success rates [72, 73]. It supplies a practical R&D system for individualized preclinical assessment of drug efficacy [74]. This model tumor constructed for OSCC has shown high resemblance in pathological histomorphology by retaining the molecular biological features and aggressive growth potential of the original tumor as seen in immunohistochemistry findings [70]. PDX model use is limited for early-stage cancers due to their reduced take-up rate. Also some cancers are unable to produce PDX models [75]. Due to the immunodeficiency of the host, it is difficult to evaluate the effects of the immune system on the tumor model [76]. However, this limitation has been solved to a certain extent with the advent of humanized models. PDX models emerged in oncology research and drug screening as valuable, but the expensive nature and requirement for equipped laboratories are drawbacks [77]. Creation of an acceptable metastatic model is still another challenge. With PDX models, the possibility of a transplanted tumor triggering an immune response against the host causing graft versus host disease (GVHD) can be delayed by using NSG mice lacking major histocompatibility complex I (MHC-I). Due to these models having broader applications in cancer biology-related clinical trials, the development of anti-cancer drugs for personalized medicine, and immunotherapy, many nations and regional institutes have taken initiatives to establish PDX biobanks and PDX libraries by spending expenditure to produce this source [78].

AI disclosure statement: The author confirms that no artificial intelligence (AI)-generated content or AI-assisted writing tools were used in the preparation of this chapter (including summaries and the abstract). All text, analysis, and conclusions are the result of the author's original work.

References

1. de Carvalho, A.B.G., Rahimnejad, M., Oliveira, R.L.M.S., *et al.*, Personalized bioceramic grafts for craniomaxillofacial bone regeneration. *Int. J. Oral Sci.*, 16, 62, 2024.
2. Roberts, T.T. and Rosenbaum, A.J., Bone grafts, bone substitutes and orthobiologics: the bridge between basic science and clinical advancements in fracture healing. *Organogenesis*, 8, 4, 114–24, 2012 Oct-Dec.
3. Carragee, E.J., Chu, G., Rohatgi, R., Hurwitz, E.L., Weiner, B.K., Yoon, S.T., Comer, G., Kopjar, B., Cancer risk after use of recombinant bone morphogenetic protein-2 for spinal arthrodesis. *J. Bone Joint Surg. Am.*, 95, 17, 1537–45, 2013 Sep 4.
4. DeCicco, D., Colella, G., Tartaro, G., Zerbinati, N., Fragola, R., Rauso, R., Wide Anterior Maxillary Reconstruction with Equine Bone Xenograft: A Case Report of 24-Month Follow-Up. *Case Rep. Surg.*, 2020, 8890935, 8, 2020.
5. Campana, V., Milano, G., Pagano, E., Barba, M., Cicione, C., Salonna, G., Lattanzi, W., Logroscino, G., Bone substitutes in orthopaedic surgery: from basic science to clinical practice. *J. Mater. Sci. - Mater. Med.*, 25, 10, 2445–61, 2014 Oct.
6. Pistilli, R., Signorini, L., Pisacane, A., Lizio, G., Felice, P., Case of severe bone atrophy of the posterior maxilla rehabilitated with blocks of equine origin bone: histological results. *Implant Dent.*, 22, 1, 8–15, 2013.
7. Robling, A.G. and Turner, C.H., Mechanical signaling for bone modeling and remodeling. *Crit. Rev. Eukaryotic Gene Express*, 19, 4, 319–338, 2009, https://doi.org/10.1615/CritRevEukarGeneExpr.v19.i4.50, 2-s2.0-70349974398, 198 17708.
8. Bauermeister, A. and Maatz, R., A method of bone maceration results of animal experiments. *J. Bone Joint Surg. Am.*, 39, 1, 153–166, 1957.
9. Pountos, I. and Giannoudis, P.V., Is there a role of coral bone substitutes in bone repair? *Injury*, 47, 12, 2606–13, 2016 Dec 1.
10. Vaia, E., Nicolò, M., Iorio-Siciliano, V., Isola, G., Ramaglia, L., Alveolar Ridge Preservation with Deproteinized Bovine Bone Mineral and Xenogeneic Collagen Matrix: A 12-Month Clinical and Histomorphometric Case Series. *Int. J. Periodontics Restorative Dent.*, 41, 3, 2021 May 1.
11. Jensen, S.S. and Terheyden, H., Bone augmentation procedures in localized defects in the alveolar ridge: clinical results with different bone grafts and bone-substitute materials. *Int. J. Oral Maxillofac. Implants*, 24, Suppl, 218–236, 2009.
12. Dumitrescu, A.L., Bone grafts and bone graft substitutes in periodontal therapy, in: *Chemicals in surgical periodontal therapy*, p. 92, Springer, Berlin, 2011.

13. Haggerty, C.J., Vogel, C.T., Fisher, G.R., Simple bone augmentation for alveolar ridge Defects. *Oral Maxillofac. Surg. Clin. North Am.*, 27, 2, 203–26, 2015 May.
14. Amid, R., Kadkhodazadeh, M., Kheiri, A., Esfandiari, S., Comparison of the healing process of xenografts with three different sources in critical-size bone defects: An *in vivo* study. *J. Adv. Periodontol. Implant Dent.*, 16, 1, 22–29, 2024 Mar 16.
15. Gashtasbi, F., Hasannia, S., Hasannia, S., Mahdi Dehghan, M., Sarkarat, F., Shali, A., Comparative study of impact of animal source on physical, structural, and biological properties of bone xenograft. *Xenotransplantation*, 27, 6, e12628, 2020 Nov.
16. Battistella, E., Mele, S., Foltran, I., Lesci, I.G., Roveri, N., Sabatino, P., Rimondini, L., Cuttlefish bone scaffold for tissue engineering: A novel hydrothermal transformation, chemical-physical, and biological characterization. *J. Appl. Biomater. Funct. Mater.*, 10, 99–106, 2012.
17. Mondal, S., Pal, U., Dey, A.J.C.I., Natural origin hydroxyapatite scaffold as potential bone tissue engineering substitute. *Ceram. Int., 42,* 18338–18346, 2016.
18. Bharatham, B.H., Bakar, A., Zuki, M., Perimal, E.K., Yusof, L.M., Hamid, M.J.B.R.I., Development and characterization of novel porous 3D alginate-cockle shell powder nanobiocomposite bone scaffold. *Biomed Res. Int., 2014,* 146723, 2014.
19. Neacsu, I.A., Serban, A.P., Nicoara, A.I., Trusca, R., Ene, V.L., Iordache, F.J.P., Biomimetic Composite Scaffold Based on Naturally Derived Biomaterials. *Polymers, 12,* 1161, 2020.
20. Ramírez Fernández, M.P., Mazón, P., Gehrke, S.A., Calvo-Guirado, J.L., De Aza, P.N., Comparison of Two Xenograft Materials Used in Sinus Lift Procedures: Material Characterization and *In Vivo* Behavior. *Materials (Basel),* 10, 6, 623, 2017 Jun 7.
21. Naomi, R., Ridzuan, P.M., Bahari, H., Current Insights into Collagen Type I. *Polymers (Basel),* 13, 16, 2642, 2021 Aug 9.
22. Bružauskaitė, I., Bironaitė, D., Bagdonas, E., Bernotienė, E., Scaffolds and cells for tissue regeneration: different scaffold pore sizes—different cell effects. *Cytotechnology*, 68, 3, 355–69, 2016 May.
23. Block, M.S., The processing of xenografts will result in different clinical responses. *J. Oral Maxillofac. Surg.*, 77, 4, 690–7, 2019.
24. Amini, A.R., Laurencin, C.T., Nukavarapu, S.P., Bone tissue engineering: recent advances and challenges. *Crit. Rev. Biomed. Eng.*, 40, 5, 363–408, 2012.
25. Karageorgiou, V. and Kaplan, D., Porosity of 3D bio-material scaffolds and osteogenesis. *Biomaterials*, 26, 27, 5474–5491, 2005.
26. Takauti, C.A., Futema, F., Brito Junior, R.B., Abrahão, A.C., Costa, C., Queiroz, C.S., Assessment of bone healing in rabbit calvaria grafted with three different biomaterials. *Braz. Dent. J.*, 25, 5, 379–84, 2014.

27. da Silva Brum, I., Frigo, L., Lana Devita, R., da Silva Pires, J.L., Hugo Vieira de Oliveira, V., Rosa Nascimento, A.L., de Carvalho, J.J., Histomorphometric, Immunohistochemical, Ultrastructural Characterization of a Nano-Hydroxyapatite/Beta-Tricalcium Phosphate Composite and a Bone Xenograft in Sub-Critical Size Bone Defect in Rat Calvaria. *Materials (Basel)*, 13, 20, 4598, 2020 Oct 15.
28. Vasileva, R. and Chaprazov, T., Bone Healing of Critical-Sized Femoral Defects in Rats Treated with Erythropoietin Alone or in Combination with Xenograft. *Vet. Sci.*, 10, 3, 196, 2023.
29. Kakar, A., Rao, S., Bappanadu, H., Deshpande, N., Hegde, S., Kohli, A., Patney, A., Mahajan, H., Osteotome-Mediated Sinus Floor Elevation using an *In Situ* Hardening Biphasic Calcium Phosphate Bone Graft Substitute Compared to Xenograft: A Randomized Controlled Clinical Trial. *Indian J. Dent. Res.*, 32, 1, 61–68, Jan–Mar 2021.
30. Klijn, R.J., Meijer, G.J., Bronkhorst, E.M., Jansen, J.A., A meta-analysis of histomorphometric results and graft healing time of various biomaterials compared to autologous bone used as sinus floor augmentation material in humans. *Tissue Eng. Part B Rev.*, 16, 5, 493–507, 2010 Oct.
31. Galindo-Moreno, P., Abril-García, D., Carrillo-Galvez, A.B., Zurita, F., Martín-Morales, N., O'Valle, F., Padial-Molina, M., Maxillary sinus floor augmentation comparing bovine versus porcine bone xenografts mixed with autogenous bone graft. A split-mouth randomized controlled trial. *Clin. Oral Implants Res.*, 33, 524–536, 2022.
32. Li, X., Lin, S.C., Duan, S.Y., The impact of deproteinized bovine bone particle size on histological outcomes in sinus floor elevation: a systematic review and meta-analysis. *Int. J. Implant Dent.*, 9, 1, 35, 2023 Oct 2.
33. Atieh, M.A., Alsabeeha, N.H., Payne, A.G., Ali, S., Faggion, C.M., Esposito, M., Interventions for replacing missing teeth: alveolar ridge preservation techniques for dental implant site development. *Cochrane Database Syst. Rev.*, 4, 2021.
34. Shakibaie, B., Blatz, M.B., Sabri, H., Jamnani, E.D., Barootchi, S., Effectiveness of Two Differently Processed Bovine-Derived Xenografts for Alveolar Ridge Preservation with a Minimally Invasive Tooth Extraction Approach: A Feasibility Clinical Trial. *Int. J. Periodontics Restorative Dent.*, 43, 5, 540–549, 2023 Sep-Oct.
35. Lai, V.J., Michalek, J.E., Liu, Q., Mealey, B.L., Ridge preservation following tooth extraction using bovine xenograft compared with porcine xenograft: A randomized controlled clinical trial. *J. Periodontol.*, 91, 3, 361–368, 2020 Mar.
36. Issa, D.R., Elamrousy, W., Gamal, A.Y., Alveolar ridge splitting and simvastatin loaded xenograft for guided bone regeneration and simultaneous implant placement: randomized controlled clinical trial. *Clin. Oral Investig.*, 28, 1, 71, 2024 Jan 4.

37. Polymeri, A., Anssari-Moin, D., van der Horst, J., Wismeijer, D., Laine, M.L., Loos, B.G., Surgical treatment of peri-implantitis defects with two different xenograft granules: A randomized clinical pilot study. *Clin. Oral Implants Res.*, 31, 11, 1047–1060, 2020 Nov.
38. Guler, B., Uraz, A., Yalım, M., Bozkaya, S., The Comparison of Porous Titanium Granule and Xenograft in the Surgical Treatment of Peri-Implantitis: A Prospective Clinical Study. *Clin. Implant Dent. Relat. Res.*, 19, 2, 316–327, 2017 Apr.
39. Khalifah, M.A., Elgendy, A.M.A., Elgendy, E., Untreated Mineralized Dentin Grafts (UMDGs) vs Xenografts Around Immediately Placed Dental Implants in the Mandibular Anterior Region: A Randomized Controlled Clinical Trial. *Int. J. Oral Maxillofac. Implants*, 3, 381–388, 2024 Jun 21.
40. Aghazadeh, A., Rutger Persson, G., Renvert, S., A single-centre randomized controlled clinical trial on the adjunct treatment of intra-bony defects with autogenous bone or a xenograft: results after 12 months. *J. Clin. Periodontol.*, 39, 7, 666–73, 2012 Jul.
41. Borgia, G.S., Pebé, P., Barbot, R., Haas, A.N., Immediate implants with buccal defects filled with bone from the tuberosity or a xenograft: 1-year randomized trial. *Braz. Oral Res.*, 36, e102, 2022 Jul 11.
42. Suman, T., Enhancing facial esthetics by other modalities. *Int. J. Dent.*, 2011, 513957, 2011.
43. Salloum, A., Bazzi, N., Squires, S., Chu, T., Benedetto, P., Benedetto, A., Comparing the application of various engineered xenografts for skin defects: A systematic review. *J. Cosmet. Dermatol.*, 22, 921–931, 2023.
44. Wong, S.K., Yee, M.M.F., Chin, K.Y., Ima-Nirwana, S., A Review of the Application of Natural and Synthetic Scaffolds in Bone Regeneration. *J. Funct. Biomater.*, 14, 5, 286, 2023 May 20.
45. Shahabipour, F., Mahdavi-Shahri, N., Matin, M.M., Tavassoli, A., Zebarjad, S.M., Scaffolds derived from cancellous bovine bone support mesenchymal stem cells' maintenance and growth. *In Vitro Cell. Dev. Biol. Anim.*, 49, 6, 440–8, 2013 Jun.
46. Bianco, J.E.R., Rosa, R.G., Congrains-Castillo, A., Joazeiro, P.P., Waldman, S.D., Weber, J.F., Saad, S.T.O., Characterization of a novel decellularized bone marrow scaffold as an inductive environment for hematopoietic stem cells. *Tissue Cell*, 7, 1516–1528, 2019.
47. Moest, T., Wehrhan, F., Lutz, R., *et al.*, Extra-oral defect augmentation using autologous, bovine and equine bone blocks: A preclinical histomorphometrical comparative study. *J. Craniomaxillofac. Surg.*, 43, 559–66, 2015.
48. Huang, X., Lou, Y., Duan, Y., Liu, H., Tian, J., Shen, Y., Wei, X., Biomaterial scaffolds in maxillofacial bone tissue engineering: A review of recent advances. *Bioact. Mater.*, 33, 129–156, 2024.
49. Aranaz, I., Alcántara, A.R., Civera, M.C., Arias, C., Elorza, B., Heras Caballero, A., Acosta, N., Chitosan: An Overview of Its Properties and Applications. *Polymers, 13*, 3256, 2021.

50. Du, D., Asaoka, T., Ushida, T., Furukawa, K.S., Fabrication and perfusion culture of anatomically shaped artificial bone using stereolithography. *Biofabrication*, 6, 045002, 2014.
51. Berglundh, T. and Lindhe, J., Healing around implants placed in bone defects treated with Bio-Oss. An experimental study in the dog. *Clin. Oral Implants Res.*, 8, 2, 117–24, 1997 Apr.
52. Klinge, B., Alberius, P., Isaksson, S., Jönsson, J., Osseous response to implanted natural bone mineral and synthetic hydroxylapatite ceramics in the repair of experimental skull bone defects. *J. Oral Maxillofac. Surg.*, 50, 241–249, 1992.
53. Wetzel, A.C., Stich, H., Caffesse, R.G., Bone apposition onto oral implants in the sinus area filled with different grafting materials. A histological study in beagle dogs. *Clin. Oral Implants Res.*, 6, 155–163, 1995.
54. Smiler, D.G., Johnson, P.W., Lozada, J.L., Misch, C., Rosenlicht, J.L., Tatum, H., Wagner, J.R., Sinus lift grafts and endosseous implants. Treatment of the atrophic posterior maxilla. *Dent. Clin. North Am.*, 36, 151–186, 1992.
55. Hing, K.A., Best, S.M., Bonfield, W., Characterization of porous hydroxyapatite. *J. Mater. Sci. - Mater. Med.*, 10, 3, 135–145, 1999.
56. Barone, A., Todisco, M., Ludovichetti, M., Gualini, F., Aggstaller, H., Torres-Lagares, D., Kenealy, J., A prospective, randomized, controlled, multicenter evaluation of extraction socket preservation comparing two bovine xenografts: Clinical and histologic outcomes. *Int. J. Periodontics Restorative Dent.*, 33, 6, 795–802, 2013.
57. Renvert, S., Roos-Jansaker, A.M., Persson, G.R., Surgical treatment of peri-implantitis lesions with or without the use of a bone. 20182018.
58. Sapoznikov, L., Haim, D., Zavan, B., Scortecci, G., Humphrey, M.F., A novel porcine dentin-derived bone graft material provides effective site stability for implant placement after tooth extraction: a randomized controlled clinical trial. *Clin. Oral Investig.*, 27, 6, 2899–2911, 2023 Jun, doi: 10.1007/s00784-023-04888-5. Epub 2023 Feb 24. PMID: 36826514; PMCID: PMC10264522.
59. Munday, W.R., Klett, Z., McNiff, J.M., Ko, C., Foreign body giant cell reaction to tarSys™ xenograft. *J. Cutaneous Pathol.*, *41*, 10, 771–774, 2014, https://doi.org/10.1111/cup.12374.
60. Sicari, B.M., Johnson, S.A., Siu, B.F., *et al.*, The effect of source, animal age upon the *in vivo* remodeling characteristics of an extracellular matrix scaffold. *Biomaterials*, 33, 5524, 2012.
61. Laurencin, C.T. and El-Amin, S.F., Xenotransplantation in orthopaedic surgery. *J. Am. Acad. Orthop. Surg.*, 16, 1, 4–8, 2008, doi: 10.5435/00124635-200801000-00002. [DOI] [PubMed] [Google Scholar].
62. Artiz, Z., Tal, H., Dayan, D., Porous bovine bone mineral in healing of human extraction sockets. Part 1: histomorphometric evaluations at 9 months. *J. Periodontol.*, 71, 1015–1023, 2000.

63. Artiz, Z., Tal, H., Dayan, D., Porous bovine bone mineral in healing of human extraction sockets. Part 2: histochemical observations at 9 months. *J. Periodontol.*, 72, 152–159, 2001.
64. Lee, D.W., Pi, S.H., Lee, S.K., Kim, E.C., Comparative histomorphometric analysis of extraction sockets healing implanted with bovine xenografts. Irradiated cancellous allografts and solvent-dehydrated allografts in humans. *Int. J. Oral Maxillofac. Implants*, 24, 609–615, 2009.
65. Piattelli, Favero, G.A., Scarano, A., *et al.*, Bone reactions to anorganic bovine bone (Bio-Oss) used in sinus augmentation procedures: a histologic long-term report of 20 cases in humans. *Int. J. Oral Maxillofac. Implants*, 14, 6, 835–840, 1999.
66. Carmagnola, Adriaens, P., Berglundh, T., Healing of human extraction sockets filled with Bio-Oss. *Clin. Oral Implants Res.*, 14, 137–143, 2003.
67. George, A.J., Ethics, virtues and xenotransplantation. *Perfusion*, 39, 2, 334–343, 2024, doi: 10.1177/02676591221140767.
68. Barbeck, M., Udeabor, S.E., Lorenz, J., *et al.*, Induction of multinucleated giant cells in response to small sized bovine bone substitute (Bio-Oss™) results in an enhanced early implantation bed vascularization. *Ann. Maxillofac. Surg.*, 4, 150–7, 2014.
69. ten Harkel, B., Schoenmaker, T., Picavet, D.I., Davison, N.L., de Vries, T.J., Everts, V., The foreign body giant cell cannot resorb bone, but dissolves hydroxyapatite like osteoclasts. *PLoS One*, 10, 10, e0139564, 2015.
70. He, F., Zhou, X., Huang, G., Jiang, Q., Wan, L., Qiu, J., Establishment and Identification of Patient-Derived Xenograft Model for Oral Squamous Cell Carcinoma. *J. Oncol.*, 2022, 3135470, 2022 Sep 5.
71. Wang, D., Pham, N.A., Tong, J., *et al.*, Molecular heterogeneity of non-small cell lung carcinoma patient-derived xenografts closely reflect their primary tumors. *Int. J. Cancer*, 140, 3, 662–673, 2017.
72. Garralda, E., Paz, K., López-Casas, P.P., *et al.*, Integrated next-generation sequencing and avatar mouse models for personalized cancer treatment. *Clin. Cancer Res.*, 20, 9, 2476–2484, 2014 May 1.
73. Ding, L., Ellis, M.J., Li, S., *et al.*, Genome remodelling in a basal-like breast cancer metastasis and xenograft. *Nature*, 464, 7291, 999–1005, 2010.
74. Izumchenko, E., Paz, K., Ciznadija, D., *et al.*, Patient-derived xenografts effectively capture responses to oncology therapy in a heterogeneous cohort of patients with solid tumors. *Ann. Oncol.*, 28, 10, 2595–2605, 2017.
75. Abdolahi, S., Ghazvinian, Z., Muhammadnejad, S., *et al.*, Patient-derived xenograft (PDX) models, applications and challenges in cancer research. *J. Transl. Med.*, 20, 206, 2022, https://doi.org/10.1186/s12967-022-03405-8.
76. Cassidy, J.W., Caldas, C., Bruna, A., Maintaining tumor heterogeneity in patient-derived tumor xenografts. *Cancer Res.*, 75, 15, 2963–8, 2015.

77. Jin, K., *et al.*, Patient-derived human tumour tissue xenografts in immunodeficient mice: a systematic review. *Clin. Transl. Oncol.*, 12, 7, 473–80, 2010.
78. Karamboulas, C., Meens, J., Ailles, L., Establishment and Use of Patient-Derived Xenograft Models for Drug Testing in Head and Neck Squamous Cell Carcinoma. *STAR Protoc.*, 1, 1, 100024, 2020 Jun 3, doi: 10.1016/j.xpro.2020.100024. PMID: 33111077; PMCID: PMC7580210.

9
Alloplastic Bone Graft

Randa A. Alfotawi

Department of Oral and Maxillofacial Surgery, College of Dentistry, King Saud University, Riyadh, Saudi Arabia

Abstract
Early in the 1960s, alloplastic materials became available, and three generations of alloplastic have since been developed. The most widely utilized alloplastic materials for bone regeneration and craniofacial area construction are compiled in this chapter. Injectable cements, mineral composites, bioactive glass, and many ceramic types are described. This chapter only provides a few instances of their therapeutic use and limitations and up-to-date evidence from literature.

Keywords: Bioactivity, osteoconduction, biomaterials, ceramic, bioactive glass, silica–calcium phosphate, polymers, PEEK

9.1 Introduction

Alloplastic bone grafts are synthetic materials designed to replace or augment bone tissue without the use of biological donor sources. Their use in oral and maxillofacial reconstruction has increased due to unlimited availability, absence of disease transmission risk, and the ability to tailor material properties to specific clinical requirements. Clinical performance depends on material composition, resorption characteristics, and interaction with the host biological environment.

There is a clinical need for biomaterials to be used in certain clinical situations, ranged from small ridge defect to a critical-size bone defect situation. The third generation of biomaterials was developed for the purpose of restoring bone defects (Table 9.1). The primary required characteristics

Email: ralfotawei@ksu.edu.sa

Randa A. Alfotawi (ed.) Oro-Facial Bone Grafts and Biomaterials, (175–192) © 2026 Scrivener Publishing LLC

Table 9.1 Material characteristics of the different generations of bone substitute biomaterials and examples.

Generation	Material characteristics and *in vivo* responses	Examples
1st generation (1960–1999)	Inert—induce fibrous tissue encapsulation	Titanium
2nd generation (1980–2000)	Responsive—bioactive, osteoconductive, degradable	Bioglass
3rd generation (2002–present)	Bioactive, osteoconductive, osteoinductive, angiogenesis, drug delivery, degradable	Biomimetic biomaterials, smart biomaterials, tissue-engineered biomaterials

Table 9.2 Definitions of properties of 3rd-generation bone substitute materials (1987–2008).

Property	Definition
Biocompatibility	The capacity to act with a suitable host response in a particular circumstance [4]
Bioactivity	The capacity to establish a direct chemical bond with bone, resulting in an exceptionally robust contact between biomaterial and bone [5]
Osteointegration	The healing process of implants placed within the bone [6]
Osteoconduction	The ability to direct bone-forming tissue into pores or onto a surface [7]
Biodegradability	The capacity to progressively vanish and make room for the creation of new tissue without impeding the process of regeneration [8]
Osteoinduction	The ability to influence stem cells' differentiation or maturation into bone-forming cells in order to stimulate bone development [7]

of bone substitute materials are the capacity to provide acceptable mechanical qualities in addition to biocompatibility, bioactivity, osteointegration, osteoconduction, biodegradability, and osteoinduction (Table 9.2). According to Tanner [1], none of the available scaffold materials fulfill all the required characteristics or are offered for sale yet. Many modifications are still needed before clinical application is applied, and a number of materials are presently undergoing testing. For instance, today's third-generation biomaterials, such as Copi OS Bone Void Filler [2], offer improved imaging and healing process observation because of their high porosity, interconnectivity, and high resorbability. Numerous inorganic and organic biomaterials, such as ceramics, silicon, demineralized allografts, polymers, and composites, are accessible for use in orthopedics and dentistry. Putties, pastes, gels, thick blocks, powders, and granules are some of the physical forms in which these bone substitute materials are produced. Ceramics usually play an important role in orthopedic and craniofacial applications because of their properties. According to Best *et al.* [3], ceramic materials have the potential to be both biocompatible and osteoconductive [3].

9.2 Mineral Substitute Ceramic

Mineral replacements have the ability to conduct electricity. Ceramics are produced by the process of sintering, which requires heating mineral salt to temperatures higher than 800°C. Sintering makes final goods stronger, but it decreases bone's ability to reconstruct and resorb when applied to bone or other minerals [9].

9.2.1 Ceramic

Ceramic-based alloplastic grafts are primarily composed of calcium phosphate compounds that resemble the mineral phase of bone. These materials function predominantly through osteoconduction, providing a scaffold that supports bone apposition and vascular ingrowth.

Tricalcium phosphate (TCP), hydroxyapatite (HA), or a mixture known as biphasic calcium phosphate makes up the majority of orthopedic ceramics (BCP). The tensile strength of these fragile materials is quite low. They are found in blocks with larger, linked porosities, which accelerate bone ingrowth while weakening the material. Pore diameters in the range of 150 to 500 microns are thought to be ideal [1, 10]. Porous materials can be sintered or non-sintered, with the latter having a higher rate of resorption. Cancellous bone is used to make bovine-derived porous ceramic (Endobon®, Biomet/Merck/

Lorenz Surgical, Zwijndrecht, Netherlands), which is sintered and treated to eliminate all but the mineral components. The poor remodeling capability brought on by the sintering process may compensate for the expected lack of immunogenicity. Coral has a porosity comparable to bone after being thermochemically treated with ammonium phosphate (Pro Osteon, Interpore Cross International, Irvine, CA). The heat treatment converts over 95% of the $CaCO_3$ in the coral to HA (coralline hydroxyapatite), which resorbs more slowly. On the surface of the material, osteoblasts may be detected, and in the linked pores, bone ingrowth has been observed without remodeling [11]. The formulations contain a range of pore diameters, with the larger pore size (about 500 μm) being better suited for cancellous bone abnormalities. A compressive strength of around 4 MPa has been reported for it, which is comparable to that of human cancellous bone [11, 12]. In 1992, the FDA approved Pro Osteon for the treatment of fractures; in 1998, it was authorized for general use. The 500-μm pore size formulation of this calcium phosphate–based bone substitute has numerous orthopedic applications, including stabilizing fractures of the distal radius [13, 14]. It is possible to replace the TCP salt in alpha and ß versions with HA. Their structure, especially their porosity, allows them to resorb and reconstruct more easily than HA. Resorption of the ß version is faster than that of the alpha form. The first β-TCP to be commercialized in the US was Vitoss (Orthovita, Malvern, PA, USA) in 2001. Its pore size varied from 1 to 1000 μm [15]. The range of this size is linked to increased biological activity histologically. Leukocytes and platelets that generate chemotactic cytokines are thought to settle in smaller pores, while bigger osteoclasts are thought to locate in larger pores. Furthermore, β-TCP exhibits advantageous characteristics such as hardness, fracture toughness, resistance to resorption, and a regulated rate of resorption [16].

Plaster of Paris, or calcium sulfate (CS), is made by calcining gypsum ($CaSO_4$. $2H_2O$). The resulting hemihydrate ($CaSO_4$. $1/2H_2O$) is partially dehydrated. It has been used for bone implantation for almost a century, even though it is an inert salt [17]. Osteoset (Wright Medical Technology, Inc., Arlington, TN, USA) was the first product to be released that contained calcium sulfate. Both a pellet and, more recently, an injectable substance (minimally invasive injectable graft, or MIIG) are available. Other commercially available products that contain calcium sulfate include Calceon (Synthes, USA), which comes in pellet form, and BonePlast (InterporeCross, Warsaw, USA), which comes in block, injectable, and pellet formats. Complete resorption of calcium sulfate can be seen as early as a few weeks after it occurs. However, prolonged resorption durations have been documented, contingent on the defect's location and size, the material's composition and structure, and the presence of additives. Even

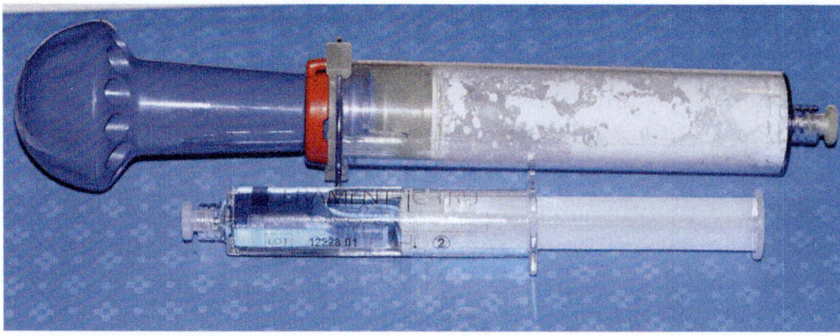

Figure 9.1 The injectable Cerament™ (Bone Support AB, Lund, Sweden).

though it has been demonstrated that replacing CS with trabecular bone promotes bone regeneration, CS rapidly resorbs through disintegration [18]. Metaphyseal faults can currently be repaired using CS. CS may provide instant stability due to its rapid resorption, but it necessitates ongoing fixation. For instance, it has been demonstrated that HA improves osteoconductivity, enables integration with the newly formed bone, and provides adequate strength during the initial healing phase when added to the injectable Cerament™ (Bone Support AB, Lund, Sweden) (Figure 9.1).

9.2.1.1 *Clinical Application*

Ceramic grafts are commonly used in ridge augmentation, sinus floor elevation, and defect filling procedures where space maintenance and gradual integration are required. Their clinical performance varies according to crystallinity, porosity, and degradation rate.

Fairbairn and Leventis [19] proposed simultaneous implant placement followed by alveolar bone augmentation employing ß-tricalcium phosphate (ß-TCP) and calcium sulfate at 4 weeks post-extraction, and loading those implants at 12 weeks, based on a multicenter clinical retrospective study of 497 patients. This resulted in a 99% overall survival rate for implants with acceptable alveolar ridge width. Similarly, Mahesh *et al.* [20] found that using calcium phosphor silicate putty mediate (BSM) for socket preservation resulted in superior bone regeneration and timely replacement of the graft with new bone than using bovine xenograft. According to histomorphometric analysis, calcium phosphor silicate grafted in extraction sockets resulted in fresh bone growth (31.7%) and residual graft material (11.4%) after 5.7 months [21]. Furthermore, alloplastic ß-TCP and HA, in conjunction with resorbable/nonresorbable barrier membranes, have been widely employed in guided bone regeneration (GBR) of intrabony periodontal abnormalities [22, 23]. Aside from allogeneic and xenogeneic bone grafts, alloplastic BSM such ß-TCP and HA are commonly employed for alveolar ridge augmentation and preservation. They also have the benefit of being readily available and posing no danger of disease transmission [24]. Clinical and histological examinations of alveolar ridges grafted with ß-TCP 4 months after grafting reveal greater alveolar ridge height and width gain, as well as improved bone quality, compared to ungrafted extraction sites [24]. Moreover, due to their inorganic nature, alloplastic BSM can be combined and used as composite bone grafts, such as HA, ß-TCP, biphasic calcium phosphate (BCP), calcium sulfate, and calcium phosphor silicate. Composite alloplastic grafts have varying consistency, desired physical properties, and a range of graft resorption times, with a faster resorption phase allowing for early bone formation and a slower resorption phase allowing for longer mineralization [25]. Mayer *et al.* [26] found that a triphasic composite alloplastic graft (HA + ß-TCP + calcium sulfate) improved clinical alveolar ridge width gain and histological bone quality within 4 months of socket preservation. Furthermore, clinical cases of extraction socket grafting with composite grafts composed of ß-TCP and biodegradable poly[lactic-co-glycolic] acid, also known as PLGA polymer, resulted in considerable alveolar ridge preservation for implant implantation [27].

Alloplastic materials, like autografts and allografts, have been clinically employed for maxillary augmentation, as well as titanium mesh scaffolds for facial contouring [28, 29]. Malik *et al.* [29] reported a nearly 5-mm increase in alveolar height using a flowable alloplastic BSM (Novabone putty), titanium mesh for vertical alveolar, and guided bone regeneration (GBR). The HA/ß-TCP composite alloplastic graft has also been used successfully in cases of maxillary sinus lift and augmentation [30]. Furthermore, only alloplastic block graft material is currently compatible with 3-D CAD/CAM technologies, allowing for the creation and utilization of patient-specific grafts for maxillary and mandibular alveolar augmentation [31]. Machtei *et al.* [32] found that alloplastic bone replacements produced equivalent or better results in alveolar GBR compared to composite alloplastic graft (HA/ß-TCP) and bovine xenograft. They also detected a higher level of left-over graft material with xenograft at the time of implant insertion. It has also been histologically documented that using nano-HA with ß-TCP as a graft material for GBR resulted in significant cellular activity and increased bone matrix formation [28–30]. Based on a study, Tomas *et al.* [33] reported four clinical investigations on alveolar GBR utilizing injectable alloplastic BSM in the recent decade. According to them, using injectable alloplastic materials increases volume gain in the grafted region, allows for the grafting of complex bone defects, and has the potential to be the preferred approach for severely resorbed maxillary and mandibular ridges.

Additionally, 14 patients had secondary orbital construction using a customized ceramic (Bioverit) orbital implant, and three patients had maxillary reconstruction. The findings demonstrated that a significant orbital volume overcorrection yielded both functional and aesthetically pleasing outcomes [34, 35].

9.3 Bioactive Glass

Bioactive glass materials interact chemically with surrounding tissues, forming a surface layer that facilitates bonding with bone. This bioactivity may support early bone formation at the graft interface while maintaining structural stability.

A carbonated apatite link is created between the host tissue and implant *via* bioactive glass, which is a silica-based material mixed with a biocompatible component like calcium phosphate. In rabbit tibial deformities, Novabone (US Biomaterials Corporation, Alachua, FL, USA) has shown quick replacement with natural bone after 2 weeks, as opposed to 12 weeks for HA replacement. Bioactive glass found in a composite polymeric cement called Cortoss (Orthovita, Malvern, PA, USA) creates a bond with bone without resorbing. It was accessible in Europe, and a pilot trial was conducted in the United States to assess its efficacy in treating spinal fractures [9]. Bioactive glasses may be useful for osteoporotic fractures (such as spinal compression fractures) and mechanical augmentation in osteoporotic bone.

9.3.1 Silica-Calcium Phosphate Composite (SCPS)

A commercially accessible, porous, bioactive, and resorbable alternative is silica–calcium phosphate composite (SCPC). However, due to its unique characteristics, this material can release sodium, phosphate, silicate, and calcium ions over time at quantities that support bone mineralization and vascularization, restrict osteoclast activity, and encourage osteoblast function [36].

9.3.1.1 Clinical Application

These materials have been applied in periodontal defects, ridge preservation, and localized bone augmentation, where controlled interaction with host bone is desired.

A study examined how applying SCPC or xenograft material affected the quality of the bone in the maxillary sinus. The scientists came to the conclusion that, in comparison to the Bio-Oss group, the SCPC group recipients' preserved bone height appears to be due to greater new bone production and maturation [37]. SCPC was evaluated as a bioactive alloplastic bone transplant in a clinical experiment to examine socket preservation. According to the study's findings, the material resorption rate was found to be correlated with bone development. Additionally, SCPC promotes bone maturation and production by stimulating bone cell function [38].

9.3.2 Polymers

Synthetic polymers used as alloplastic grafts provide structural flexibility and radiolucency, with biological performance dependent on surface characteristics and mechanical stability.

Originally used to repair unstable distal radius fractures, poly(methyl methacrylate) (PMMA) bone cement is now often employed in vertebroplasty [39]. Due to its potential for both local and systemic toxicity, it is not a common option for treating the distal radius now that there are substitute materials available.

9.3.2.1 High-Density Polyethylene

This thermoplastic material is semi-crystalline, biocompatible, and non-biodegradable. It has exceptional mechanical qualities that make it ideal for non-load-bearing applications involving facial augmentation [40]. Since the 1970s, MEDPOR® implants have been the most often used.

It has been used to treat abnormalities such as orbital floor reconstruction, nasal tip correction, cheek bone deformities, and hemifacial microsomia (a condition in which one half of the face is underdeveloped).

9.3.2.2 Clinical Application

In order to restore bone volume and contour, synthetic biomaterials are frequently employed in facial rejuvenation and augmentation procedures. However, their use is associated with several common problems, such as exposure from fibrous capsule development and infection [41, 42]. A review of the literature found that sitting-related maxilla, ear, and nose implant failure occurred in 18 out of 285 cases (6.3%) [43]. "Medpore implants reported infection" (3–4%) [44]. Blepharoptosis, exposure, and infection were the most frequent complications with orbital implants, accounting for 10.5% of cases [45]. Extrusion rates can range from 3.1% to 21% [46, 47]. "Infection cases were the only issues directly associated with the use of this biomaterial" [48, 49]. There was a reported 12.5% infection rate (Malar, mandibular angle) [50].

9.3.3 Polyetheretherketone (PEEK)

PEEK is a sub-member of a family of thermoplastic composites, called polyaryletherketone (PAEK) polymers, and has the best performance [51]. Another prevalent sub-members of the PAEK family is polyetherketoneketone (PEKK). Both PEEK and PAEK were introduced in the engineering community in the 1980s [52]. PEEK has exceptional qualities, chemical resistance, and ultrahigh performance [53]. PEEK gained a lot of attention in the medical and dental fields as a result of these astounding results. One benefit of PEEK is that it causes fewer allergic and hypersensitivity reactions [54]. Additionally, PEEK is more aesthetically pleasing when compared to Ti due to its radiolucency, and it has minimal to no effect on magnetic resonance imaging artifacts [54]. Additionally, PEEK's mechanical and physical characteristics are comparable to those of bone.

9.3.3.1 Clinical Application

PEEK's custom-made implant (PSI) technology is addressing the problem of incorrectly using pre-bent plates to restore medial or distal support when

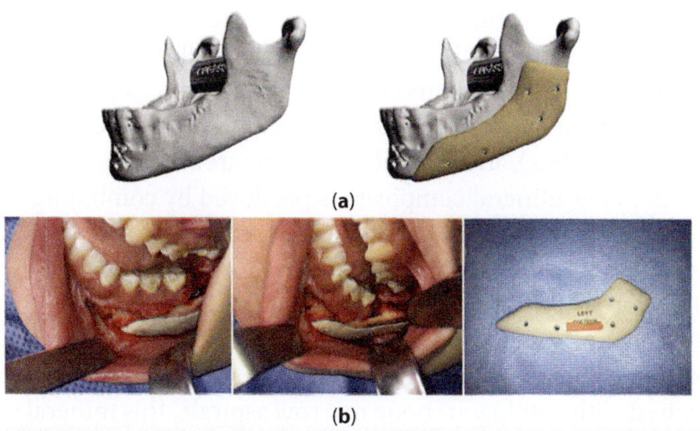

Figure 9.2 Patient-specific implant for manibulas body and angle construction using peek P. The image is reprinted from mineral composites publication: Maxillofacial plastic reconstruction surgery by Alasseri N, Alasaj A. Patient specific implants for maxillofacial defects: challenges and solution 2020;24(15), copyright (2020) with permission from Springer open.

the orbital ledge and/or intra-orbital buttress are damaged. There are limited reports on the clinical use of peek material for orbital reconstruction, despite its reputation for cranial bone reconstruction. According to Gander *et al.* [55], PEEK PSI is preferable to manually bent titanium mesh implants because it enables perfect orbital fracture restoration utilizing a full digital procedure. Similarly, PEEK PSI showed more clinical efficacy in repairing the volume and form of the injured orbit walls, according to Chepurnyi *et al.* [56]. Numerous case studies show that a 3D-printed, patient-specific PEEK implant was successfully used to repair a maxillary defect following trauma; the study found that the implant's function and appearance were satisfactory [57]. In another case study, nine patients with post-traumatic, post-oncology, and orthognathic surgery deformities were rebuilt employing PSI peek. Eight patients reported successful reconstruction [58]. The authors of a review paper on PSI PEEK for effective reconstruction of the craniofacial region, including the mandible, cranial, orbital, and zygomatic bones, came to the conclusion that using titanium or PSI PEEK resulted in higher patient satisfaction and fewer complications. Its high price is its primary disadvantage (Figure 9.2) [59].

9.4 Mineral Composites

Mineral composites when combined with DBM, cancellous bone, and mineral replacements offer potential osteoinduction and osteoconduction. Opteform that contains cancellous bone (Exatech, Alachua, Florida, USA) and DBM (using Osteofil, RTI) is customized to the requirements of the bone defect. In addressing bone abnormalities, Allomatrix (Allosource + Wright Medical), which is marketed as a DBM and calcium sulfate combination, is comparatively safe and effective [18]. Putty ("Custom"), block ("DR" for distal radius), and injectable versions are all available for this combination. Another mineral composite is produced by combining hydroxyapatite, tricalcium phosphate, and bovine collagen matrix (Collagraft, Zimmer, Inc., Warsaw, IN, USA and NeuColl, Campbell, CA, USA). The FDA approved the use of this combination in 1993, making it one of the first bone substitutes [9]. It was authorized to treat abnormalities of the diaphyseal and metaphyseal bones in order to promote osteoconduction. When paired with autologous bone marrow aspirate, this mineral composite demonstrated osteoconductive and osteoinductive qualities, potentially even osteogenesis. However, according to Scaglione and Buchman [60], this material is structurally unsound. Clinical applications of composite ceramic and polymer combinations have been identified [61].

9.4.1 Clinical Application

Composite grafts are utilized in defects requiring prolonged structural support with gradual biological integration.

Li *et al.* [61] investigated the development and implantation of a mandibular condyle in a 27-year-old woman who had an unintentional condyle removal during an osteotomy procedure using rapid prototyping of nanoscale hydroxyapatite/polyamide (n-HA/PA) and computer-aided design/computer-aided manufacturing (CAD/CAM). The patient's symmetrical facial shape and occlusion had recovered following condyle implantation at the 24-month follow-up. There was just a 5-mm variation from the maximum mouth opening of 39 mm.

Gorla *et al.* [62] evaluated the effects of autogenous bone versus composite mineral (ChronOS; DePuy Syntheses) coupled with autogenous bone for sinus floor lift in a randomized control trial. The volume of regenerated tissue at the time of implant implantation did not change, according to the authors' findings. The histological investigation of the composite bone mineral of autogenous bone transplant and α-TCP was examined in another case series study. They discovered that the mixture formed granules and lamellar bone with all the cell types needed for bone remodeling. For up to a year post graft, granules of the α-TCP were still embedded in bone trabeculae [63].

A satisfactory outcome was reported for the management of an anterior vertebral fracture using Nano-HAp/polyamide 66 composites [64]. In a controlled trial for patients with cleft alveolar bone and palate, a combination of hydroxyapatite agarose composite gel and autologous bone was utilized; the study found no difference with autogenous bone [65]. A good outcome was reported from a randomized clinical trial that examined the use of a composite mixture of polymers and nano-hydroxyapatite in the treatment of periodontal bone deficiencies [66].

9.5 Injectable Cement

Skeletal Regeneration System (SRS) (Norian, Synthes USA, Paoli, PA, USA) is the first injectable biological cement that the FDA approved in 1998. It is a powdered mixture of calcium carbonate and calcium phosphate with soluble sodium phosphate [9]. After treating distal radius fractures, it was first authorized for use in general orthopedics to treat metaphyseal abnormalities. One advantage of injectable mineral cement over pellets, blocks, and granules is that it requires a less invasive technique and permits a customized infill of the defect. The calcium phosphate cement Bone Source (Howmedica Leibinger Inc. Dallas, Texas, USA) is authorized for craniofacial anomalies. In a multicenter FDA-monitored study including 38 patients, Bone Source was shown to be as effective as autografted bone in repairing metaphyseal fractures in a range of open and closed injuries [67]. In contrast to SRS, it necessitates a dry setting medium, which may be challenging in a fracture setting. Alpha BSM, another calcium phosphate cement, has been approved for use in dentistry (ETEX Inc., Cambridge, MA, USA) [68]. In Europe, malleable Biobon and Calcibon (Biomet/Merck) have received approval for orthopedic use.

9.5.1 Clinical Application

A degradable carbonated apatite injectable cement (NORIAN SRS) was used in different maxillofacial region, orbit, frontal bone, cranium, and mandible to overcome post-traumatic or cysts defects in 27 patients with a mean of 29 months follow-up period. Injectable carbonated apatite, according to the author, is a good bone mineral alternative for cranio-maxillofacial surgery, particularly for moderately sized abnormalities [69]. Following extraction and implant insertion, 16 patients received PD VitalOs Cement, which contains β-tricalcium phosphate and monocalcium phosphate monohydrate, to bridge the coronal gap between the bone and the implant. After a year, the 16 implants were radiographically assessed, and the mean peri-implant bone loss was 0.48–0.20 mm [70]. Sverzut *et al.* [71], on the other hand, assessed the use of injectable calcium phosphate (BoneSource(®), BS|) for sinus lift in 10 patients; however, they reported unsatisfactory clinical outcomes to allow for the subsequent insertion of implants.

In a review by Lio *et al.* [72] about the injectable bone cement in cranio-maxillofacial bone, it was concluded that injectable calcium phosphate cements (CPCs) are highly promising solution for many maxillofacial bone defects. However, not all clinical indications have conclusive data supporting the successful application of CPC. The development of ideal connectivity porosity to improve vascularity inside injectable cement, mechanical stability, optimal degradable time, and the addition of an antibacterial agent to the mix are some areas that require attention [72].

9.6 Conclusion

Even though the gold standard for bone augmentation is autogenous bone, scientists are still trying to develop the perfect biomaterial that could replace it in order to prevent donor side effects and overcome autogenous bone's common disadvantage when used solely for facial augmentation, i.e., to obtain volume. However, the major problem is the clinical requirement, such as the anatomical condition, such as injecting the materials in a less invasive manner or using sculpture to reshape the contour of the deficit region. Material resorption should occur concurrently with bone remodeling. In terms of mechanical properties, the material modulus of elasticity should be comparable to that of bone, such as PEEK. Currently, hardened CPCs are superior to hydrogel or putty forms of other inorganic salt compounds, but still fall short of bone tissue or highly sintered calcium phosphate ceramics.

AI disclosure statement: The author confirms that no artificial intelligence (AI)-generated content or AI-assisted writing tools were used in the preparation of this chapter (including summaries and the abstract). All text, analysis, and conclusions are the result of the author's original work.

References

1. Tanner, K.E., Bioactive composites for bone tissue engineering. *Proc. Inst. Mech. Eng. Part H-J. Eng. Med.*, 224, 1359–72, 2010.
2. Bongio, M., van den Beucken, J.J., Leeuwenburgh, S.C., Jansen, J.A., Development of bone substitute materials: From 'biocompatible' to 'instructive'. *J. Mater. Chem.*, 20, 8747–59, 2010.
3. Best, S.M., Porter, A.E., Thian, E.S., Huang, J., Bioceramics: Past, present and for the future. *J. Eur. Ceram. Soc.*, 28, 1319–27, 2008.
4. Williams, D.F., *Definitions in biomaterials: Proceedings of a consensus conference of the European Society for Biomaterials, Chester, UK*, 3–5 March 1986, 4th ed., Elsevier Science Ltd, Oxford, 1987.
5. Cao, W. and Hench, L.L., Bioactive materials. *Ceram. Int.*, 22, 493–507, 1996.
6. Gerds, T.A. and Vogeler, M., Endpoints and survival analysis for successful osseointegration of dental implants. *Stat. Methods Med. Res.*, 12005, 4, 579–90, 2005.
7. Wilson-Hench, J., Osteoinduction, in: *Definition in Biomaterial*, 4th ed., D. Williams (Ed.), pp. 8–29, Elsevier, Amsterdam, 1987.
8. Navarro, M., Michiardi, A., Castano, O., Planell, J., Biomaterials in orthopaedics. *J. R. Soc. Interface*, 5, 1137–1158, 2008.
9. Ilan, D.I. and Ladd, A.L., Bone graft substitutes. *Operative Tech. Plast. Reconstr. Surg.*, 9, 151–60, 2002.
10. Truumees, E. and Herkowitz, H., Alternative to autologous bone harvest in spine surgery. *Univ. Pa. Orthop. J.*, 12, 77–88, 1999.

11. Shors, E.C., Coralline bone graft substitutes. *Orthop. Clin. North Am.*, 30, 599–608, 1999.
12. McCalden, R.W., McGeough, J.A., CourtBrown, C.M., Age-related changes in the compressive strength of cancellous bone—The relative importance of changes in density and trabecular architecture. *J. Bone Joint Surg.-Am.*, 79A, 421–27, 1997.
13. Bucholz, R.W., Carlton, A., Holmes, R., Interporous Hydroxyapatite as a Bone Graft Substitute in Tibial Plateau Fractures. *Clin. Orthop. Relat. Res.*, 240, 53–62, 1989.
14. Wolfe, S.W., Pike, L., Slade, J.F., Katz, L.D., Augmentation of distal radius fracture fixation with coralline hydroxyapatite bone craft substitute. *J. Hand Surg.-Am.*, 24A, 816–27, 1999.
15. Resnick, D.K., Vitoss bone substitute. *Neurosurgery*, 50, 1162–64, 2002.
16. Viswanath, B., Raghavan, R., Gurao, N., Ramamurty, U., Ravishankar, N., Mechanical properties of triCalcium Phosphate single crystals grown by molten salt synthesis. *Acta Biomater.*, 4, 1448–54, 2008.
17. Dreesman, H., Ueber Knochenplombierung. *Bietr. Klin. Chir.*, 9, 804–10, 1892.
18. Kelly, C.M., The use of a surgical grade Calcium sulphate as a bone graft substitute: Results of a multicentre trial. *Clin. Orthop.*, 382, 42–50, 2001.
19. Fairbairn, P. and Leventis, M., Protocol for Bone Augmentation with Simultaneous Early Implant Placement: A Retrospective Multicenter Clinical Study. *Int. J. Dent.*, 589135, 2015.
20. Mahesh, L., Venkataraman, N., Shukla, S., Prasad, H., Kotsakis, G.A., Alveolar ridge preservation with the socket-plug technique utilizing an alloplastic putty bone substitute or a particulate xenograft: A histological pilot study. *J. Oral Implantology*, 41, 178–83, 2015.
21. Kotsakis, G.A., Joachim, F.P., Saroff, S.A., Mahesh, L., Prasad, H., Rohrer, M.D., Histomorphometric evaluation of a Calcium-phosphoSilicate putty bone substitute in extraction sockets. *Int. J. Periodontics Restorative Dent.*, 34, 233–9, 2014.
22. Queiroz, L.A., Santamaria, M., Casati, M., Silverio, K., Nociti-Junior, F., Sallum, E., Enamel matrix protein derivative plus synthetic bone substitute for the treatment of mandibular Class II furcation defects: A case series. *Quintessence Int.*, 46, 199–205, 2015.
23. Mansour, A., Al-Hamed, F.S., Torres, J., Marino, F.T., Chapter 3—Alveolar bone grafting: Rationale and clinical applications, in: *Dental Implants and Bone Grafts*, H. Alghamdi and J. Jansen (Eds.), Woodhead Publishing Swaston, UK, 2020.
24. Joshi, C.P., Dani, N.H., Khedkar, S.U., Alveolar ridge preservation using autogenous tooth graft versus ß-triCalcium Phosphate alloplast: A randomized, controlled, prospective, clinical pilot study. *J. Indian Soc. Periodontol.*, 20, 429–34, 2016.

25. Fairbairn, P., Leventis, M., Mangham, C., Horowitz, R., Alveolar Ridge Preservation Using a Novel Synthetic Grafting Material: A Case with Two-Year Follow-Up. *Case Rep. Dent.*, 6412806, 2018.
26. Mayer, Y., Zigdon-Giladi, H., Machtei, E.E., Ridge Preservation Using Composite Alloplastic Materials: A Randomized Control Clinical and Histological Study in Humans. *Clin. Implant Dent. Relat. Res.*, 18, 1163–1170, 20162016.
27. Saito, H., Shiau, H.J., Prasad, H., Reynolds, M.A., Evaluation of a Poly(Lactic-Co-Glycolic) Acid-Coated β-TriCalcium Phosphate Bone Substitute for Alveolar Ridge Preservation: Case Series. *Clin. Adv. Periodontics*, 7, 190–94, 2017.
28. Alagl, A.S. and Madi, M., Localized ridge augmentation in the anterior maxilla using titanium mesh, an alloplast, and a nano-bone graft: A case report. *J. Int. Med. Res.*, 46, 2001–7, 2018.
29. Malik, R., Gupta, A., Bansal, P., Sharma, R., Sharma, S., Evaluation of Alveolar Ridge Height Gained by Vertical Ridge Augmentation Using Titanium Mesh and Novabone Putty in Posterior Mandible. *J. Maxillofac. Oral Surg.*, 19, 32–39, 2020.
30. Salviano, S.H., Lopes, A.J.C., Brum, I.D.S., Frigo, L., Dos Santos, M.J., Consonni, S.R., De Carvalho, J.J., Histomorphometric Evaluation of Bone-Guided Regeneration in Maxillary Sinus Floor Augmentation Using Nano-Hydroxyapatite/ß-TriCalcium Phosphate Composite Biomaterial: A Case Report. *Int. Med. Case Rep. J.*, 14, 697–706, 2021.
31. Yen, H.H. and Stathopoulou, P.G., CAD/CAM and 3D-Printing Applications for Alveolar Ridge Augmentation. *Curr. Oral Health Rep.*, 5, 127–32, 2018.
32. Machtei, E.E., Mayer, Y., Horwitz, J., Zigdon-Giladi, H., Prospective randomized controlled clinical trial to compare hard tissue changes following socket preservation using alloplasts, xenografts vs no grafting: Clinical and histological findings. *Clin. Implant Dent. Relat. Res.*, 21, 14–20, 2019.
33. Tomas, M., Čandrlić, M., Juzbašić, M., Ivanišević, Z., Matijević, N., Včev, A., Cvijanović Peloza, O., Matijević, M., Perić Kačarević, Z., Synthetic Injectable Biomaterials for Alveolar Bone Regeneration in Animal and Human Studies. *Materials*, 14, 2858, 2021.
34. Falkhausen, R., Mitsimponas, K., Adler, W., Brand, M., von Wilmowsky, C., Clinical outcome of patients with orbital fractures treated with patient specific CAD/CAM ceramic implants–a retrospective study. *J. Craniomaxillofac. Surg.*, 149, 6, 468–79, 2021.
35. Gebel, A., Eichhorn, S., Kim, J., Jae-Hyun Park, J., Midface reconstruction using customized Bioverit implant. *Laryngorhinootologie*, 101, S 02, S223, 2022.
36. Aniket, Y.A., Young, A., Marriott, I., El-Ghannam, A., Promotion of pro-osteogenic responses by a bioactive ceramic coating. *J. Biomed. Mater. Res. A*, 100, 3314–3325, 2012.

37. Kudsi, R., Dawson, D.R., Gonzalez, O.A., Kutkut, A., Tucci, M.A., Porras-Aguilar, R., Momox, A.E., Al-Sabbagh, M., Relationship between bone quality and shrinkage in maxillary sinus augmentation using synthetic alloplast versus xenograft. *J. Periodontal Implant Sci.*, 55, e5, 2024, https://doi.org/10.5051/jpis.2401320066.
38. Adel-Khattab, D., Afifi, N.S., Abu El Sadat, S.M., Aboul-Fotouh, M.N., Tarek, K., Horowitz, R.A., Bone regeneration and graft material resorption in extraction sockets grafted with bioactive silica-calcium phosphate composite (SCPC) versus non-grafted sockets: clinical, radiographic, and histological findings. *J. Periodontal Implant Sci.*, 50, 6, 418–434, 2020, doi: 10.5051/jpis.2000040002. PMID: 33350181; PMCID: PMC7758298.
39. Jensen, M.E., Evans, A.J., Mathis, J.M., Kallmes, D.F., Cloft, H.J., Dion, J.E., Percutaneous polymethylmethacrylate vertebroplasty in the treatment of osteoporotic vertebral body compression fractures: Technical aspects. *AJNR Am. J. Neuroradiol.*, 18, 1897–904, 1997.
40. Rai, A., Datarkar, A., Arora, A., Adwani, D.G., Utility of high density porous polyethylene implants in maxillofacial surgery. *J. Maxillofac. Oral Surg.*, 13, 1, 42–46, 2014, DOI: 10.1007/s12663-012-0459-2. PMID: 24644395; PMCID: PMC3955470.
41. Stelter, K., Strieth, S., Berghaus, A., Porous polyethylene implants in revision rhinoplasty: chances and risks. *Rhinology*, 45, 4, 325–331, 2007, PMID: 18085029.
42. Salgado, P.C., Sathler, P.C., Castro, H.C., Alves, G.G., de Oliveira, A.M., de Oliveira, R.C., Maia, M.D.C., Rodrigues, C.R., Coelh, P.G., Fuly, A., Cabral, L.M., Granjeiro, J.M., Bone Remodeling, Biomaterials and Technological Applications: Revisiting Basic Concepts Biocompatible materials; Bone remodeling; Hydroxyapatite; Therapeutic risks. *J. Biomater. Nanobiotechnol.*, 2, 3, 2011.
43. Cenzi, R., Farina, A., Zuccarino, L., Carinci, F., Clinical outcome of 285 Medpor grafts used for craniofacial reconstruction. *J. Craniofac. Surg.*, 16, 4, 526–30, 2005, doi: 10.1097/01.scs.0000168761.46700.dc. PMID: 16077294.
44. Berghaus, A. and Stelter, K., Alloplastic materials in rhinoplasty. *Curr. Opin. Otolaryngol. Head Neck Surg.*, 14, 4, 270–7, 2006, doi: 10.1097/01.moo.0000233599.14671.4a. PMID: 16832185.
45. Jung, S., Cho, W., Paik, J., *et al.*, Long-term surgical outcomes of porous polyethylene orbital implants: a review of 314 cases. *Br. J. Ophthalmol.*, 96, 494–498, 2012.
46. Peled, Z.M., Warren, A.G., Johnston, P., Yaremchuk, M.J., The Use of Alloplastic Materials in Rhinoplasty Surgery: A Meta-Analysis. *Plast. Reconstr. Surg.*, 121, 3, 85e–92e, 2008, DOI: 10.1097/01.prs.0000299386.73127.a7.
47. Kim, H.S., Park, S.S., Kim, M.H., Kim, M.S., Kim, S.K., Lee, K.C., Problems associated with alloplastic materials in rhinoplasty. *Yonsei Med. J.*, 55, 6, 1617–23, 2014.

48. de Moraes Ferreira, A.CR., Muñoz, X.M.J.P., Okamoto, R., Pellizer, E.P., Garcia Jr., I.R., Postoperative Complications in Craniomaxillofacial Reconstruction With Medpor. *J. Craniofac. Surg.*, 27, 2, 425–428, 2016, DOI: 10.1097/SCS.0000000000002325.
49. Storck, K., Kotz, S., Riedel, F., Veit, J., Complications associated with alloplastic materials in rhinoplasty and their operative management. *Facial Plast. Surg.*, 40, 04, 485–492, 2024, DOI: 10.1055/s-0043-1772846.
50. Khorasani, M., Janbaz, P., Rayati, F., Maxillofacial reconstruction with Medpor porous polyethylene implant: a case series study. *J. Korean Assoc. Oral Maxillofac. Surg.*, 44, 3, 128–35, 2018.
51. Suphangul, S., Rokaya, D., Kanchanasobhana, C., Rungsiyakull, P., Chaijareenont, P., PEEK Biomaterial in Long-Term Provisional Implant Restorations: A Review. *J. Funct. Biomater.*, 13, 2, 33, 2022, https://doi.org/10.3390/jfb13020033.
52. Huang, B., Qian, J., Wang, G., Cai, M., Synthesis and properties of novel copolymers of poly(ether ketone diphenyl ketone ether ketone ketone) and poly(ether amide ether amide ether ketone ketone). *Polym. Eng. Sci., 54,* 1757–1764, 2014.
53. Najeeb, S., Zafar, M.S., Khurshid, Z., Siddiqui, F., Applications of polyetheretherketone (PEEK) in oral implantology and prosthodontics. *J. Prosthodont. Res.*, 60, 1, 12–9, 2016.
54. Lee, W.T., Koak, J.Y., Lim, Y.J., Kim, S.K., Kwon, H.B., Kim, M.J., Stress shielding and fatigue limits of poly-ether-ether-ketone dental implants. *J. Biomed. Mater. Res. B Appl. Biomater., 100,* 1044–1052, 2012.
55. Gander, T., Essig, H., Metzler, P., Lindhorst, D., Dubois, L., Rücker, M., Schumann, P., Patient specific implants (PSI) in reconstruction of orbital floor and wall fractures. *J. Craniomaxillofac. Surg.*, 43, 1, 126–130, 2015.
56. Chepurnyi, Y., Chernogorskyi, D., Kopchak, A., Petrenko, O., Clinical efficacy of peek patient-specific implants in orbital reconstruction. *J. Oral Biol. Craniofac. Res.*, 10, 2, 49–53, 2020.
57. Hamsho, R., Mahardawi, B., Assi, H., Alkhatib, H., Polyetheretherketone (PEEK) Implant for the Reconstruction of Severe Destruction in the Maxilla: Case Report. *Plast. Reconstr. Surg. Glob. Open*, 10, 8, e4473, 2022, doi: 10.1097/GOX.0000000000004473. PMID: 35999877; PMCID: PMC9390812.
58. Abdullakutty, A., Madhavarajan, S., Collyer, J., Sneddon, K., Uses of PEEK in maxillofacial reconstruction: a 6-year review of cases. *Br. J. Oral Maxillofacial Surg.*, 50, S39–40, 2012.
59. Alasseri, N. and Alasraj, A., Patient-specific implants for maxillofacial defects: challenges and solutions. *Maxillofac. Plast. Reconstr. Surg.*, 42, 15, 2020, https://doi.org/10.1186/s40902-020-00262-7.
60. Scaglione, P.H. and Buchman, M.T., Collagraft bone substitute in upper extremity fractures: A preliminary study. *Surg. Forum*, 48, 563–65, 19971997.
61. Li, J., Hsu, Y., Luo, E., Khadka, A., Hu, J., Computer-Aided Design and Manufacturing and Rapid Prototyped Nano-scale Hydroxyapatite/Polyamide

(n-HA/PA) Construction for Condylar Defect Caused by Mandibular Angle Ostectomy. *Aesthet. Plast. Surg.*, 35, 636–40, 20112011.
62. Gorla, L.D., Spin-Neto, R., Boos, F.B., Pereira, R.D., Garcia-Junior, I.R., Hochuli-Vieira, E., Use of autogenous bone and ß-tricalcium phosphate in maxillary sinus lifting: a prospective, randomized, volumetric computed tomography study. *Int. J. Oral Maxillofac. Surg.*, 44, 12, 1486–91, 2015.
63. Chappard, D., Guillaume, B., Mallet, R., Pascaretti-Grizon, F., Basle, M.F., Libouban, H., Sinus lift augmentation and β-TCP: A microCT and histologic analysis on human bone biopsies. *Micron.*, 41, 4, 321–6, 2010.
64. Wang, G.J., Wang, Q., Yang, J., Wang, S., Zhong, D.J., Xu, S., Nanohydroxyapatite/polyamide 66 composite vertebrae repair anterior cervical vertebral fractures. *Chin. J. Tissue Eng.*, 20, 3, 397–401, 2016.
65. Iwai, S., Shimizu, H., Suzawa, Y., Akashi, M., Yura, Y., Hydroxyapatite agarose composite gels as a biochemical material for the repair of alveolar bone defects due to cleft lip and palate. *J. Oral Maxillofac. Surg. Med. Pathol.*, 27, 5, 637–644, 2015.
66. Dayashankar, C.P., Deepika, P.C., Siddaramaiah, B., Clinical and radiographic evaluation of citric acid-based nano hydroxyapatite composite graft in the regeneration of intrabony defects-a randomized controlled trial. *Contemp. Clin. Dent.*, 8, 3, 380–386, 2017.
67. Dickson, K.F.M., Friedman, J.M., Buchholz, J.G.M., Flandry, F.D.M., The Use of BoneSource Hydroxyapatite Cement for Traumatic Metaphyseal Bone Void Filling. *J. Trauma-Injury Infect. Crit. Care*, 53, 1103–8, 2002.
68. Knaack, D., Goad, M.E.P., Aiolova, M., Rey, C., Tofighi, A., Chakravarthy, P., Lee, D.D., Resorbable Calcium Phosphate bone substitute. *J. Biomed. Mater. Res.*, 43, 399–409, 1998.
69. Wolff, K.D., Swaid, S., Nolte, D., Böckmann, R.A., Hölzle, F., Müller-Mai, C., Degradable injectable bone cement in maxillofacial surgery: indications and clinical experience in 27 patients. *J. Craniomaxillofac. Surg.*, 32, 2, 71–9, 2004, doi: 10.1016/j.jcms.2003.12.002. PMID: 14980585.
70. Taschieri, S., Rosano, G., Weinstein, T., Del Fabbro, M., Replacement of vertically root-fractured endodontically treated teeth with immediate implants in conjunction with a synthetic bone cement. *Implant Dent.*, 19, 6, 477–486, 2010.
71. Sverzut, A.T., Rodrigues, D.C., Lauria, A., Armando, R.S., de Oliveira, P.T., Moreira, R.W., Clinical, radiographic, and histological analyses of calcium phosphate cement as filling material in maxillary sinus lift surgery. *Clin. Oral Implants Res.*, 26, 6, 633–8, 2015, doi: 10.1111/clr.12346. Epub 2014 Feb 6. PMID: 24502772.
72. Liao, H., Hoekstra, J.W., Wolke, J., Leeuwenburgh, S., Jansen, J., Injectable Calcium Phosphate Cements for the Reconstruction/Repair of Oral and Cranio-maxillofacial Bone Defects: Clinical Outcome and Perspectives, in: *Organ Tissue Engineering*, pp. 355–72, 2021.

10

Commercially Available Graft Materials FDA Approved and the Supporting Studies

Randa A. Alfotawi

Department of Oral and Maxillofacial Surgery, College of Dentistry, King Saud University, Riyadh, Saudi Arabia

Abstract

This chapter provides an overview of the various inorganic and organic biomaterials, including ceramics, demineralized allograft, polymers, and composites, that are accessible for orthopedic and dental applications. These bone substitutes come in a variety of physical forms, including solid blocks, putties, pastes, gels, granules, powders, and porous scaffolds. Due to their qualities, ceramics are typically used in orthopedic and craniofacial applications. The primary bone substitutes are currently on the market, which are either FDA or non-FDA-approved form; both natural and artificial sources are presented.

Keywords: FDA, bone grafts, xenograft, allograft, alloplasts, bone substitutes, ceramics, composite

10.1 Introduction

Commercially available bone graft materials approved by regulatory authorities have become integral to contemporary oral and maxillofacial reconstructive practice. Regulatory approval provides assurance regarding safety and manufacturing standards; however, clinical performance remains dependent on material properties, biological behaviour, and appropriate clinical application. This chapter reviews FDA-approved graft materials and the evidence supporting their use, with emphasis on scientific validity rather than commercial comparison. The third generation of biomaterials was developed

Email: ralfotawei@ksu.edu.sa

in response to the need for regeneration of bone defect, and specifically for use in clinically compromised situations such as those with immunocompromised states or scenarios of critical-size defect. Osteointegration and capability to achieve sufficient mechanical qualities are the main required characteristics of bone substitute materials. There are currently no commercially available scaffold materials because the ideal ones have not yet been produced. A number of materials are presently undergoing testing, and numerous advancements are still required before clinical application is practical. Current third-generation biomaterials, such as Copi OS Bone Void Filler, have excellent porosity, interconnectivity, and resorbability, which provide improved imaging and visualization of the healing process. The FDA-approved and non-FDA-approved bone grafts materials available on the market, such as Bio-Oss, are covered in this chapter.

10.2 What is FDA Approved

FDA approval indicates that a medical device or biomaterial has met regulatory requirements for safety, quality, and intended use. Approval does not imply clinical superiority or universal applicability across all indications. Bone graft materials are typically cleared through pathways such as premarket notification or premarket approval, depending on classification and risk profile. It is a procedure for approving bone grafts to ensure their safety and ability to regenerate bone. The FDA is in charge of the approval process, which varies depending on the type of grafting device and the graft. Obtaining complete FDA approval for bone grafts involves four major steps.

Table 10.1 Summary of medical devices' classification and their definitions according to FDA.

Classification	Definition	Example
I	Medical devices are those that, in the event of a malfunction, are unlikely to harm people [4].	Blood pressure cuffs, tongue depressors, and crutches
II	Devices that, in the event of a malfunction, are unlikely to cause absurd physical injury [4].	Surgical drapes, cardiac monitors
III	Devices that are meant to drastically alter patient health but carry a high risk of harm [5].	Defibrillators and pacemakers

Table 10.2 Summary of all the bone graft materials which are FDA-approved and available in the market for clinical applications.

Type	Commercial name	Company	Composition	Uses	Advantages	Disadvantages
Alloplast	Bonesave™ [7]	Stryker	Hydroxyapatite cement	Bone filler	Higher compression and tensile strength than tricalcium phosphate, and highly biocompatible	Slow graft resorption
	Bonesoure® [8]	Stryker	Hydroxyapatite cement	Bone filler	Higher compression and tensile strength than tricalcium phosphate, and highly biocompatible	Slow graft resorption
	Norian SRS® [9]	Synthesis	Injectable calcium phosphate	Bone-void filler. Recommended for the calcaneal, distal radius, tibial plateau	Higher compression and tensile strength than tricalcium phosphate, and highly biocompatible	Poor mechanical strength

(Continued)

Table 10.2 Summary of all the bone graft materials which are FDA-approved and available in the market for clinical applications. (*Continued*)

Type	Commercial name	Company	Composition	Uses	Advantages	Disadvantages
	Osstic™ [10]	(Gpbio)	Combining the amino acid phosphoserine with tricalcium phosphate	Bioceramic glue	The amino acid causes quick (minutes) bonding, which strengthens the fixation between tissues and biomaterials (Pujari-Palmer), a functionalized bone cement synthetic graft that is the "Gold Standard" of synthetic grafts and has the most compositional similarity to bone	Unpredictably degrades, making it unsuitable for load-bearing areas
	Cortoss® [11]	Orthovita, Inc	Bioactive glass	Treatment of vertebral compression fractures (VCFs)	Forms connections with bone and tissue, turns on genes that regulate osteogenesis, and has antimicrobial qualities	Limited range of SiO_2 content for graft bioactivity

(*Continued*)

Table 10.2 Summary of all the bone graft materials which are FDA-approved and available in the market for clinical applications. (*Continued*)

Type	Commercial name	Company	Composition	Uses	Advantages	Disadvantages
	MIIG® X3 [12]	Wright Medical, Inc	Calcium sulfate	Introduced into open bone cavities or gaps that are not necessary for the skeletal system's bony structure to remain stable, resulting in osseous defects or osseous defects brought on by damage to the bone	Easy to prepare and inexpensive to produce	Lacks mechanical strength, resorbs more quickly than bone dissolves, and poses a major risk of wound drainage
	Bonesource® [13]	Stryker Nederland B.V.	Calcium phosphate	Reconstruction of craniofacial defects	They are easily molded by the temperature dissolution–precipitation reaction	Low mechanical strength, their lack of compressive strength, and their failure to allow osteoinduction

(*Continued*)

Table 10.2 Summary of all the bone graft materials which are FDA-approved and available in the market for clinical applications. (*Continued*)

Type	Commercial name	Company	Composition	Uses	Advantages	Disadvantages
	Calcibon® [14]	Biomet Europe	Calcium phosphate	Bone void filler after benign and low-grade malignant bone tumors have been cured	They are easily molded by the temperature dissolution–precipitation reaction	Low mechanical strength, their lack of compressive strength, and their failure to allow osteoinduction delayed resorption
	Chronos® Inject [15]	Synthes, Inc	Injectable calcium phosphate	Designed to be used as a filler for the metaphyseal bone void in order to treat bone deformities.	They are easily molded by the temperature dissolution–precipitation reaction	Low mechanical strength, their lack of compressive strength, and their failure to allow osteoinduction delayed resorption

(*Continued*)

Table 10.2 Summary of all the bone graft materials which are FDA-approved and available in the market for clinical applications. (*Continued*)

Type	Commercial name	Company	Composition	Uses	Advantages	Disadvantages
	Eurobone® [16]	Surgical Concepts	Injectable calcium phosphate	Filling of defect following resection of benign tumor, additional bioactive mechanical filling of defect in revision arthroplasty	Easy to prepare and inexpensive to produce	Lacks mechanical strength, resorbs more quickly than bone dissolves, and poses a major risk of wound drainage
	Ostim® [17]	Hereaus	Nanocrystalline hydroxyapatite paste	Periodontal surgery, cement for bone fractures	Mechanically and biologically efficient and safe	Cannot resorb the form of regenerated bone
	Allogran-R [18]	Biocomposites	Fully absorbable B tri-calcium phosphate F	Bone void	The "Gold Standard" of synthetic grafts is the one whose composition is most like that of bone	Unpredictably degrades, making it unsuitable for load-bearing areas

(*Continued*)

Table 10.2 Summary of all the bone graft materials which are FDA-approved and available in the market for clinical applications. (*Continued*)

Type	Commercial name	Company	Composition	Uses	Advantages	Disadvantages
	Cellplex™ [19]	Wright Medical Technology	Tricalcium phosphate	Packed gently into the skeletal system's bone voids or gaps, such as the spine, pelvis, and extremities	The "Gold Standard" of synthetic grafts is the one whose composition is most like that of bone	Unpredictably degrades, making it unsuitable for load-bearing areas
	Cerasorb®M [20]	Curasan	Pure B -tricalcium phosphate (>99%)	Used as a filler of oral and maxillofacial surgery bone defects	The large, highly coarse surface area provides for increased osteoconductivity	Unpredictably degrades, making it unsuitable for load-bearing areas
	Chron OS™ [21]	Syntheses	B -tricalcium phosphate	Fills in iatrogenic and traumatic bone deficiencies as well as reconstruction-related deformities. Use is mentioned in: spinal fusion or open-wedge osteotomies	The "Gold Standard" of synthetic grafts is the one whose composition is most like that of bone	Limited mechanical properties

(*Continued*)

Table 10.2 Summary of all the bone graft materials which are FDA-approved and available in the market for clinical applications. (*Continued*)

Type	Commercial name	Company	Composition	Uses	Advantages	Disadvantages
	Vitoss Scaffold Foam [22]	(Orthovita)	-Tricalcium phosphate and collagen type I		For solids or spaces that are not essential to the bony structure stability, use as a bone void filler. Both medically generated osseous defects and osseous defects resulting from acute bone injury can be treated using Vitoss scaffold foam.	Not indicated in large defect limited mechanical properties

(*Continued*)

Table 10.2 Summary of all the bone graft materials which are FDA-approved and available in the market for clinical applications. (*Continued*)

Type	Commercial name	Company	Composition	Uses	Advantages	Disadvantages
	Boneceramic® [23]	(Straumann)	Hydroxyapatite & B-tricalcium phosphate	Sinus floor augmentation. Provide a strong foundation for a dental implant while supporting and promoting natural bone growth over time	A robust matrix for long-term bone volume preservation, 60% hydroxyapatite (HA) inhibits excessive resorption and maintains bone volume. 40% ß-Tricalcium phosphate (ß-TCP) for a quick initial response of bone-forming cells for quicker resorption and natural bone replacement	Limitation of mechanical strength based on mixture of graft
	Osteoset [24]	(Wright Medical Technology)	Calcium sulfate hemihydrate	Filling osseous flaws and controlling dead space with 7-mm custom-molded beads	Dependable, regulated resorption rate that closely resembles the rate at which bone grows naturally	Low mechanical strength and the possibility of severe wound drainage

(*Continued*)

Table 10.2 Summary of all the bone graft materials which are FDA-approved and available in the market for clinical applications. (*Continued*)

Type	Commercial name	Company	Composition	Uses	Advantages	Disadvantages
	Boneplast® [25]	(Biomet)	**Calcium Sulfate**	Filling osseous defects and managing dead space with custom molded, 7 mm beads	Easy to prepare and inexpensive to produce	Lacks mechanical strength, resorbs more quickly than bone dissolves, and poses a major risk of wound drainage
	Stimulan® [26]	(Biocomposites)	**Calcium Sulfate**	Filling osseous flaws and controlling dead space with 7 mm custom-molded beads	Easy to prepare and inexpensive to produce	Lacks mechanical strength, resorbs more quickly than bone dissolves, and poses a major risk of wound drainage

(*Continued*)

Table 10.2 Summary of all the bone graft materials which are FDA-approved and available in the market for clinical applications. (*Continued*)

Type	Commercial name	Company	Composition	Uses	Advantages	Disadvantages
	Altapore Shape [27]	(Baxter International)	Silica-substitute calcium phosphate	Fill up the skeletal system's bony gaps or holes	Forms connections with bone and tissue, turns on genes that regulate osteogenesis, antibacterial properties, promotes early vascularization, increases cellular activity, and enhances bone growth as demonstrated in pre-clinical and *in vitro* studies	Limited range of SiO_2 content for graft bioactivity
	Signafuse [28]	(Bioventus Surgical)	Bioglass and a biphasic mineral (60% hydroxyapatite, 40% B-tricalcium phosphate)	Cervical and lumber fusion/deformity correction	Helps accelerate cellular activity and kickstart osteogenesis	Limited range of SiO_2 content for graft bioactivity

(*Continued*)

Table 10.2 Summary of all the bone graft materials which are FDA-approved and available in the market for clinical applications. (*Continued*)

Type	Commercial name	Company	Composition	Uses	Advantages	Disadvantages
	CEMEX® [29]	(Exactech)	Polymethylmethacrylate (PMMA) bone cement	For the fixation of plastic and metal joint prostheses to host bone	Secures orthopedic implants firmly in place	Lack of inherent adhesive qualities, heat sensitivity, the possibility of bone cement implantation syndrome, cement fragmentation, and implants may deteriorate and come loose due to foreign body reaction

(*Continued*)

Table 10.2 Summary of all the bone graft materials which are FDA-approved and available in the market for clinical applications. (*Continued*)

Type	Commercial name	Company	Composition	Uses	Advantages	Disadvantages
	Gentac-Ment® [30]	(Leader Biomedical)	Polymethylmethacrylate (PMMA) bone cement and gentamicin	Guided bone and tissue regeneration Spinal fusion adhesion control and prevention deferring osteoarthritis vertebroplasty Deferring osteoarthritis osteotomy	Secures orthopedic implants in place. The crucial task of cement is to disperse the impacting forces as equally as feasible, low harding heat generation, release of antibiotics	Lack of inherent adhesive qualities, heat sensitivity, the possibility of bone cement implantation syndrome, cement fragmentation, and implants may deteriorate and come loose due to foreign body reaction
	Divergence-L® [31]	Medtronic	Polyetheretherketone (PEEK)	Oblique lateral interbody fusion		

(*Continued*)

Table 10.2 Summary of all the bone graft materials which are FDA-approved and available in the market for clinical applications. (*Continued*)

Type	Commercial name	Company	Composition	Uses	Advantages	Disadvantages
	Pivox™ [32]	Medtronic	Polyetheretherketone (PEEK)	Oblique lateral spine Divergence—lateral interbody fusion	Resistance to degradation (Resistance to chemical anti-allergic reaction). Modulus of elasticity is similar to bone	Very expensive, has less surface energy, therefore it has less surface adhesion. It can degrade in the body, difficulty in manufacturing
	Augment® Bone Graft [33]	Wright Medical Group	Combines a bioresorbable synthetic bone matrix (beta-tricalcium phosphate, or B-TCP) with a recombinant human platelet-derived growth factor B homodimer (Rhpdgf-BB).	Osteoinductive, osteoconduction	In two clinical trials involving patients undergoing ankle or hindfoot arthrodesis and transforaminal lumbar or lateral interbody fusion, respectively, both devices encouraged bone ingrowth without the need for autograft harvesting, causing less discomfort than autograft with comparable outcomes	Not studied long term, expensive

(*Continued*)

Table 10.2 Summary of all the bone graft materials which are FDA-approved and available in the market for clinical applications. (*Continued*)

Type	Commercial name	Company	Composition	Uses	Advantages	Disadvantages
	Healos [34]	Depuy Synthes Spine	Collagen+HA	Used with bone marrow aspirate	Posterolateral lumbar fusion in spine fusion	Slow resorption of graft, risk of disease transmission or unfavorable immune response
	SCPC50® [35]	Shefabone [35]	Silica calcium phosphate nanocomposite	Socket preservation, ridge augmentation, sinus lift	Creates bonds with bone and tissue, turns on genes that regulate osteogenesis, and has antimicrobial qualities	Limited range of SiO_2 content for graft bioactivity, long resorption rate that reaches >4 months [68]

(*Continued*)

Table 10.2 Summary of all the bone graft materials which are FDA-approved and available in the market for clinical applications. (*Continued*)

Type	Commercial name	Company	Composition	Uses	Advantages	Disadvantages
	Cerament ™ [36]	Spine and bone support	Csh 60%/ Ha 40%	Mal-union of the bone, vertebroplasty, bone voids filling from surgically debriding a persistent infection, and vertebral augmentation of osteoporotic collapses	Injectable cement that assumes the shape of any defect, non-invasive surgery	Orthotopic site, low mechanical strength

(*Continued*)

Table 10.2 Summary of all the bone graft materials which are FDA-approved and available in the market for clinical applications. (*Continued*)

Type	Commercial name	Company	Composition	Uses	Advantages	Disadvantages
	HERAFILL® Beadsg) [37]	Heraeus Medical.	Hydrogenated triglycerides, calcium carbonate, calcium sulfate dihydrate, and gentamicin	Recommended to fill bone voids caused by surgically debriding hematogenic, post-traumatic, chronic, and post-operative osteomyelitis/osteitis, as well as infected pseudoarthrosis and infected osteosynthesis in patients	The presence of calcium carbonate and radio-opaque balances pH in the event of infection, and osteoconduction, drug delivery, and full absorption in a few months	Limited application to the infection site, little structural support, and a lengthy resorption period
	Calcibon® [38]	Biomet LTD,	Precipitated hydroxyapatite, calcium carbonate, calcium hydrogen phosphate, and alpha-tri-calcium phosphate	Metaphyseal filling, cancellous bone defects, distal radius fractures, and tibial head fractures fractures of the calcaneus	Osteoconductive, malleable paste, compressive strength (up to 60 MPa), *in situ* hardening, and cellularly mediated biodegradation	Fixation, stability, and precise repositioning; Longer absorption time

(*Continued*)

Table 10.2 Summary of all the bone graft materials which are FDA-approved and available in the market for clinical applications. (*Continued*)

Type	Commercial name	Company	Composition	Uses	Advantages	Disadvantages
	Proosteon® [39]	Interpore Cross International, Irvine, CA	Calcium carbonate combined with biologic hydroxyapatite	Mostly used to fill metaphyseal abnormalities; gradual resorption with varying strength; interconnected channels permit tissue ingrowth	Osteoconductive, porosity	Slow resorption rate, absence of osteoinductive action, and lack of structural support
	Triosite® [40]	Zimmer Pty Ltd	60% Ha/40% Tcp	Bone graft with high tibial osteotomy and posterior spinal fusion	It might be combined with bone marrow	Material found after a lengthy (4 years) follow-up (Hooper, 2013)
	Jectos (Orthopedic List.Com) [41]	Kasios (Injectable Bone Substitute)	55%Dcpd (Brushite), 45%Tcp	Bone gap filling in cases of trauma, including wedge osteotomy, distal radius malunion, tibial and calcaneus fractures, and radius	Injectable cement	Long resorption rate (4–6 years) and insufficient strength requiring external fixing

(*Continued*)

Table 10.2 Summary of all the bone graft materials which are FDA-approved and available in the market for clinical applications. (*Continued*)

Type	Commercial name	Company	Composition	Uses	Advantages	Disadvantages
	Jectos+ (Orthopedic List.Com) [42]	Wright Medical Technology	Zirconia as a radiopacifier and calcium phosphate	The vertebral body after kyphoplasty on young patients that are stable after recent traumatic vertebral body fracture	Radiopaque injectable bone cement synthetic	Not recommended in compression vertebra fracture
	PRO-STIM™ [43]	Wright Medical Technology	10% calcium phosphate, 40% DBM, and 50% C calcium sulfate	Bone filler material	Osteinductive, osteoconductive, flowable, composite bone graft	Human origin. Absence of structural support in injectable and putty form
	Genex (Orhopedic List.Com) [44]	Biocomposites Lt.	Calcium sulfate and tri-calcium phosphate in a ratio of 1:1	Refilling the defect following the removal of the tumor	Osteoinduction and osteoconduction	Inflammation and destruction of soft tissue [44]

(*Continued*)

Table 10.2 Summary of all the bone graft materials which are FDA-approved and available in the market for clinical applications. (*Continued*)

Type	Commercial name	Company	Composition	Uses	Advantages	Disadvantages
Xenograft	Creos™ xenoprotect [45]	Nobel Biocare™ (Wessing B)	Resorbable collagen membrane	GBR	Geistlich Bio-Gide®'s smooth side acts as a scaffold for fibroblast attachment and stops soft tissue from developing into the defect. Geistlich Bio-Gide®'s rough, open-pored layer side provides a framework for blood vessels and bone cells	Transmissible spongiform encephalopathies (TSE) and bovine spongiform encephalopathy (BSE) x
	Bioguide® [46]	Geistlich	Natural collagen	Guided bone regeneration	Geistlich Bio-Gide®'s smooth side acts as a scaffold for fibroblast attachment and stops soft tissue from developing into the defect. Geistlich Bio-Gide®'s rough, open-pored layer side provides a framework for blood vessels and bone cells	Transmissible spongiform encephalopathies (TSE) and bovine spongiform encephalopathy (BSE) X

(*Continued*)

Table 10.2 Summary of all the bone graft materials which are FDA-approved and available in the market for clinical applications. (*Continued*)

Type	Commercial name	Company	Composition	Uses	Advantages	Disadvantages
	Mineross ®Cancellous [47]	Biohorizons [47]	Cancellous bone	Ridge and sinus augmentation socket grafting periodontal defects grafting for implant placement	Without a second surgical site, there is a lower chance of infection and no more pain	Hazard of disease spread or adverse immunological reaction
	Mineross ®Cortical [47]	Biohorizons [47]	Cortical bone	Ridge and sinus augmentation socket grafting periodontal defects grafting for implant placement	Without a second surgical site, there is a lower chance of infection and no more pain	Hazard of disease spread or adverse immunological reaction
	DBX® [48]	DePuy synthesis	Demineralized bone matrix	Augmentation of alveolar ridge in maxilla and mandible	Contains growth factors making it osteoinductive	Growth factors in varying concentrations from various manufacturers and batches

(*Continued*)

Table 10.2 Summary of all the bone graft materials which are FDA-approved and available in the market for clinical applications. (*Continued*)

Type	Commercial name	Company	Composition	Uses	Advantages	Disadvantages
	Dynagraft® Putty And Gel [49]	Sterigenics Radiation Technologies, LLC	Demineralized bone matrix	As a bone graft extender (for the spine, pelvis, and extremities) and as a bony void filler for the spine and pelvis, it should be carefully packed into bony gaps in the skeletal system	Contains growth factors making it osteoinductive, hardens at body temperature moldable and easily shaped to pack into any defect resists irrigation to minimize migration from site	Growth factors in varying concentrations from various manufacturers and batches
	Osteolife [50]	Biomedical	Mineralized freeze-dried bone (FDBA)	Socket preservation Ridge augmentation	Contains growth factors making it osteoinductive	Growth factors in varying concentrations from various manufacturers and batches
	Collagraft [51]	Zimmer/Neucoll	Tricalcium phosphate (TCP), HA, and bovine collagen	Long bone fracture grafting and traumatic defect filling	When combined with bone marrow, osteoconductive and osteoinductive	Difficult to restrict to the intended site and requires aspirated marrow

(*Continued*)

Table 10.2 Summary of all the bone graft materials which are FDA-approved and available in the market for clinical applications. (*Continued*)

Type	Commercial name	Company	Composition	Uses	Advantages	Disadvantages
	tarSys™	(IOP Ophthalmics, Costa Mesa, California, USA)	Decellularized small intestinal submucosa	Nasal septal perforation structural integrity to the eyelid	Demonstrated favorable clinical outcomes in cases of lagophthalmos and Graves ophthalmopathy	Foreign body reaction
Xenograft	Osseo-Seal	Osseoshap. USA	Bovine bone derivative	Bone graft	Purified osteoconductive mineral structure	Transmissible spongiform encephalopathies (TSE) and bovine spongiform encephalopathy (BSE) X
Xenograft	Zyplast	Zyderm; Inamed Corporation, Santa Barbara, California	Bovine collagen fillers cross-linked with glutaraldehyde	Specifically strengthen the collagen fibers	GBR	Transmissible spongiform encephalopathies (TSE) and bovine spongiform encephalopathy (BSE) X

(*Continued*)

Table 10.2 Summary of all the bone graft materials which are FDA-approved and available in the market for clinical applications. (*Continued*)

Type	Commercial name	Company	Composition	Uses	Advantages	Disadvantages
Xenograft	Gen-Os	OsteoBiol by Tecnoss Dental, Torino-Italy	Cortico-cancellous heterologous bone mix	Alveolar ridge preservation, periodontal regeneration of deep infrabony pockets and for lateral maxillary sinus lift approach	The cortico-cancellous nature allows for the progressive resorption of graft material	Transmissible spongiform encephalopathies (TSE) and bovine spongiform encephalopathy (BSE) X
Xenograft	Endobon® (EB)	Zimmer Biomet	Bovine bone with hydroxyapatite ceramic	Socket preservation, management of defects in peri-implantitis		Transmissible spongiform encephalopathies (TSE) and bovine spongiform encephalopathy (BSE) X
Xenograft	OsteoBiol® mp3	Osteobiol (Italy)	Pre-hydrated cortico-cancellous bone mix with 10% collagen gel	Horizontal and vertical augmentation Peri-implant defects Periodontal	Easily applied	Slow resorption

(*Continued*)

Table 10.2 Summary of all the bone graft materials which are FDA-approved and available in the market for clinical applications. (*Continued*)

Type	Commercial name	Company	Composition	Uses	Advantages	Disadvantages
Xenograft	Cerabone and Cerabone plus	Botiss Biomateriaks, Germany	Bovine bone grafts combined with hyaluronic acid	Horizontal and vertical augmentation Peri-implant defects Periodontal intrabony defects Socket and ridge preservation Sinus lift Furcation defects (class I and II)	A sticky bone material upon hydration, easy handling for delivery	Transmissible spongiform encephalopathies (TSE) and bovine spongiform encephalopathy (BSE) X
Xenograft	Ivory dentin graft:	Ivory graft,	Porcine tooth-derived product	Socket preservation	Greater amount of new bone formation	Contraindicated acute inflammation hypersensitivity and immunologic disorders

(*Continued*)

Table 10.2 Summary of all the bone graft materials which are FDA-approved and available in the market for clinical applications. (*Continued*)

Type	Commercial name	Company	Composition	Uses	Advantages	Disadvantages
Allograft+ Alloplast	Allomatrix [51]	Allosource + Wright Medical	Calcium Sulfate + DBM as carrier: block (DR) injectable putty (custom)	Periarticular fractures (DR), metaphyseal abnormalities, and nonunion, delayed, and perhaps delayed unions	Potentially osteoinductive and osteoconductive potential stability with DR form potentially better carrier (inert, nonprotein) compared to other carriers for DBM	Human origin. Absence of structural support in injectable and putty form
	Healos [51]	Orquest	HA coated bovine collagen sponge, approved in Europe	Autograft or autograft extender replacement for spinal fusion	Osteoinductive when combined with marrow	Potential immunogenicity, no structural support, needs aspirated marrow
	Copios (Bone Void Filler) [52]	Zimmer, Personla Fit, Renewal Life.	Cap +Type I Collagen+BMP in DICAL	Found in paste and sponge, this substance is utilized as bone filler	Capable of being combined with bone marrow	Cannot be used in places that are subject to stress

These include Regenerative Medicine Advanced Therapy (RMAT), 510K clearance, Investigational Device Exemption/Premarket Approval (IDE/PMA), and human cells, tissues, and cellular and tissue-based products (HTC/P). A premarket submission known as the 510K procedure assesses if a device's safety and effectiveness are significantly equivalent to those of a product that is legally marketed [1]. The experimental device can be utilized in clinical research to gather efficacy and safety data because of IDE/PMA. The Premarket Approval is thereafter be supported by these data [2]. The Center for Biologics Evaluation and Research regulates HCT/Ps [2]. However, RMATs require an Investigational New Drug (IND) application, either new or current. Certain xenogeneic cell products and human gene treatments fall under this category [3]. Additionally, according to the FDA, medical devices are divided into three classes; Table 10.1 defines each type.

The following procedures apply to bone grafts, including synthetic, autologous cellular, and demineralized grafts used as fillers for bone void: For 510K clearance, minimal clinical investigations and animal or benchwork tests are needed [6]. Human clinical trial Level I IDE is necessary for premarket approval in order to approve grafts that fall within the category of Class III combinations of medical drugs and devices, such as P-15 (a synthetic amino-acid peptide), recombinant bone morphogenetic protein-2 (rhBMP-2), and rhBMP-2. However, the FDA does not conduct a premarket evaluation for HCT/P for bone grafts, and only some clinical and preclinical research is needed. Nonstructural and cellular-based allografts are two examples of transplant materials. Regenerative medicine devices, which are characterized as human cell and tissue products, therapeutic tissue engineering goods, cell therapy, or any combination product utilizing such products or therapies, are exempt from the RMAT pathway [3]. The currently available and registered bone graft from all types are presented in Table 10.2.

10.3 Enhancing Bone Regeneration with Bioactive Material

In 2002, Infuse BMP-2 was approved by the FDA for anterior lumbar interbody fusion [53], and in 2004, it was granted approval for treatment of tibial nonunion [54]. In 2007, the FDA approved its used as a substitute for autogenous bone grafts for sinus augmentations and targeted alveolar ridge augmentations for extraction socket defects [55]. The study found that employing BMP-2 produced better results than autografts and improved bone repair in smokers. While off-label use may cause edema and obstruct the patient's airway, there is also a danger of ectopic bone development.

Table 10.3 Summary of non-FDA commercially available bone graft and commonly used in Europe.

Type	Commercial name	Source	Potential risks
Xenograft	Geistlich's Bio-Oss [61]	Bovine bone	Bovine spongiform encephalopathy (BSE) X and transmissible spongiform encephalopathies (TSE) [62]
Xenograft	A-OSS	A deproteinized bovine bone graft	Bovine spongiform encephalopathy (BSE) X and transmissible spongiform encephalopathies (TSE)
Xenograft	Biotek's Bio-Gen	Equine bone graft	No known disease that humans can contract from horses
xenograft	MatrixOss CREST BIOLOGIC, Banglor	Porcine particulate materials with carbonate apatite	Transmissible spongiform encephalopathies (TSE) and bovine spongiform encephalopathy
Alloplast	Stryker's Hydroset [63–65]	Self-setting, calcium phosphate cement	Limited resorption rate
Xenograft+ Alloplast	IBI Smartbone® [66]	Bovine mineral bone matrix with bioresorbable polymers and collagen fragments	Bovine spongiform encephalopathy (BSE) X and transmissible spongiform encephalopathies (TSE)
Allograft	Osteocel Plus (ACE Southern [67]	Bone matrix that preserves osteoprogenitor cells and natural mesenchymal stem cells	Inflammatory side effects from off-label applications, varying levels of growth factors from various batches and manufacturers, and high costs

OP-1 (BMP 7): This device was approved for use in early 2000; however, the FDA approval was revoked in 2014. It was approved as a substitute to autograft in recalcitrant long bone non-unions if autograft is not practicable and other therapies have failed [56]. In 2004, it was approved for revision posterolateral lumbar fusion [57].

Augment bone graft is made up of beta-tricalcium phosphate and rhPDGF-BB. In 2015, it was authorized by the FDA for surgical ankle fusion (tibiotalar joint) and/or hindfoot (containing calcaneocuboid, subtalar, and talonavicular joints) [58].

GEM 21S: is likewise a combination of tricalcium phosphate and rhPDGF-Bb graft. In 2005, it was approved by the FDA for periodontal abnormalities like 1) furcation periodontal defects, 2) gingival recession linked to periodontal problems, and 3) intrabony periodontal defects [59].

iFactor is composed of P-15 suspended in a hydrogel carrier and adsorbed onto inorganic bone mineral [60]. The FDA has approved it in November 2015 for the reconstruction of a single-level cervical disc that has deteriorated from C3–C4 to C6–C7 following a single-level discectomy for intractable radiculopathy (arm pain and/or neurological deficit) when conservative treatment has failed.

Many products are utilized in Europe and around the world but are not approved in the United States. Approved products in Europe are termed Conformit é Europ éenne, which means European Conformity. One example of graft material that is popular worldwide but not in the United States is Geistlich's Bio-Oss product, which is detailed in Table 10.3. A-OSS, a deproteinized bovine bone graft, is another European conformity graft not commonly utilized in the US. In Europe, equine bone grafts like Biotek's Bio-gen have also been approved [61].

10.4 Conclusion

The chapter describes over 50 commercially available products that can be used as bone grafts or as adjuvant and bioactive materials. Although most generally available products are FDA approved, several products that are commonly used were approved in Europe but are not FDA approved.

AI disclosure statement: The author acknowledges the use of AI-based tools for minor language editing or grammatical correction. However, all intellectual contributions, analyses, and conclusions presented in this chapter are entirely the author's own.

References

1. U.S.Food.&.Drug Adminstration, Premarket notification 510(k)[July2, 2020]; Available from: https://www.fda.gov/medical-devices/premarket-submissions/premarke t-notification-510k, 2020.
2. U.S.Food.&.Drug Adminstration, Investigational device exemption (IDE) [July 2, 2020]; Available from: https://www.fda.gov/medical-devices/how-study-and-market- your-device/investigational-device-exemption-ide, 2019.
3. Vaggelas, and Seimetz, D., Expediting drug development: FDA's new regenerative medicine advanced therapy designation. *Ther. Innov. Regul. Sci.*, 53, 3, 364–373, 2019.
4. Gupta, S.K., Medical device regulations: a current perspective. *J. Young Pharm.*, 8, 1, 2016.
5. Schlauderaff, and Boyer, K.C., An overview of Food and Drug Administration medical device legislation and interplay with current medical practices. *Cureus*, 11, 5, e4627, 2019.
6. Abjornson, Brecevich, A., Callanan, T., Dowe, C., Cammisa, F.P., Lorio, M.P., ISASS recommendations and coverage criteria for bone graft substitutes used in spinal surgery. *Int. J. Spine Surg.*, 12, 6, 757–771, 2018.
7. Kapur, R.A., Amirfeyz, R., Wylde, V., *et al.*, Clinical outcomes and fusion success associated with the use of BoneSave in spinal surgery. *Arch. Orthop. Trauma Surg.*, 130, 641–647, 2010, https://doi.org/10.1007/s00402-009-0936-3.
8. Dickson, Kyle, F., *et al.*, The use of BoneSource hydroxyapatite cement for traumatic metaphyseal bone void filling. *J. Trauma*, 53, 6, 1103–8, 2002, doi: 10.1097/00005373-200212000-00012.
9. Cassidy, C., *et al.*, Norian SRS cement compared with conventional fixation in distal radial fractures. A randomized study. *J. Bone Joint Surg. Am.*, 85, 11, 2127–37, 2003, doi: 10.2106/00004623-200311000-00010.
10. Procter, P., Hulsart-Billström, G., Alves, A., Pujari-Palmer, M., Wenner, D., Insley, G., Engqvist, H., Larsson, S., Gluing Living Bone Using a Biomimetic Bioadhesive: From Initial Cut to Final Healing. *Front. Bioeng. Biotechnol.*, 9, 728042, 2021 Nov 8, doi: 10.3389/fbioe.2021.728042. PMID: 34820360; PMCID: PMC8606677.
11. Gilula, L. and Persenaire, M., Subsequent fractures post–vertebral augmentation: Analysis of a prospective randomized trial in osteoporotic vertebral compression fractures. *Am. J. Neuroradiol.*, 34, 1, 221–7, 2013 Jan 1.
12. Zhou, H. and Yu, B., Using of injectable bio-degradable calcium sulfate as bone graft substitute in the treatment of periarticular fractures. *Int. J. Clin. Exp. Med.*, 9, 11, 21645–53, 2016 Jan 1.
13. Yao, J. and Ho, A.M., Bone graft substitutes in the treatment of distal radius and upper limb injuries. *Oper. Tech. Orthop.*, 19, 2, 77–87, 2009 Apr 1.
14. Grafe, I.A., Baier, M., Nöldge, G., *et al.*, Calcium-Phosphate and Polymethylmethacrylate Cement in Long-term Outcome after Kyphoplasty

of Painful Osteoporotic Vertebral Fractures. *Spine*, 33, 11, 1284–1290, May 15, 2008, DOI: 10.1097/BRS.0b013e3181714a84.

15. Arora, R., Milz, S., Sprecher, C., Sitte, I., Blauth, M., Lutz, M., Behaviour of ChronOS™ Inject in metaphyseal bone defects of distal radius fractures: Tissue reaction after 6–15 months. *Injury*, 43, 10, 1683–8, 2012 Oct 1.
16. Van Lieshout, E.M., Van Kralingen, G.H., El-Massoudi, Y., Weinans, H., Patka, P., Microstructure and biomechanical characteristics of bone substitutes for trauma and orthopaedic surgery. *BMC Musculoskelet. Disord.*, 12, 1–4, 2011 Dec.
17. Huber, F.X., Belyaev, O., Hillmeier, J., Kock, H.J., Huber, C., Meeder, P.J., Berger, I., First histological observations on the incorporation of a novel nanocrystalline hydroxyapatite paste OSTIM® in human cancellous bone. *BMC Musculoskelet. Disord.*, 7, 1–4, 2006 Dec.
18. Bhattacharjee, A., Kuiper, J.H., Roberts, S., Harrison, P.E., Cassar-Pullicino, V.N., Tins, B., Bajada, S., Richardson, J.B., Predictors of fracture healing in patients with recalcitrant nonunions treated with autologous culture expanded bone marrow-derived mesenchymal stromal cells. *J. Orthop. Res.*,® 37, 6, 1303–9, 2019 Jun.
19. Kucera, T., *et al.*, Histological assessment of tissue from large human bone defects repaired with β-tricalcium phosphate. *Eur. J. Orthop. Surg. Traumatol. Orthop. Traumatol.*, 24, 8, 1357–65, 2014, doi: 10.1007/s00590-013-1329-4.
20. Zijderveld, S.A., Zerbo, I.R., van den Bergh, J., Schulten, E., Bruggenkate, C.M., Maxillary Sinus Floor Augmentation Using a β3-Tricalcium Phosphate (Cerasorb) Alone Compared to Autogenous Bone Grafts. *Int. J. Oral Maxillofac. Implants*, 20, 3, 432–40, 2005 May 1.
21. Bonardi, J.P., dos Santos Pereira, R., Lima, F.B., Faverani, L.P., Griza, G.L., Okamoto, R., Hochuli-Vieira, E., Prospective and randomized evaluation of ChronOS and Bio-Oss in human maxillary sinuses: histomorphometric and immunohistochemical assignment for RUNX 2, vascular endothelial growth factor, and osteocalcin. *J. Oral Maxillofac. Surg.*, 76, 2, 325–35, 2018 Feb 1.
22. Meadows, G.R., Adjunctive use of ultraporous β-tricalcium phosphate bone void filler in spinal arthrodesis. *Orthopedics*, 25, 5 Suppl., s579–s584, 2002.
23. Frenken, J.W., Bouwman, W.F., Bravenboer, N., Zijderveld, S.A., Schulten, E.A., Ten Bruggenkate, C.M., The use of Straumann® Bone Ceramic in a maxillary sinus floor elevation procedure: a clinical, radiological, histological and histomorphometric evaluation with a 6-month healing period. *Clin. Oral Implants Res.*, 21, 2, 201–8, 2010 Feb.
24. Zgoda, M., Osman, M.K., Thornhill, C., Calcium sulphate pellets (Osteoset®) improve bone graft incorporation, but not femoral head sphericity after shelf acetabuloplasty for Perthes' disease. *J. Orthop. Trauma Rehab.*, 31, 2, 207–15, 2024 Dec.
25. Clayer, M., Injectable form of calcium sulphate as treatment of aneurysmal bone cysts. *ANZ J. Surg.*, 78, 5, 366–70, 2008 May.

26. Müller-Goebel, J.M., Bächinger, D., Röösli, C., Huber, A., Dalbert, A., Efficacy of Calcium Sulfate Antibiotic Carriers in the Treatment of Severe Infections of the Temporal Bone. *Otol. Neurotol. Open*, 4, 3, e061, 2024 Sep 1.
27. Bolger, C., Jones, D., Czop, S., Evaluation of an increased strut porosity silicate-substituted calcium phosphate, SiCaP EP, as a synthetic bone graft substitute in spinal fusion surgery: a prospective, open-label study. *Eur. Spine J.*, 28, 1733–1742, 2019, https://doi.org/10.1007/s00586-019-05926-1.
28. Krause, K.L., DeDeaux, C., Jung, E., Than, K.D., Two-level reverse Bohlman transsoseous approach for treatment of symptomatic pseudarthrosis. *Br. J. Neurosurg.*, 33, 1, 84–7, 2019 Jan 2.
29. Jiranek, W.A., Hanssen, A.D., Greenwald, A.S., Antibiotic-loaded bone cement for infection prophylaxis in total joint replacement. *JBJS*, 88, 11, 2487–500, 2006 Nov 1.
30. Wähnert, D., Grüneweller, N., Gueorguiev, B., Vordemvenne, T., Gehweiler, D., Removal of cement-augmented screws in distal femoral fractures and the effect of retained screws and cement on total knee arthroplasty: a biomechanical investigation. *J. Orthop. Traumatol.*, 22, 1–8, 2021 Dec.
31. Theologis, A.A., Patel, S., Burch, S., Radiographic comparison of L5–S1 lateral anterior lumbar interbody fusion cage subsidence and displacement by fixation strategy: anterior plate versus integrated screws. *J. Neurosurg. Spine*, 38, 1, 126–30, 2022 Sep 2.
32. Nath, C. and Naskar, S., Lumbar and Lumbo-Sacral Spine Implants, in: *Handbook of Orthopaedic Trauma Implantology*, pp. 1–30, Springer Nature Singapore, Singapore, 2022 Nov 26.
33. DiGiovanni, C.W., Baumhauer, J., Lin, S.S., *et al.*, Prospective, Randomized, Multi-Center Feasibility Trial of rhPDGF-BB versus Autologous Bone Graft in a Foot and Ankle Fusion Model. *Foot Ankle Int.*, 32, 4, 344–354, 2011.
34. Carter, J.D., Swearingen, A.B., Chaput, C.D., Rahm, M.D., Clinical and radiographic assessment of transforaminal lumbar interbody fusion using HEALOS collagen-hydroxyapatite sponge with autologous bone marrow aspirate. *Spine J.*, 9, 6, 434–438, 2009.
35. Elshafey, M.M., Tarek, Z.M., Fahmy, R.A., Piezosurgical Buccal Plate Repositioning Technique: A Modified Surgical Approach for the Horizontal Augmentation of Atrophied Mandibles. *Int. J. Oral Maxillofac. Implants*, 39, 1, 57–64, 2024 Feb 27, doi: 10.11607/jomi.10427. PMID: 37910834.
36. Masala, S., Nano, G., Marcia, S., Muto, M., Fucci, F.P.M., Simonetti, G., Osteoporotic vertebral compression fractures augmentation by injectable partly resorbable ceramic bone substitute (CERAMENT (™)|SPINE SUPPORT): a prospective nonrandomized study. *Neuroradiology*, 54, 6, 589–596, 2012, available at: WOS:000304399700007.
37. Franceschini, M., Di Matteo, A., Âsebeck, H., Bchner, H., Vogt, S., Treatment of a chronic recurrent fistulized tibial osteomyelitis: administration of a novel antibiotic-loaded bone substitute combined with a pedicular muscle

flap sealing. *Eur. J. Orthop. Surg. Traumatol.*, 22, 1, 245–249, 2012, available at: http://dx.doi.org/10.1007/s00590-012-0956-5.
38. Khan, S.N., Fraser, J.F., Sandhu, H.S., Cammisa, F.P., Girardi, F.P., Lane, J.M., Use of osteopromotive growth factors, demineralized bone matrix, and ceramics to enhance spinal fusion. *J. Am. Acad. Orthop. Surg.*, 13, 2, 129–137, 2005, available from: WOS:000228355000006.
39. Bostrom, M.P.G. and Lane, J.M., Future directions - Augmentation of osteoporotic vertebral bodies. *Spine*, 22, 24, 38S–42S, 1997, available at: WOS:000071145000007.
40. Ransford, A.O., Morley, T., Edgar, M.A., Webb, P., Passuti, N., Chopin, D., Morin, C., Michel, F., Garin, C., Pries, D., Synthetic porous ceramic compared with autograft in scoliosis surgery - A prospective, randomised study of 341 patients. *J. Bone Joint Surg.-Br.*, 80B, 1, 13–18, 1998, available at: WOS:000071622000004.
41. Obert, L., Lepage, D., Gasse, N., Rochet, S., Garbuio, P., Extra-articular distal radius malunion: The phosphate cement alternative. *Orthop. Traumatol.-Surg. Res.*, 96, 5, 574–578, 2010, available at: WOS:000282592000013.
42. Heo, H.D., Cho, Y.J., Sheen, S.H., Kuh, S.U., Cho, S.M., Oh, S.M., Morphological changes of injected calcium phosphate cement in osteoporotic compressed vertebral bodies. *Osteoporos. Int.*, 20, 12, 2063–2070, 2009.
43. Teufack, S., Harrop, J., Prasad, S., Bone Graft Extenders, in: *Minimally Invasive Spinal Deformity Surgery*, M.Y. Wang, *et al.* (Eds.), pp. 337–345, Springer Vienna, 2014. https://scholar.google.com/scholar?hl=en&as_sdt=0%2C5&q=-Teufack%2C+S.%2C+Harrop%2C+J.%2C+Prasad%2C+S.%2C+-Bone+Graft+Extenders%2C+in%3A+Minimally+Invasive+Spinal+Deformity+Surgery%2C+M.Y.+Wang%2C+et+al.+%28Eds.%29%2C+pp.+337%E2%80%93345%2C+Springer+Vienna%2C+2014.&btnG=.
44. Friesenbichler, J., Maurer-Ertl, W., Sadoghi, P., Pirker-Fruehauf, U., Bodo, K., Leithner, A., Adverse Reactions of Artificial Bone Graft Substitutes: Lessons Learned From Using Tricalcium Phosphate geneX®. *Clin. Orthop. Relat. Res.*, 472, 3, 976–982, March 2014. DOI: 10.1007/s11999-013-3305-z.
45. Wessing, B., Emmerich, M., Bozkurt, A., Horizontal ridge augmentation with a novel resorbable collagen membrane: a retrospective analysis of 36 consecutive patients. *Int. J. Periodontics Restorative Dent.*, 36, 2, 179–187, 2016.
46. Li, S.T., Yuen, D., Martin, D., Lee, N.S., A comparative study of a new porcine collagen membrane to Bio-Gide®. Science, Technology, Innovation, pp. 1–5, 2015.
47. Nevins, M., Parma-Benfenati, S., Janke, U.W., Kleyer, A., Rasperini, G., Tinti, C., Schupbach, P., Kim, D.M., The efficacy of mineralized allograft cortical and cancellous chips in maxillary sinus augmentations. *Int. J. Periodontics Restorative Dent.*, 34, 6, 789–93, 2014 Nov-Dec, doi: 10.11607/prd.1720. PMID: 25411734.

48. Jo, S.H., Kim, Y.-K., Choi, Y.-H., Histological Evaluation of the Healing Process of Various Bone Graft Materials after Engraftment into the Human Body. *Materials, 11*, 714–721, 2018, https://doi.org/10.3390/ma11050714.
49. Khorsand, A., Soleimani Shayesteh, Y., Pour, T., Negaresh, A.H., A clinical and radiographical evaluation on the treatment of grade II furcation involvement of mandibular molars by demineralized bone matrix (Dynagraft) as compared with coronally positioned flap (CPF). *J. Dent. Med.*, 17, 1, 19–25, 2004 Apr 10.
50. Shapiro, S.A., Case Presentation: Full Mouth Implant Treatment *Via* a Trio of Modalities. *Dent. Implantol. Update*, 22, 12, 81–8, 2011.
51. Ilan, D.I. and Ladd, A.L., Bone graft substitutes. *Operative Tech. Plast. Reconstr. Surg.*, 9, 4, 151–60, 2002 Nov 1.
52. Bongio, M., van den Beucken, J.J., Leeuwenburgh, S.C., Jansen, J.A., Development of bone substitute materials: from 'biocompatible' to 'instructive'. *J. Mater. Chem.*, 20, 40, 8747–8759, 2010, available at: WOS:000282518200003.
53. Carreira, A.C., Lojudice, F.H., Halcsik, E., Navarro, R.D., Sogayar, Granjeiro, J.M., Bone morphogenetic proteins: facts, challenges, and future perspectives. *J. Dent. Res.*, 93, 4, 335–345, 2014.
54. James, W., LaChaud, G., Shen, J., Asatrian, G., Nguyen, V., Zhang, X., Ting, K., Soo, C., A review of the clinical side effects of bone morphogenetic protein-2. *Tissue Eng. B Rev.*, 22, 4, 284–297, 2016.
55. Suárez-López Del Amo, F., Monje, A., Padial-Molina, M., Tang, Z., Wang, H.L., Biologic Agents for Periodontal Regeneration and Implant Site Development. *Biomed Res. Int.*, 2015, 957518, 2015, doi: 10.1155/2015/957518. Epub 2015 Oct 5. PMID: 26509173; PMCID: PMC4609805.
56. Ong, K.L., Villarraga, M.L., Lau, E., Carreon, L.Y., Kurtz, S.M., Glassman, S.D., Off- label use of bone morphogenetic proteins in the United States using administrative data. *Spine (Phila Pa 1976)*, 35, 19, 1794–1800, 2010. DOI: 10.1097/BRS.0b013e3181ecf6e4. https://journals.lww.com/spinejournal/abstract/2010/09010/off_label_use_of_bone_morphogenetic_proteins_in.10.aspx.
57. White, A.P., Vaccaro, A.R., Hall, J.A., Whang, P.G., Friel, B.C., McKee, M.D., Clinical applications of BMP-7/OP-1 in fractures, nonunions and spinal fusion. *Int. Orthop.*, 31, 6, 735–741, 2007.
58. Augment bone graft summary of safety and effectiveness data (SSED), Available at: https://www.accessdata.fda.gov/cdrh_docs/pdf10/p100006b.pdf, June 26, 2020.
59. Hench, L.L. and West, J.K., *Biological Applications of Bioactive Glasses*, Harwood Academic Publishers, 1996.
60. Arnold, P.M., Sasso, R.C., Janssen, M.E., Fehlings, M.G., Heary, R.F., Vaccaro, A.R., Kopjar, B., I-factor bone graft vs. autograft in anterior cervical discectomy and fusion: 2-year follow-up of the randomized single-blinded

Food and Drug Administration investigational device exemption study. *Neurosurgery*, 83, 3, 377–384, 2018.
61. Gokhale, S.T. and Dwarakanath, C.D., The use of a natural osteoconductive porous bone mineral (Bio-Oss) in infrabony periodontal defects. *J. Indian Soc. Periodontol.*, 16, 2, 247–252, 2012.
62. Kim, Y., Nowzari, H., Rich, S.K., Risk of prion disease transmission through bovine- derived bone substitutes: a systematic review. *Clin. Implant Dent. Relat. Res.*, 15, 5, 645–653, 2013.
63. Moroni, A., Hoang-Kim, A., Lio, V., Giannini, S., Current augmentation fixation techniques for the osteoporotic patient. *Scand. J. Surg.*, 95, 2, 103–109, 2006.
64. Sallent, I., Capella-Monsonís, H., Procter, P., Bozo, I.Y., Deev, R.V., Zubov, D., Vasyliev, R., Perale, G., Pertici, G., Baker, J., Gingras, P., Bayon, Y., Zeugolis, D.I., The few who made it: commercially and clinically successful innovative bone grafts. *Front. Bioeng. Biotechnol.*, 8, 952, 2020.
65. DeKeyser, G.J., Kellam, P.J., Haller, J.M., Locked plating and advanced augmentation techniques in osteoporotic fractures. *Orthop. Clin. North Am.*, 50, 159–169, 2019, doi: 10.1016/j.ocl.2018.12.002.
66. Taschieri, S., Ofer, M., Corbella, S., Testori, T., Dellavia, C., Nemcovsky, C., Canciani, E., Francetti, L., Del Fabbro, M., Tartaglia, G., The Influence of Residual Alveolar Bone Height on Graft Composition after Maxillary Sinus Augmentation Using Two Different Xenografts: A Histomorphometric Comparative Study. *Materials*, 13, 5093, 2020, https://doi.org/10.3390/ma13225093.
67. Grabowski, G. and Robertson, R.N., Bone allograft with mesenchymal stem cells: A critical review of the literature. *Hard Tissue*, 2, 2, 20–29, 2013 Mar 22.
68. Kudsi, R., Dawson, D.R., Gonzalez, O.A., Kutkut, A., Tucci, M.A., Porras-Aguilar, R., Momox, A.E., Al-Sabbagh, M., Relationship between bone quality and shrinkage in maxillary sinus augmentation using synthetic alloplast versus xenograft. J Periodontal Implant Sci., 55, 4, 306–320, 2025 Aug. doi: 10.5051/jpis.2401320066. Epub 2024 Dec 2. PMID: 40047187; PMCID: PMC12411137.

11

Graft Materials Used for Facial Rejuvenation and the Evidence

Hourya Alnofaie[1]* and Nasser Asiri[2]

[1]*Oral and Maxillofacial Surgery Division, Basic Dental Sciences Department, College of Dentistry, Princess Nourah Bint Abdulrahman University, Riyadh, Saudi Arabia*
[2]*Oral and Maxillofacial Surgery, Sama Poly Clinic, Riyadh, Saudi Arabia*

Abstract
Facial rejuvenation often necessitates restoring facial contours and volume lost due to aging, trauma, or congenital anomalies. Onlay bone grafts have become a cornerstone in craniofacial reconstruction, offering structural support and aesthetic enhancement. This chapter provides an in-depth analysis of various onlay bone graft materials—including titanium, porous polyethylene (Medpor), polysiloxane, and polyetheretherketone (PEEK)—evaluating their clinical efficacy, levels of evidence, FDA approval status, advantages, disadvantages, and associated complications. The discussion is supported by a comprehensive review of current literature, encompassing clinical studies, systematic reviews, and case series.

***Keywords*:** Facial rejuvenation, onlay bone grafts, facial implant, silicone, PEEK

11.1 Introduction

Restoration of facial structures and functions following trauma, tumor resection, infection, or congenital skeletal deformities remains a cornerstone of maxillofacial surgical practice. In addition to functional rehabilitation, aesthetic enhancement particularly in the context of age-related changes has become increasingly significant. Common age-associated concerns such as volume depletion, disharmony in facial proportions,

**Corresponding author*: Hsalnofaie@pnu.edu.sa

Randa A. Alfotawi (ed.) Oro-Facial Bone Grafts and Biomaterials, (229–246) © 2026 Scrivener Publishing LLC

and diminished contour definition can be effectively addressed through augmentation techniques utilizing autologous tissue, allogeneic grafts, or synthetic implants. These aesthetic alterations often stem from well-documented skeletal changes, notably a reduction in anterior projection and volume loss in the maxilla and mandible [1].

For aesthetic enhancement, facial implants are most frequently utilized to augment key skeletal regions including the malar prominence, chin, and the mandibular angle or ramus [2]. The types of onlay bone graft for facial rejuvenation or reconstructions divide largely into two main sections, which are (1) autologous tissues such as bone, cartilages, and fat; and (2) alloplastic materials. Facial rejuvenation using alloplastic materials has gained prominence as a preferred alternative to autologous grafting, owing to their favorable safety profile and the elimination of donor site morbidity and associated complications. They include a variety of materials, including metals, ceramics such as hydroxyapatite, and several classes of polymers. Frequently used polymeric materials include polysiloxane (silicone), porous polyethylene (Medpor), polytetrafluoroethylene (Gore-Tex), and polymethylmethacrylate (PMMA) [3]. Of these options, silicone and Medpor implants are among the most widely adopted in contemporary practice [2, 4]. While autologous grafts have long been considered the gold standard guided by the principle of replacing "like with like", they carry notable disadvantages [4]. These include donor site morbidity, longer operative durations, and the potential for graft resorption or remodeling, which may negatively affect the durability and predictability of aesthetic outcomes [4].

Historically, facial reconstruction has been grounded in the use of autologous bone grafts, which were considered the gold standard due to their inherent osteoconductive, osteoinductive, and osteogenic properties [5]. Common donor sites included the rib, iliac crest, and calvarium [5]. Despite their biological advantages, autografts presented several drawbacks, including donor site morbidity, variable and often unpredictable resorption rates, and prolonged operative times [6]. These limitations prompted the search for alternative materials with fewer complications and more predictable outcomes. By the 1980s, synthetic and alloplastic substitutes began to gain traction [7–10]. Titanium, one of the earliest metals adopted, was valued for its mechanical strength, excellent biocompatibility, and integration [10]. This was followed by the introduction of porous polyethylene (Medpor) in the 1990s and polyetheretherketone (PEEK) in the early 2000s [11–13]. Each of these materials contributed uniquely to the advancement of facial skeletal reconstruction, with growing emphasis on long-term durability, radiologic visibility, ease of contouring, and improved aesthetic integration.

Alloplastic facial implants have been well established in the literature as a dependable method for enhancing facial skeletal contours and restoring symmetry. They offer a predictable and effective approach to facial augmentation, with a relatively low incidence of complications reported across a range of implant materials [14]. This consistent safety and efficacy profile has contributed to their widespread acceptance in both reconstructive and aesthetic facial surgery.

The objective of this chapter is to provide a comprehensive review of the currently available alloplastic materials utilized in facial rejuvenation procedures. Each material will be examined with respect to its regulatory status, including U.S. Food and Drug Administration (FDA) approval, as well as its clinical indications, contraindications, and biomechanical and aesthetic advantages. Potential disadvantages and limitations associated with each material will also be critically discussed, with the aim of guiding clinicians in selecting the most appropriate graft type based on patient-specific anatomical and aesthetic needs.

11.2 Types of Alloplastic Graft Materials

11.2.1 Titanium

Titanium remains one of the most widely used materials in craniofacial surgery, effectively replacing earlier materials such as stainless steel and cobalt–chromium alloys [15]. This shift is largely attributed to titanium's optimal balance of mechanical strength, biocompatibility, integrability, and imaging compatibility, particularly its reduced artifact production on computed tomography and its safety in magnetic resonance imaging environments [15]. A key feature of titanium is its natural resistance to corrosion, which results from the formation of a stable oxide layer upon exposure to oxygen [15]. This thin film of titanium oxide acts as a protective shield, preserving the implant's integrity once placed within the body [15]. Furthermore, titanium exhibits the unique capacity for osseointegration, allowing for direct molecular interaction and bonding with adjacent bone tissue [16]. This property significantly enhances titanium implant stability and long-term success in reconstructive procedures [16], which makes it suitable for structural facial support, orbital floor reconstruction, malar augmentation, and mandibular reconstruction [17–19].

Considering its rigidity and stability characterized by an elastic modulus significantly higher than that of native bone that makes titanium ideal for rigid fixation in craniofacial trauma and reconstruction, this makes it ideal for load-bearing applications [20]. However, these same mechanical properties render it less suitable for facial augmentation in aesthetic applications [21]. The use of titanium hardware in craniofacial surgery has been extensively studied, with complication rates varying based on the anatomical site. For example, titanium plates used in mandibular reconstruction exhibit relatively high complication rates, including a 14% incidence of infection and up to 20% requiring plate removal [3]. One notable drawback is the potential for a "stress shielding" effect, whereby the implant's rigidity reduces the physiological load on the surrounding bone [22]. This can result in progressive resorption and weakening of the native bone, potentially leading to implant loosening over time [22]. Despite its favorable attributes, titanium may become visible beneath thin skin, particularly in regions such as the periorbital area, leading to undesirable aesthetic outcomes [23]. Additional limitations include patient-reported discomfort due to thermal sensitivity, as titanium's high thermal conductivity can cause a persistent sensation of cold in the implant area, often necessitating its removal [23]. Titanium implants are FDA-approved and extensively validated through both experimental and clinical studies [24].

11.2.2 Silicone

Silicone remains one of the most extensively used materials in facial implantology due to its favorable biocompatibility and ease of use [21]. It is described as polydimethylsiloxane, smooth, nonporous. The behavior and characteristics of silicone polymers vary depending on the degree of polymerization and the extent of crosslinking between polymer chains [21]. Through vulcanization, a process that enhances chain length and crosslinking density, silicone can be converted into more viscous and structurally stable forms [21]. As a result, it is available in multiple consistencies, including solid, gel, and liquid, each tailored to specific surgical applications [21]. Solid silicone implants have gained widespread acceptance in facial reconstructive and aesthetic surgery due to their long-term biocompatibility, structural stability, and versatility in contour augmentation [25]. Unlike injectable silicone—which is explicitly disapproved by the U.S. Food and Drug Administration (FDA) for cosmetic use due to its association with serious adverse outcomes including granuloma formation, soft tissue necrosis, embolization, and systemic inflammatory responses—solid silicone implants have been cleared for clinical use under the FDA's 510(k) regulatory framework [26]. These medical-grade silicone elastomer implants are manufactured in standardized and patient-specific forms, allowing for tailored augmentation of the chin, malar regions, nasal dorsum, and other facial subunits [27]. Silicone implants offer several advantages including a greater degree of augmentation, ease of carving and removal, lower early risk of infection, and affordability [3, 28]. However, disadvantages include the potential for chronic inflammatory response with capsule formation, implant mobility leading to seroma or chronic peri-implantitis, risk of extrusion, bone resorption, and an increased likelihood of late infection [3, 28]. When implanted, silicone tends to become encapsulated within a fibrous capsule rather than integrating into host tissues. While this encapsulation facilitates straightforward implant removal when needed, it can also contribute to complications such as seroma formation, implant displacement, extrusion, and unsatisfactory aesthetic outcomes [21]. These same properties, however, have made silicone particularly suitable for procedures like breast reconstruction, where removability and contour flexibility are advantageous. In the context of facial augmentation, complications associated with silicone implants include implant migration, pressure-induced bony resorption, and soft tissue visibility of the fibrous capsule [2]. A review examining silicone use for malar, chin, and mandibular augmentation reported a complication rate of 5%, with infection occurring in 2.2% of cases and bone resorption noted in up to 55% of patients [2]. Approximately 4.1% required reoperation for implant removal [2]. A broader meta-analysis involving 443 patients demonstrated an infection rate of just 1.6%, with an overall low incidence of adverse outcomes [14]. Silicone also showed a relatively low rate of unsatisfactory cosmetic results of 2.7% when compared to other materials like Medpor [14]. However, data from Rubin and Yaremchuk revealed that silicone implants had a higher rate of removal due to complications, with an incidence of 11.7%, compared to 0.5% for porous polyethylene and 1.3% for hydroxyapatite implants [4].

Notable FDA-cleared devices include the Perma Facial Implant® by SurgiSil and the Customized Contour Implant series by Implantech Associates, both of which are indicated for soft tissue augmentation and correction of congenital or acquired craniofacial deficiencies [29, 30]. It is imperative that clinicians distinguish between approved solid implants and liquid silicone injections, the latter of which remains prohibited for aesthetic indications due to unacceptably high complication rates and lack of regulatory approval [26]. Example of solid silicone used for facial rejuvenation is shown in Figures 11.1 and 11.2.

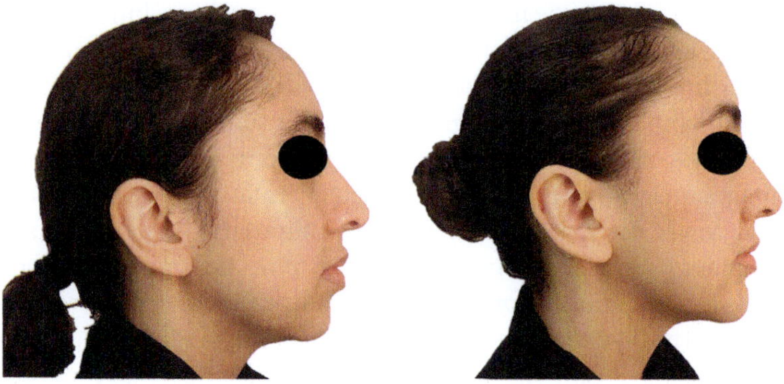

(a) (b)

Figure 11.1 Chin deficiency case managed with chin silicone implant. (a) Preoperative photograph of the patient. (b) Postoperative photograph of the patient.

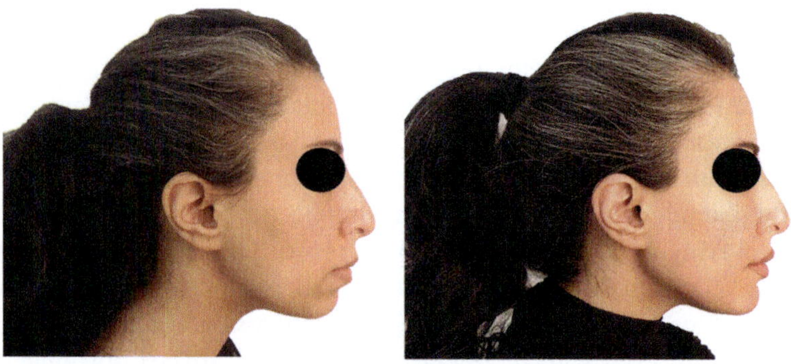

(a) (b)

Figure 11.2 Case of malar hypoplasia, chin deficiency with undefined facial features managed with malar and mandibular angle silicone implants in addition to genioplasty. (a) Preoperative photograph of the patient. (b) Postoperative photograph of the patient.

11.2.3 Porous Polyethylene (PE) [Medpor]

Polyethylene is a commonly used polymer in facial rejuvenation, offering a range of consistencies and mechanical strength depending on its formulation [25]. Polyethylene (Medpor, Porex Surgical, Inc.) is a high-density porous polyethylene implant characterized by relatively large pore sizes (100–300 μm), which facilitate substantial fibrous tissue ingrowth over time [31]. Unlike silicone, Medpor's pore structure promotes tissue integration rather than fibrous encapsulation, resulting in improved implant stability [32]. A key benefit is its flexibility and ability to be tailored, enabling surgeons to adapt it precisely to the patient's anatomical structure [32]. Clinical studies show high patient satisfaction and low complication rates when Medpor is used in well-vascularized areas [32]. However, there is reported complication.

Porous polyethylene implants, such as medpor most used in microtia reconstruction, chin, and malar augmentation [2]. It can be shaped intraoperatively to meet patient-specific needs and is usually secured with screws [32]. However, due to tissue ingrowth, their removal is more challenging than that of silicone implants—a characteristic that is advantageous in applications like microtia reconstruction [33]. Medpor offers several advantages in facial reconstruction, most notably its ability to support fibrous tissue ingrowth, which promotes stable integration with the surrounding anatomy [2]. Its radiolucent properties also make it compatible with postoperative imaging, including CT and MRI, without causing significant artifact [2]. However, these same features can present challenges [2]. The porous structure that allows for incorporation can make implant removal technically difficult, particularly in revision cases [2]. Additionally, some patients may experience thermal sensitivity due to the material's conductivity, which can lead to discomfort in certain environments [2].

When used in areas such as the cheeks, chin, and jawline, Medpor implants demonstrated a low complication profile, with infection occurring in only 0.7% of cases [14]. Approximately 5% of patients required implant removal or revision surgery, and 3.9% experienced noticeable or excessive prominence—slightly higher than the 1.4% reported for silicone in comparable sites [14]. Eighteen out of 285 cases (6.3%) reported Medpor implant failure when it is placed in the nose, maxilla, and ear [34]. Also, infection rate was 3–4% in rhinoplasty cases involving Medpor [35]. Su-kyung Jung *et al.* reported that the most common complication for orbital implants was blepharoptosis at 10.5% when grafted with Medpor, followed by exposure and infection [36]. Similarly, extrusion rates ranging from 3.1% to as high as 21% were reported [37, 38]. Additionally, 12.5% infection was reported when Medpor implant is used for zygoma and angle of mandible [39]. A larger meta-analysis examining outcomes across all facial zones reported an overall infection rate of 1.2%, while suboptimal aesthetic results were observed in about 5% of patients [14].

Medpor implants are FDA-cleared for various facial reconstructive applications. These include augmentation and restoration of craniofacial defects, such as post-traumatic or congenital deformities, and specific uses like chin prostheses, orbital floor repair, and prevention of temporal hollowing [40]. For instance, the Stryker CMF MEDPOR Customized Implant was cleared under FDA 510(k) number K153508, and the MEDPOR TITAN 3D Orbital Floor Implant was cleared under K142568 [40, 41]. These approvals confirm Medpor's regulatory status for facial skeletal use.

11.2.4 Polyetheretherketone (PEEK)

Polyetheretherketone (PEEK) is a durable polymer that has gained widespread use in craniofacial, spinal, and cranial vault surgeries. It is favored for its excellent biocompatibility, strong mechanical properties, and minimal artifact production on CT and MRI imaging due to its radiolucent nature. Personalized, computer-designed PEEK implants have shown high success rates in cranial applications, with consistently low rates of postoperative complications [42]. Evidence from smaller clinical studies has demonstrated that PEEK onlay implants may gradually integrate with surrounding bone, showing early signs of osseointegration in some cases [43]. Experimental data also suggest that titanium-coated PEEK implants offer enhanced bone integration compared to uncoated forms, indicating a promising direction for improving implant–host interaction [43]. Clinically, customized PEEK devices have been used to correct a variety of facial defects [44]. However, infection rates in some reports have reached 8%, which is slightly higher than rates seen with alternative materials [45]. This may be due to PEEK's tendency to promote bacterial colonization and biofilm development [22]. A study by Sarfraz *et al.* compared microbial adhesion on PEEK versus titanium surfaces, both with and without salivary exposure. Results revealed that salivary coating facilitated bacterial binding in general, with PEEK demonstrating a higher affinity for bacterial attachment than titanium [22]. In clinical practice, surface modification strategies have been adopted to counter this, and therefore, it became one of the most used implant materials nowadays. Coating PEEK with hydroxyapatite has improved both osseointegration and fixation outcomes [46]. Other promising bioactive coatings—such as bioglass (calcium sodium phosphosilicate) and β-tricalcium phosphate—are also under evaluation for their ability to enhance implant integration [47].

A special advantage of PEEK is its radiolucency, which refers to radiological imaging transparency [48]. This provides a definite postoperative assessment, which frees the artefacts typically presented by metallic implants. In biomechanics, the elastic modulus of PEEK is reproductive of cortical bone [48]. This congruence reduces the implant–implant stress shielding and adjacent bony structures, the path towards increased osseointegration and long-term stability [48]. One of the major advantages of PEEK is that it is extremely user-friendly in surgery [48]. In comparison to most implant materials characterized by their inherent stiffness, PEEK allows for intraoperative flexibility [48]. This flexibility allows for precision individualized to the particular anatomical variation of the patient, thereby enabling technique for better aesthetic and functional results [48].

Tissue compatibility-wise, PEEK implants in my experience have exhibited very good biocompatibility, with little inflammation or foreign body reactions in surrounding tissue [48]. Briefly, PEEK possesses some distinctive characteristics and is supported by clinical evidence and a superior option for craniofacial surgical use [48]. Its imaging strengths, biomechanical compatibility, intraoperative pliability, and tissue tolerance highlight its superiority as an option of preference in this context [48]. It became more popular due to its ability to be fabricated specifically to the patient's defect, also known as, patient-specific implants (PSIs), where it provides accuracy and satisfaction [43, 44]. PEEK has received FDA approval for its use in medical applications [49]. Examples of PEEK to reconstruct facial defects in syndromic patients are shown in Figures 11.3 and 11.4.

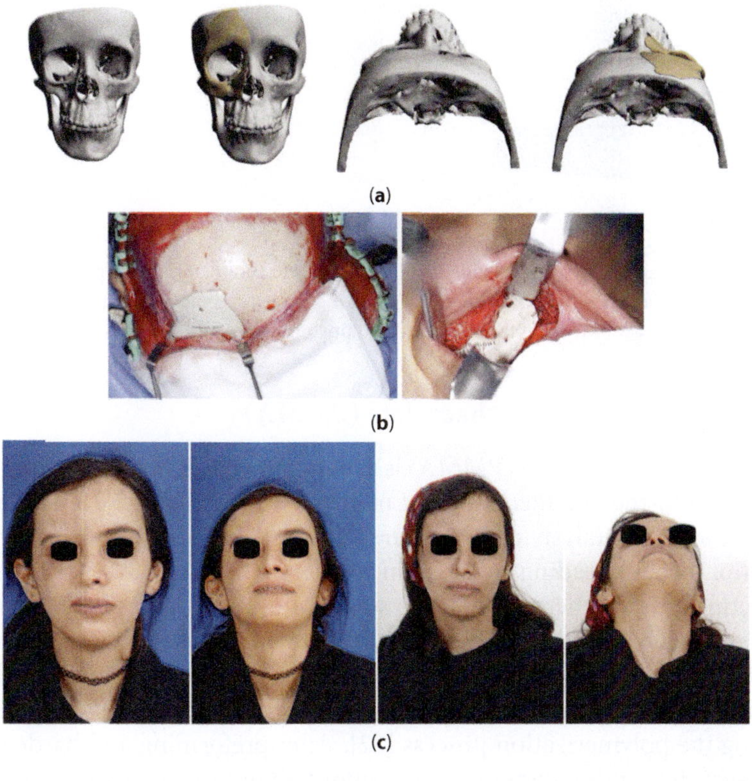

(a)

(b)

(c)

Figure 11.3 Parry–Romberg syndrome case managed with polyetheretherketone (PEEK) patient-specific implant (PSI). (a) 3D reconstruction of the CT showing the defects and the planned implants. (b) Intraoperative views of the implants. (c) Pre- and postoperative photographs of the patient.

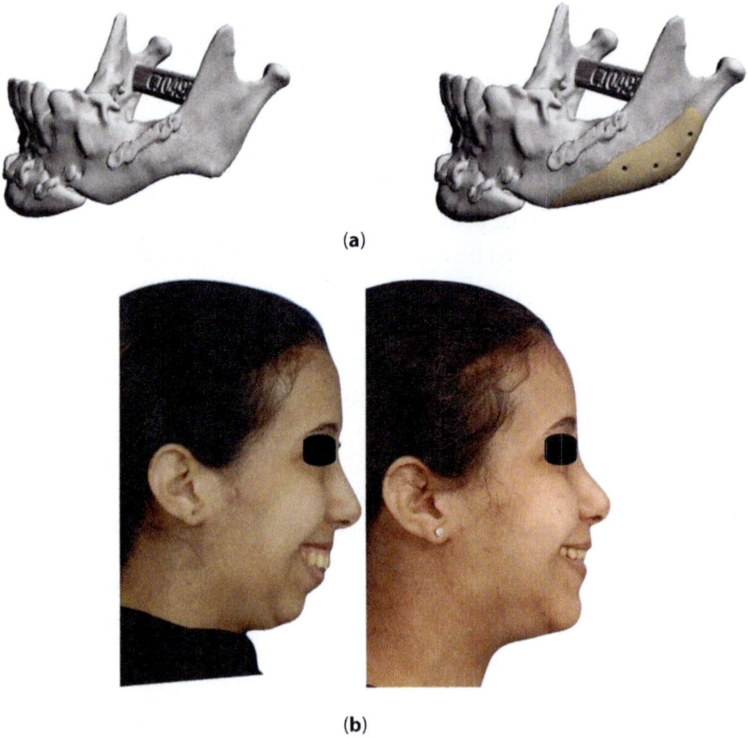

Figure 11.4 Hemifacial case managed with polyetheretherketone (PEEK) patient-specific implant (PSI). (a) 3D reconstruction of CT showing defect and planned implant. (b) Intraoperative view of the implant. (c) Pre- and postoperative photographs of the patient.

11.2.5 Polymethylmethacrylate (PMMA)

Polymethylmethacrylate (PMMA) is a high-strength, rigid acrylic polymer produced by the polymerization of methyl methacrylate [32]. It is synthesized through catalysis of a powdered mixture, in which an exothermic reaction occurs, leading to a rise in temperatures up to 80°C and hence inflicting a risk of thermal injury to surrounding soft tissues [32]. As such, it is necessary that the material should be handled carefully and temporarily withdrawn from tissues while molding [32]. PMMA is highly biocompatible and minimally toxic, and it can be intraoperatively molded during the polymerization process [32]. After preforming and hardening, however, its rigidity compromises conformability to irregular bony contours [50]. To overcome this, PMMA implants can be preoperatively custom-fabricated from computed tomography (CT) imaging, enabling exact anatomical matching to suit individual patient requirements [50]. Solid

PMMA implants are FDA-approved for certain medical uses, specifically orthopedic and cranial surgery [51]. PMMA is also widely used for bone cement in joint arthroplasty and cranioplasty [51]. These are both established evidence-based uses. However, solid PMMA implants are not FDA-approved for aesthetic facial rejuvenation [51]. While PMMA fillers like Bellafill are approved for the nasolabial folds, it is only for injectable products and not for solid implants [52]. Thus, their application in solid PMMA for facial aesthetics would be off-label and should be carefully considered [51]. Physicians who are considering using solid PMMA implants for facial rejuvenation must weigh the risks and benefits carefully and alert patients to the off-label application. Additional study and regulatory review are necessary to determine the safety and effectiveness of the implants for use in cosmetic surgery.

11.2.6 Polytetrafluorethylene and Expanded Polytetrafluorethylene

Expanded polytetrafluoroethylene (ePTFE), known commercially as Gore-Tex (W.L. Gore and Associates), which is widely employed in reconstructive facial surgery, was originally developed for application in vascular surgery [53]. In comparison to its predecessor, pure polytetrafluoroethylene (PTFE), though it is susceptible to mechanical degradation with possible consequences including inflammation, fibrous capsule formation, infection, and explantation risk [32], the ePTFE has improved biological properties. The expanded version possesses a porous structure of intermediate pore sizes (10–30 μm), permitting some degree of fibrous tissue invasion without causing any notable inflammatory or fibrotic reactions [31]. This feature facilitates easier removal when required and improves its application in both subcutaneous augmentation procedures and custom implant designs adhering to individual anatomical specifications [32]. While ePTFE is more compatible than the older PTFE and has been associated with fewer complications than such materials as MedPor or silicone, as Peled *et al.* point out in a meta-analysis [37], it is not without complication. A variety of complications, including infection, extrusion, shrinkage, migration, and scarring, have been described in several reports [31]. Indeed, non-expanded PTFE has proved to work substantially worse both experimentally and clinically, with greater vulnerability to infection and poorer integration compared to MedPor [35]. The facial application mean rate of infection in the case of mixed Gore-Tex implants was estimated at about 2.2% [3]. However, in certain applications—such as secondary rhinoplasty small-volume augmentations—Hsieh TY have noted infection and rejection rates of up to 10.6% [32]. Additional research by Yang *et al.* demonstrates that when ePTFE contacts blood intraoperatively, the edges can become stiffened, resulting in a palpable implant and potential implant separation from the underlying bone. This can result in over-contouring, hematoma, or seroma [54]. In addition, the cost of Gore-Tex is a limitation, as it is generally more expensive than commonly used alternatives such as silicone, Medpor, or Mersilene. It is important to note that Gore-Tex products are not specifically approved as safe and effective for wrinkles, lip augmentation, or other types of "facial rejuvenation," and the long-term dangers have not been studied. ePTFE (K201153) has been cleared by the FDA 510(k) under the brand name Tisuthes for facial skeletal augmentation, i.e., for use in the chin, mandible, and malar areas [55]. This clearance means that the device has been found to be substantially equivalent to legally marketed predicate devices for use in these anatomical sites [55].

11.2.7 Calcium Phosphate

Calcium phosphate cements and ceramics, such as hydroxyapatite-based cements, are utilized on a daily basis as bone graft substitutes in craniofacial reconstructive surgery [8, 56]. Although it is known as osteoconductive bone graft, in facial augmentation, their role is to provide a positive scaffold such that bone deposition by the surrounding tissues is facilitated or as a filler material. An example of one such product is Hydroset, an injectable, self-setting calcium phosphate cement for bone substitution. After it is set, it has osteoconductive and osteointegrative capabilities due to its porous microstructure and crystalline nature. It can be used in granular form for alveolar ridge augmentation and in block form for interpositional grafting in osteotomy [9]. In spite of these properties, the brittleness of the material and its poor ability to conform to irregular surfaces limit its application in onlay or contour augmentation [32]. Also, its low tensile and compressive strength makes it unsuitable for use in load-bearing areas. However, it has a potential to be shaped with accuracy, which makes it a viable option for cranioplasty procedures [32]. HydroSet, a self-setting calcium phosphate cement manufactured by Stryker, has received FDA clearance for specific craniofacial applications [57]. According to the FDA 510(k) summary (K161447), HydroSet is indicated for use in the repair of neurosurgical burr holes, contiguous craniotomy cuts, and other cranial defects, as well as in the augmentation or restoration of bony contour in the craniofacial skeleton [57]. This clearance encompasses reconstructive procedures involving the craniofacial skeleton [57]. However, it is important to note that the FDA approval does not explicitly include cosmetic facial rejuvenation procedures [57]. Therefore, the use of HydroSet for purely aesthetic purposes would be considered off-label. Recently, compact and porous silicon carbide (SiC) was investigated for craniofacial bone augmentation; the material showed tendency to integrate with underling bone [58, 59].

11.2.8 Composite Implants

Composite implants represent an area of growing interest in facial implantology to increase the potential of single-material devices. Composite implants are designed through the combination of two or more biomaterials to take advantage of their complementary properties and to obtain better integration, stability, and aesthetical results. For instance, ePTFE composite face implants (Implantech, Ventura, CA) combine expanded polytetrafluoroethylene (ePTFE) and silicone, the biocompatibility and soft-tissue interface of ePTFE with the structural stability and contour retention of silicone [50]. The combination improves handling and postoperative outcome. Ongoing improvement in composite implant design still strives for an optimal balance among mechanical behavior, biocompatibility, and cost-effectiveness in clinical use [50]. Earlier composite materials were reported as promising graft for craniofacial augmentation made of calcium sulfate polyethylene [60]. Recently, an experimental construct made of silicon calcium phosphate injected into biomimetic scaffold was assessed as a potential surgical procedure for facial augmentation [61].

11.3 Conclusion

A wide range of implants are available for enhancing and reconstructing the craniofacial skeleton. While autologous grafts remain an option, their use is often limited by factors such as inconsistent outcomes, prolonged operative time, donor site morbidity, and fast resorption rate of 50% of the given volume. As a result, alloplastic materials have become the preferred choice for facial contouring and structural augmentation. To date, no single implant material has consistently demonstrated superior short- or long-term outcomes in the literature. Nevertheless, certain materials carry specific limitations that must be considered. Custom-designed implants made from titanium, hydroxyapatite (HaP), and polyetheretherketone (PEEK) have shown promising results in patient-specific applications. Moving forward, large-scale, ideally randomized controlled studies are needed to provide more definitive data regarding the long-term safety and efficacy profiles of these materials.

AI disclosure statement: The author acknowledges the use of AI-based tools for minor language editing or grammatical correction. However, all intellectual contributions, analyses, and conclusions presented in this chapter are entirely the author's own.

References

1. Wong, C.-H. and Mendelson, B., Newer Understanding of Specific Anatomic Targets in the Aging Face as Applied to Injectables. *Plast. Reconstr. Surg.*, 136, 44S–48S, Nov. 2015, doi: 10.1097/PRS.0000000000001752.
2. Rojas, Y.A., Sinnott, C., Colasante, C., Samas, J., Reish, R.G., Facial Implants: Controversies and Criticism. A Comprehensive Review of the Current Literature. *Plast. Reconstr. Surg.*, 142, 4, 991–999, Oct. 2018, doi: 10.1097/PRS.0000000000004765.
3. Rubin, P.J. and Yaremchuk, M.J., Complications and Toxicities of Implantable Biomaterials Used in Facial Reconstructive and Aesthetic Surgery: A Comprehensive Review of the Literature. *Plast. Reconstr. Surg.*, 100, 5, 1336–1353, Oct. 1997, doi: 10.1097/00006534-199710000-00043.
4. Yaremchuk, M.J., *Atlas of Facial Implants*, 2nd ed., Elsevier Health Sciences, London, 2019.
5. Burchardt, H., The biology of bone graft repair. *Clin. Orthop. Relat. Res.*, 174, 28–42, Apr. 1983.
6. Ozaki, W. and Buchman, S.R., Volume maintenance of onlay bone grafts in the craniofacial skeleton: micro-architecture versus embryologic origin. *Plast. Reconstr. Surg.*, 102, 2, 291–9, Aug. 1998, doi: 10.1097/00006534-199808000-00001.
7. Sela, M. and Taicher, S., Restoration of movement to the upper eyelid in facial palsy by an individual gold implant prosthesis. *J. Prosthet. Dent.*, 52, 1, 88–90, Jul. 1984, doi: 10.1016/0022-3913(84)90188-4.
8. Alexander, H., Calcium-based ceramics and composites in bone reconstruction. *CRC Crit. Rev. Biocompatibility*, 4, 43–77, 1987.
9. Salyer, K.E. and Hall, C.D., Porous Hydroxyapatite as an Onlay Bone-Graft Substitute for Maxillofacial Surgery. *Plast. Reconstr. Surg.*, 84, 2, 236–244, Aug. 1989, doi: 10.1097/00006534-198908000-00008.
10. Raveh, J., Stich, H., Sutter, F., Greiner, R., Use of the titanium-coated hollow screw and reconstruction plate system in bridging of lower jaw defects. *J. Oral Maxillofac. Surg.*, 42, 5, 281–294, May 1984, doi: 10.1016/0278-2391(84)90108-3.
11. Romano, J.J., Iliff, N.T., Manson, P.N., Use of Medpor Porous Polyethylene Implants in 140 Patients with Facial Fractures. *J. Craniofac. Surg.*, 4, 3, 142–147, Jul. 1993, doi: 10.1097/00001665-199307000-00007.

12. Toth, J.M., Wang, M., Estes, B.T., Scifert, J.L., Seim, H.B., Turner, A.S., Polyetheretherketone as a biomaterial for spinal applications. *Biomaterials*, 27, 3, 324–334, Jan. 2006, doi: 10.1016/j.biomaterials.2005.07.011.
13. Kim, M.M., Boahene, K.D.O., Byrne, P.J., Use of Customized Polyetheretherketone (PEEK) Implants in the Reconstruction of Complex Maxillofacial Defects. *Arch. Facial Plast. Surg.*, 11, 1, 53–57, Jan. 2009, doi: 10.1001/archfaci.11.1.53.
14. Oliver, J.D., *et al.*, Alloplastic Facial Implants: A Systematic Review and Meta-Analysis on Outcomes and Uses in Aesthetic and Reconstructive Plastic Surgery. *Aesthet. Plast. Surg.*, 43, 3, 625–636, Jun. 2019, doi: 10.1007/s00266-019-01370-0.
15. Morehead, J.M. and Holt, G.R., Soft-tissue response to synthetic biomaterials. *Otolaryngol. Clin. North Am.*, 27, 1, 195–201, Feb. 1994.
16. Costantino, P.D., Friedman, C.D., Lane, A., Synthetic biomaterials in facial plastic and reconstructive surgery. *Facial Plast. Surg.*, 9, 1, 1–15, Jan. 1993, doi: 10.1055/s-2008-1064591.
17. Sugar, A.W., Kurlakose, M., Walshaw, N.D., Titanium mesh in orbital wall reconstruction. *Int. J. Oral Maxillofac. Surg.*, 21, 3, 140–144, Jun. 1992, doi: 10.1016/S0901-5027(05)80780-5.
18. Lee, Y.-W., You, H.-J., Jung, J.-A., Kim, D.-W., Mandibular reconstruction using customized three-dimensional titanium implant. *Arch. Craniofac. Surg.*, 19, 2, 152–156, Jun. 2018, doi: 10.7181/acfs.2018.01830.
19. Blake, G.B., MacFarlane, M.R., Hinton, J.W., Titanium in reconstructive surgery of the skull and face. *Br. J. Plast. Surg.*, 43, 5, 528–535, Sep. 1990, doi: 10.1016/0007-1226(90)90115-G.
20. Kreppel, M., Kauke, M., Grandoch, A., Safi, A.-F., Nickenig, H.-J., Zöller, J., Evaluation of Fronto-Orbital Advancement Using Titanium-Based Internal Fixation for Corrective Pediatric Craniofacial Surgery. *J. Craniofac. Surg.*, 29, 6, 1542–1545, Sep. 2018, doi: 10.1097/SCS.0000000000004689.
21. Quatela, V.C. and Chow, J., Synthetic Facial Implants. *Facial Plast. Surg. Clin. North Am.*, 16, 1, 1–10, Feb. 2008, doi: 10.1016/j.fsc.2007.09.002.
22. Sarfraz, S., *et al.*, Comparison of Titanium and PEEK Medical Plastic Implant Materials for Their Bacterial Biofilm Formation Properties. *Polymers (Basel)*, 14, 18, 3862, Sep. 2022, doi: 10.3390/polym14183862.
23. Pan, Z. and Patil, P.M., Titanium osteosynthesis hardware in maxillofacial trauma surgery: to remove or remain? A retrospective study. *Eur. J. Trauma Emerg. Surg.*, 40, 5, 587–591, Oct. 2014, doi: 10.1007/s00068-013-0348-5.
24. U.S. Food and Drug Administration, Medical Device Material Performance Study: Titanium (Ti) Safety Profile, FDA, Maryland, 2022.
25. Yaremchuk, M.J., Facial skeletal reconstruction using porous polyethylene implants. *Plast. Reconstr. Surg.*, 111, 6, 1818–27, May 2003, doi: 10.1097/01.PRS.0000056866.80665.7A.

26. U.S. Food and Drug Administration (FDA), FDA warns about illegal use of injectable silicone for body contouring and associated health risks, https://www.fda.gov/news-events/press-announcements/fda-warns-about-illegal-use-injectable-silicone-body-contouring-and-associated-health-risks.
27. Brandt, M.G. and Moore, C.C., Implants in facial skeletal augmentation. *Curr. Opin. Otolaryngol. Head Neck Surg.*, 21, 4, 396–9, Aug. 2013, doi: 10.1097/MOO.0b013e32836385d1.
28. Morera Serna, E., Scola Pliego, E., Mir Ulldemolins, N., Martínez Morán, A., Treatment of chin deformities. *Acta Otorrinolaringol. Esp.*, 59, 7, 349–58, 2008.
29. U.S. Food and Drug Administration (FDA), 510(k) Summary: SurgiSil Perma Facial Implant® (K071823), FDA, Maryland, 2007.
30. U.S. Food and Drug Administration (FDA), 510(k) Summary: Implantech Customized Contour Implants (K200610), FDA, Maryland, 2020.
31. Tantawi, D., Eberlin, S., Calvert, J., Midface implants: surgical and nonsurgical alternatives. *Clin. Plast. Surg.*, 42, 1, 123–7, Jan. 2015, doi: 10.1016/j.cps.2014.09.005.
32. Hsieh, T., Dhir, K., Binder, W.J., Hilger, P.A., Alloplastic Facial Implants. *Facial Plast. Surg.*, 37, 06, 741–750, Dec. 2021, doi: 10.1055/s-0041-1725088.
33. Romo, T. and Reitzen, S., Aesthetic Microtia Reconstruction with Medpor. *Facial Plast. Surg.*, 24, 1, 120–128, Feb. 2008, doi: 10.1055/s-2008-1037453.
34. Cenzi, R., Farina, A., Zuccarino, L., Carinci, F., Clinical outcome of 285 Medpor grafts used for craniofacial reconstruction. *J. Craniofac. Surg.*, 16, 4, 526–30, Jul. 2005, doi: 10.1097/01.scs.0000168761.46700.dc.
35. Berghaus, A. and Stelter, K., Alloplastic materials in rhinoplasty. *Curr. Opin. Otolaryngol. Head Neck Surg.*, 14, 4, 270–277, Aug. 2006, doi: 10.1097/01.moo.0000233599.14671.4a.
36. Jung, S.-K., Cho, W.-K., Paik, J.-S., Yang, S.-W., Long-term surgical outcomes of porous polyethylene orbital implants: a review of 314 cases. *Br. J. Ophthalmol.*, 96, 4, 494–498, Apr. 2012, doi: 10.1136/bjophthalmol-2011-300132.
37. Peled, Z.M., Warren, A.G., Johnston, P., Yaremchuk, M.J., The Use of Alloplastic Materials in Rhinoplasty Surgery: A Meta-Analysis. *Plast. Reconstr. Surg.*, 121, 3, 85e–92e, Mar. 2008, doi: 10.1097/01.prs.0000299386.73127.a7.
38. Kim, Y.-H., *et al.*, Reconstruction of Medial Orbital Wall Fractures without Subperiosteal Dissection: The 'Push-Out' Technique. *Arch. Plast. Surg.*, 44, 6, 496–501, Nov. 2017, doi: 10.5999/aps.2017.01319.
39. Khorasani, M., Janbaz, P., Rayati, F., Maxillofacial reconstruction with Medpor porous polyethylene implant: a case series study. *J. Korean Assoc. Oral Maxillofac. Surg.*, 44, 3, 128–135, Jun. 2018, doi: 10.5125/jkaoms.2018.44.3.128.
40. U.S. Food and Drug Administration (FDA), Stryker CMF MEDPOR Customized Implant, FDA, Maryland, 2016.
41. U.S. Food and Drug Administration (FDA), Stryker MEDPOR TITAN 3D Orbital Floor Implant, FDA, Maryland, 2016.

42. Brandicourt, P., Delanoé, F., Roux, F.-E., Jalbert, F., Brauge, D., Lauwers, F., Reconstruction of Cranial Vault Defect with Polyetheretherketone Implants. *World Neurosurg.*, 105, 783–789, Sep. 2017, doi: 10.1016/j.wneu.2017.04.049.
43. Saponaro, G., *et al.*, Patient-Specific Facial Implants in Polyetheretherketone and Their Stability. *Ann. Plast. Surg.*, 90, 6, 564–567, Jun. 2023, doi: 10.1097/SAP.0000000000003527.
44. Alasseri, N. and Alasraj, A., Patient-specific implants for maxillofacial defects: challenges and solutions. *Maxillofac. Plast. Reconstr. Surg.*, 42, 1, 15, Dec. 2020, doi: 10.1186/s40902-020-00262-7.
45. Järvinen, S., *et al.*, The use of patient specific polyetheretherketone implants for reconstruction of maxillofacial deformities. *J. Craniomaxillofac. Surg.*, 47, 7, 1072–1076, Jul. 2019, doi: 10.1016/j.jcms.2019.03.018.
46. Durham, J.W., Montelongo, S.A., Ong, J.L., Guda, T., Allen, M.J., Rabiei, A., Hydroxyapatite coating on PEEK implants: Biomechanical and histological study in a rabbit model. *Mater. Sci. Eng., C*, 68, 723–731, Nov. 2016, doi: 10.1016/j.msec.2016.06.049.
47. Ma, R. and Tang, T., Current Strategies to Improve the Bioactivity of PEEK. *Int. J. Mol. Sci.*, 15, 4, 5426–5445, Mar. 2014, doi: 10.3390/ijms15045426.
48. Kauke-Navarro, M., Knoedler, L., Knoedler, S., Deniz, C., Stucki, L., Safi, A.-F., Balancing beauty and science: a review of facial implant materials in craniofacial surgery. *Front. Surg.*, 11, Jan. 2024, doi: 10.3389/fsurg.2024.1348140.
49. U.S. Food and Drug Administration (FDA), Medical Device Material Performance Study PEEK Safety Profile, FDA, Maryland, 2020.
50. Papel, I.D., *et al.* (Eds.), 4 Synthetic and Biologic Implants, in: *Facial Plastic and Reconstructive Surgery*, Georg Thieme Verlag, Stuttgart, 2016, doi: 10.1055/b-0036-135550.
51. U.S. Food and Drug Administration (FDA), Medical device material performance study: Polymethyl methacrylate Safety Profile, FDA, Maryland, 2021.
52. U.S. Food and Drug Administration, Bellafill® Instructions for Use, FDA, Maryland, 2014.
53. McAuley, C.E., Steed, D.L., Webster, M.W., Seven-year Follow-up of Expanded Polytetrafluoroethylene (PTFE) Femoropopliteal Bypass Grafts. *Ann. Surg.*, 199, 1, 57–60, Jan. 1984, doi: 10.1097/00000658-198401000-00010.
54. Yang, P., *et al.*, A Modified Technique For Expanded Polytetrafluoroethylene Shaping in Chin Augmentation. *J. Craniofac. Surg.*, 26, 2, e146–e148, Mar. 2015, doi: 10.1097/SCS.0000000000001382.
55. U.S. Food and Drug Administration (FDA), TisuthesTM e-PTFE Surgical Patch, FDA, Maryland, 2021.
56. Burstein, F.D., *et al.*, Hydroxyapatite Cement in Craniofacial Reconstruction: Experience in 150 Patients. *Plast. Reconstr. Surg.*, 118, 2, 484–489, Aug. 2006, doi: 10.1097/01.prs.0000234811.48147.64.
57. U. S. Food and Drug Administration (FDA), HydroSet XT, FDA, Maryland, 2016.

58. Alfotawi, R., Compact Silicon Carbide Bio Glass Graft Material for Bone Augmentation. *J. Craniofac. Surg.*, Apr. 2025, doi: 10.1097/SCS.0000000000011421.
59. El-Ghannam, A., *et al.*, Novel 3D printed bioactive SiC orthopedic screw promotes bone growth associated activities by macrophages, neurons, and osteoblasts. *J. Biomed. Mater. Res. A*, 113, 1, Jan. 2025, doi: 10.1002/jbm.a.37801.
60. Fouad, H., *et al.*, Porous Polyethylene Coated with Functionalized Hydroxyapatite Particles as a Bone Reconstruction Material. *Materials*, 11, 4, 521, Mar. 2018, doi: 10.3390/ma11040521.
61. Alfotawi, R., Premnath, S., El-Ghannam, A., Alsafadi, M., Mahmood, A., *In Vivo* Analysis of Porous Bioactive Silicon Carbide Scaffold for Craniofacial Bone Augmentation. *J. Craniofac. Surg.*, 35, 2, 699–704, 2024 March-April 01, doi: 10.1097/SCS.0000000000009864. Epub 2023 Nov 28. PMID: 38014939.

12

Supplementary Techniques in Bone Grafting Procedures for Jaw Bones

Reham A.L. Jasser

Department of Periodontics and Community Dentistry, College of Dentistry, King Saud University, Riyadh, Saudi Arabia

Abstract

Bone grafting in the jaw is an essential surgical procedure in periodontology that helps restore jaw contour and function after tooth loss or injury, providing a solid base for dental implants. The procedure helps restore atrophic jaws due to loss of teeth, periodontal disease, trauma, and congenital defects. An array of graft materials, including autogenous, allogeneic, alloplastic, and xenogeneic, is selected based on patient needs and clinical situations. Despite the effectiveness of these materials, achieving optimal healing and integration remains a significant challenge. Supplementary techniques, *viz.*, platelet concentrates and growth factors, aim to improve bone generation and graft integration, resulting in enhanced stability, reduced healing time, and better patient outcomes. Platelet concentrates derived from human plasma, including platelet-rich fibrin (PRF), platelet-rich plasma (PRP), and concentrated growth factor (CGF), are valuable in dental practice due to their healing properties. These concentrates are rich in platelets, growth factors, and bioactive molecules supporting regeneration of tissues. PRP, PRF, and CGF are different generations of concentrates that enhance bone regeneration, with PRP promoting osteoblast proliferation, PRF offering cost-effective preparation and improved benefits, and CGF providing a denser matrix enriched with growth factors for effective regeneration. Various growth factors, such as platelet-derived growth factor (PDGF), bone morphogenetic proteins (BMPs), transforming growth factor-beta (TGF-β), and enamel matrix derivatives (EMDs), are essential for bone regeneration. BMPs like recombinant human BMP-2 (rhBMP-2) and rhBMP-7 promote osteogenesis and graft integration, while PDGF aids in cell proliferation and angiogenesis, both crucial for successful bone grafting. TGF-β aids in the differentiation of MSCs into osteoblasts enhancing healing. EMDs, sourced from porcine tooth buds, replicate natural tooth development and enhance periodontal and bone regeneration.

Email: raljasser@ksu.edu.sa

Randa A. Alfotawi (ed.) Oro-Facial Bone Grafts and Biomaterials, (247–276) © 2026 Scrivener Publishing LLC

The clinical applications of these supplementary techniques are diverse. PRP has been used to enhance bone density and activity in sinus augmentation, while PRF has shown effectiveness in reducing inflammation and preserving alveolar sites. CGF has demonstrated benefits in vertical bone gain and osseointegration. With differing degrees of success, BMPs have been utilized for alveolar ridge preservation and for augmenting the floor of maxillary sinus. PDGF has been studied for its efficacy in periodontal and peri-implant regeneration, showing significant improvements in bone fill and clinical attachment levels (CALs). TGF-β, although less studied in clinical settings, has shown potential in preclinical models for enhancing bone healing and regeneration. EMDs have been extensively used in periodontal regeneration, improving clinical outcomes in intrabony defects and alveolar ridge preservation. Advancements in supplementary techniques for jawbone grafting have greatly enhanced reconstructive procedures by promoting healing, improving graft stability, and accelerating recovery. Innovations in bone regeneration techniques show potential for enhancing patient satisfaction in dental and maxillofacial surgeries. Future research should aim to optimize these methods and customize treatment for better patient care in dental and maxillofacial surgeries.

Keywords: Bone morphogenetic proteins, concentrated growth factor, enamel matrix derivatives, jawbone grafting, platelet concentrates, platelet-derived growth factor, platelet-rich fibrin, platelet-rich plasma

12.1 Introduction

Bone grafting in the jaw is a common surgical procedure used in periodontology to restore jaw contour and function following tooth loss, injury, or disease [1]. This procedure enhances stability and integration of the implants with the existing bone, establishing a strong foundation for their prolonged functionality [2, 3]. Additionally, bone grafting effectively addresses atrophic jaw issues from tooth loss, trauma, periodontal disease, and congenital defects [1, 4]. Bone grafting utilizes various sources such as autogenous (harvested from the patient), allogeneic (from a donor), xenogeneic (from animals), or alloplastic (synthetic materials) grafts, each offering distinct advantages tailored to the patient's needs. The selection of graft material varies based on individual clinical circumstances. A key challenge in bone grafting is achieving optimal healing and integration of bone graft with surrounding bone [5]. Supplementary techniques for jawbone grafting include adjunctive procedures or methods used to enhance the bone grafting. The primary goals of these techniques are to [6, 7].

1. **Enhance bone regeneration**: Promote healthy bone growth and regeneration

2. **Improve graft integration**: Ensure the bone graft integrates successfully with the surrounding bone tissue
3. **Increase stability**: Provide stability to the jawbone and surrounding tissues
4. **Reduce healing time**: Minimize the time required for healing and recovery
5. **Improve overall outcomes**: Achieve better overall results, including improved jaw function, aesthetics, and patient satisfaction

These supplementary techniques, when combined with other procedures, have the potential to optimize results, reduce complications, and improve patient outcomes [5]. The advent of new technologies has led to the introduction of various supplementary techniques. Two key types of supplementary techniques are often used in dental practice [8]:

1. Platelet concentrates
2. Other growth factors

12.2 Platelet Concentrates

Human-derived platelet concentrates contain platelets, growth factors, and bioactive molecules, making them valuable products for therapeutic applications. These components are crucial for promoting healing, tissue regeneration, and bone growth [9]. Since their introduction in 1954, plasma concentrates have significantly evolved and are now effectively used in periodontics and implant dentistry [10]. Platelet concentrates are optimal bone substitutes as they promote proper bone growth and create a suitable matrix for new bone tissue formation [11]. Platelet concentrates, when used alone or with other grafting procedures, enhance the effectiveness of the grafts by promoting cell growth, improving blood vessel formation, reducing inflammation, and accelerating recovery, resulting in better integration and stability of grafts [11–13]. The effectiveness of platelet concentrates in promoting bone regeneration for intraosseous periodontal defects is still debated, with multiple controlled clinical trials and systematic reviews yielding conflicting results [14–18]. Despite the variability in study designs and outcomes, platelet concentrates have shown potential benefits when used either alone or alongside other grafting materials [16, 19–25].

Three main platelet concentrate types are commonly used in dentistry (Figure 12.1):

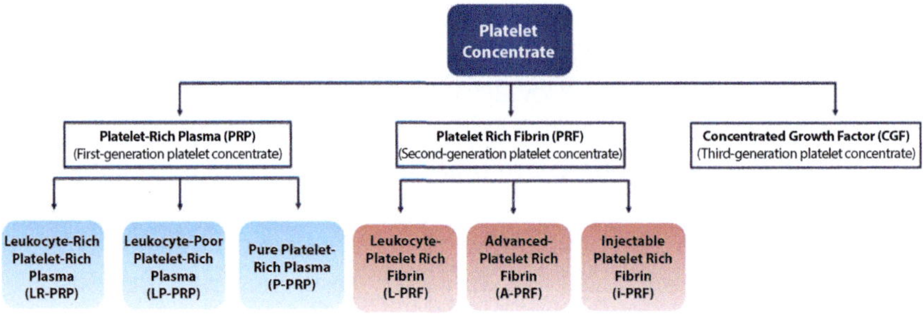

Figure 12.1 Types of platelet concentrates.

12.2.1 Platelet-Rich Plasma

Platelet-rich plasma (PRP) is a first-generation platelet concentrate containing high levels of platelet and low levels of natural fibrinogen [13]. The preparation process for platelet activation involves collecting a large blood sample, adding an anticoagulant, and centrifuging it twice to separate plasma and concentrate platelets. Activated platelets release growth factors within 3–5 days, stimulating the proliferative phase for up to 10 days [9]. Activated PRP contains over 300 bioactive molecules crucial for tissue regeneration and bone remodeling [26].

Based on leukocyte content, PRP can be categorized into three types [27]:

1. **Leukocyte-rich PRP (LR-PRP):** This has a high leukocyte concentration that stimulates inflammation and tissue repair.
2. **Leukocyte-poor PRP (LP-PRP):** This has a low leukocyte concentration, which reduces inflammation and supports tissue regeneration.
3. **Pure PRP (P-PRP):** This contains only platelets and plasma without leukocytes.

12.2.1.1 Mechanism of Action

In bone grafting, PRP activates growth factors, including bone morphogenetic proteins (BMPs), PDGF, transforming growth factor-beta (TGF-β), and vascular endothelial growth factor (VEGF), stimulating osteoblasts, osteoclasts, and stem cells for growth and differentiation. This enhances bone regeneration and graft integration by promoting angiogenesis and regulating inflammation, fostering optimal healing conditions, ultimately improving the success of bone grafting procedures [28, 29].

12.2.1.2 Clinical Applications

Since the first introduction of the PRP therapy, numerous studies have investigated the effectiveness of PRP [30–39]. Studies have primarily focused on the hypothesis that optimized bone healing can lead to improved bone mineral density. A study by Consolo and colleagues assessed the effectiveness of PRP in sinus augmentation by comparing the combination of PRP and autologous bone to those treated with autologous bone alone (n=16). PRP initially improved bone density and activity, but these benefits waned after 6–7 months, indicating short-lived regenerative effects [30, 41]. Ilgenli *et al.* found that combining PRP with demineralized freeze-dried bone allograft (DFDBA) enhanced outcomes (probing pocket depth, CAL, and defect resolution) for intrabony defect treatment compared to using PRP alone [31]. In another study that included four partially edentulous patients, implants placed in sinus grafts containing both particulate autogenous bone and PRP demonstrated a higher bone-to-implant contact rate than those in grafts of bone alone, despite similar healing patterns [32]. An randomized controlled trial (RCT) found that both PRP and bone grafts effectively improved periodontal health in treating defects, with bone grafts showing slightly better outcomes. However, these differences were not statistically significant, suggesting that both treatments are viable options for periodontal regeneration [38]. Conversely, some studies found PRP to be ineffective in bone regeneration, graft integration, and bone healing [33, 34, 37]. In one study, on bone grafting for sinus floor elevation, maxillary bone volume on PRP application did not significantly increase compared to standard treatments [33]. Similarly, another study reported a negative impact on bone density in sinus floor augmentation by PRP before implant placement, as shown by CT evaluations [34]. Raghoebar and colleagues found no significant variation of outcomes between PRP-treated and non-PRP sides in maxillary sinus augmentation with autologous bone grafts, indicating that PRP may not offer additional benefits [37]. A retrospective study revealed that long-term outcomes using PRP do not vary significantly in dental implants. Among the evaluated parameters (bleeding index, plaque index, probing depth [PD], Periotest® values, mobility grade, and radiological bone loss), 64% showed poorer results in the PRP group in comparison to the control group. This suggests that PRP may not contribute to improved long-term implant success [39]. A comparative study demonstrated that PRP significantly enhanced bone formation within 3 months post-surgery. When used in combination with autografts or allografts, PRP resulted in greater new bone growth after 6 months compared to synthetic materials [40]. While initial studies suggested potential benefits of PRP in promoting bone formation, subsequent studies revealed limited effects, thereby restricting its clinical application in dental practice [42].

Platelet-rich fibrin (PRF) promotes tissue healing by offering a simple preparation process, cost-effectiveness, and does not require any biochemical modifications [6, 9]. The PRF preparation protocol includes collecting a blood sample without anticoagulants and centrifuging it to create three layers: acellular plasma (top layer), PRF clot (middle layer), and a base of red corpuscles (bottom layer) [43, 44]. Unlike natural blood clots, PRF is homogeneous, stable, and easier to handle [55]. PRF promotes bone regeneration by stimulating osteoblast proliferation and upregulation of key bone formation genes, such as ALP, Runx2, COL1A, and OCN [45], through its growth factors [46, 47]. Moreover, PRF has proven to be effective in reducing inflammation and preserving alveolar sites, making it a valuable tool for enhancing oral health and healing. The effectiveness of PRF in repairing bone defects has led to it being one of the most studied plasma advanced PRFs (A-PRFs), which have shown promise in enhancing bone regeneration and promoting wound healing [49, 50].

12.2.1.3 Leukocyte Platelet-Rich Fibrin

Leukocyte platelet-rich fibrin (L-PRF), a first-generation PRF, is prepared by centrifugation of blood at 2700 RPM for 12 minutes, producing a matrix of fibrin rich in platelets, leukocytes, and growth factors [43, 51, 52]. The elevated levels of leukocytes and platelets in L-PRF enhance the liberation of growth factors for up to 14 days, accelerating the process of healing. The concentrated platelets and leukocytes enhance regeneration by providing cytokines and critical growth factors that support immune responses, control inflammation, facilitate wound healing, and promote bone regeneration [53]. L-PRF is particularly beneficial in ridge augmentation, sinus lifts, bone and palatal defect repair, socket preservation, and gingival recession [54], as it aids in the integration of bone grafts by offering a scaffold that fosters cellular communication and regeneration of tissues.

12.2.1.4 Advanced Platelet-Rich Fibrin

Advanced platelet-rich fibrin (A-PRF), a second-generation PRF, originated by lowering the centrifugation to 1300 RPM and the force of relative centrifugation to 200×g, following the introduction of L-PRF [55]. In comparison to L-PRF, A-PRF offers advantages such as increased concentration of growth factors, cell count, and a more open three-dimensional structure [56, 57]. While both A-PRF and L-PRF are effective in promoting bone regeneration and wound healing, the enhanced cellular properties and growth factor levels of A-PRF make it the preferred choice for reconstructive surgeries and jaw graft procedures [58–60].

12.2.1.5 *Injectable Platelet-Rich Fibrin*

Injectable platelet-rich fibrin (i-PRF) is a liquid injectable form of PRF prepared using centrifugation for 3 minutes at a speed of 700 RPM [8]. It contains high cellular content, growth factors, and cytokines aiding in effective treatment due to its direct application and high bioavailability. Its gradual release enhances tissue regeneration over time, although its degradation within 2 weeks constrains long-term use [61, 62]. It offers several key benefits in jawbone grafting, including enhanced bone regeneration, improved graft integration, and reduced bone resorption. Its minimally invasive nature, low risk of complications, and natural and biocompatible properties make it an attractive treatment option for jawbone grafting [8, 63].

12.2.1.5.1 Mechanism of Action

PRF utilizes a fibrin matrix that allows the gradual release of growth factors and cytokines, aiding a coordinated cellular response. When activated, PRF liberates growth factors including PDGF, TGF-β, VEGF, and BMPs as the fibrin matrix breaks down. The sustained release of these factors amplifies the proliferation and differentiation of bone cells, including osteoprogenitor cells, osteoblasts, and osteoclasts, thereby facilitating bone regeneration and graft integration. Additionally, this process supports angiogenesis and helps regulate inflammation, creating an ideal environment for bone healing [61, 64–66].

12.2.1.5.2 Clinical Applications

PRF has various clinical uses, including bone grafting, periodontal surgery, and oral implantology, where it promotes healing and facilitates regeneration of bone [59]. A clinical and radiographic study indicated that while DFDBA is commonly used and is considered effective for extraction socket preservation, using it alongside PRF can enhance outcomes [67]. A recent controlled study demonstrated that PRF significantly enhances alveolar bone density and promotes wound healing more than the control, suggesting its positive effect on bone and tissue healing [68]. Similarly, data from multiple controlled and real-world studies suggest that the use of PRF, either alone or with traditional regenerative treatments, improves postoperative healing. It also helps reduce the loss of alveolar width and height, while supporting socket preservation and ridge augmentation [69–75].

Several reviews and meta-analyses show that PRF can effectively aid bone regeneration and tissue healing, making it a promising option alone or combined with other therapies [48, 76–78]. A review of 25 studies reported that autologous PRF enhances regeneration in procedures such as tooth extraction and bone augmentation [76]. Similarly, a meta-analysis of 12 RCTs demonstrated that the use of PRF, either alone or as an adjunct, resulted in less bone loss and increased bone density compared to empty sockets and grafts [48]. A further examination of the literature showed that PRF with bone grafts can improve tissue and bone formation in infrabony defects, potentially accelerating bone healing in intrabony defect treatment [77]. Furthermore, evidence highlights the extensive potential of PRF and its broadening applications within oral and maxillofacial surgery [78].

12.2.2 Concentrated Growth Factor

Concentrated growth factor (CGF) is a third-generation platelet concentrate developed from autologous blood without anticoagulants and is prepared through centrifugation at variable speeds (2400 to 3000 rpm) [79]. This process results in distinct blood components: red blood cells at the base, CGF gel in the middle layer, and platelet-poor plasma on the top layer [80, 81]. Some studies, however, have described a four-layer system, which includes serum, the CGF buffy coat, a growth factor-rich liquid layer containing stem cells, and red blood cells [82–85]. Compared to PRF, CGF offers high concentrations of growth factors on a denser matrix providing enhanced support for tissue regeneration [61, 64]. Studies indicate that CGF can release growth factors for as far as 14 days, a duration longer than that of PRP and PRF [86, 87]. Additionally, CD34+ progenitor cells associated with the CGF layers, play a pivotal role in vascular maintenance and angiogenesis [88, 89].

12.2.2.1 Mechanism of Action

In bone grafting, CGF exerts its effects through various growth factors, such as PDGF, TGF-β, and VEGF, which triggers a cascade of cellular responses. Upon application, CGF stimulates osteoblasts to proliferate and differentiate, enhancing bone matrix deposition and mineralization at the graft site [79, 90, 91]. Concurrently, CGF promotes angiogenesis, enhancing blood vessel formation and perfusion to deliver oxygen, nutrients, and growth factors to graft sites [92, 93]. Furthermore, CGF plays a vital role in controlling the balance between pro-inflammatory and anti-inflammatory cytokines, thereby optimizing the inflammatory response for optimal bone healing. CGF growth factors promote bone regeneration and graft integration, and accelerate healing [93, 94].

12.2.2.2 Clinical Applications

Several studies, including case reports and case series, have highlighted the advantages of using CGF for bone regeneration [95–99]. A study found that combining CGFs with deproteinized bovine bone mineral (DBBM) reduced ridge resorption and resulted in greater new bone formation compared to using DBBM with collagen membranes, demonstrating the efficacy of CGFs in promoting bone regeneration [95]. Two studies reported favorable results in vertical bone gain following sinus augmentation with CGF as the graft material, even though different techniques were used in each study [100, 101]. Similarly, Sohn *et al.* reported rapid bone formation with CGF alone under an elevated sinus membrane, leading to significant new bone growth along the implant body [97]. The bone quality around implants indicates successful osseointegration, vital for implant success [99]. Studies suggest that CGF with implants improves bone quality, promotes faster bone formation, and enhances osteoblastic differentiation, resulting in higher osseointegration activity and increased bone volume compared to the control groups [102, 103]. Additionally, studies show that using CGF in alveolar osteitis treatment led to faster granulation tissue formation by Day 4 and reduced pain scores by Day 7 compared to control groups receiving conventional interventions or laser treatment [104, 105]. A systematic review that included 11 studies concluded that CGF enhances osseointegration, promotes bone regeneration, and increases implant stability and survival rates. Additionally, the extended release of growth factors by CGF contributes to faster and more effective bone healing [99]. Data from a meta-analysis suggest that adding CGF to grafting materials improves treatment for periodontal intrabony defects compared to using grafting materials alone [106]. Although many studies indicate that CGF is a promising option to traditional bone graft materials, there is ongoing debate about its overall therapeutic effectiveness [107–109].

12.3 Other Growth Factors

Other growth factors are natural mediators that promote bone regeneration and enhance the outcomes of dental procedures by stimulating essential cellular processes necessary for bone healing [110]. The use of growth factors has revolutionized wound healing and tissue regeneration in dentistry, particularly benefiting the restoration of periodontal and bone tissues [111, 112]. Although researchers have identified numerous growth factors, only a limited number have been utilized for bone grafting in dental practice [110, 113].

12.3.1 Bone Morphogenetic Proteins

Bone morphogenetic proteins (BMPs), which belong to the transforming growth factor (TGF-β) superfamily, can enhance outcomes when used with other growth factors in treating fractured or non-healing bones [114]. Among the identified BMPs, BMP-2 and BMP-7 are the most powerful inducers of bone and cartilage formation [115]. Recombinant human BMPs (rhBMPs), such as rhBMP-2 and rhBMP-7, play a critical role in maxillofacial surgery due to their osteoinductive properties [114, 116, 117]. Although rhBMP-2 is known to stimulate osteogenesis and bone growth, rhBMP-7 enhances bone regeneration and healing [116, 118]. BMPs, particularly rhBMP-2, are often used in dental procedures to enhance bone growth in areas with insufficient bone volume such as those prepared for dental implants [119]. These proteins are typically combined with a carrier like collagen sponge for the effective delivery of BMPs to the graft site [119]. Both rhBMP-2 and rhBMP-7 are approved by the United States food and drug administration (FDA) for clinical trials to promote bone regeneration by stimulating the differentiation and growth of bone marrow stem cells [120–122].

12.3.1.1 Mechanism of Action

BMPs attract osteoprogenitor cells to the bone defect site and enhance the cellular pool for regeneration. Upon binding to BMP receptors (BMPRs), BMPs activate serine/threonine kinase activity on target cells, resulting in suppressor of mothers against decapentaplegic (SMAD) phosphorylation. Phosphorylated SMADs form complexes that regulate osteogenesis-related gene expression by translocating to the nucleus. In addition, BMPs activate non-SMAD pathways such as MAPK, PI3K/AKT, and Wnt, which regulate cellular processes including proliferation, differentiation, and survival [123]. BMPs play a key role in jawbone grafting by fostering bone formation, enhancing the integration of grafts, and stimulating extracellular matrix production. These properties make BMPs highly valuable in clinical procedures for repairing bone defects resulting from trauma, tumors, congenital disorders, and other conditions [124–127].

12.3.1.2 Clinical Applications

In a pilot-controlled trial with nine patients, combining rhBMP-7 and a deproteinized bone substitute led to less bone formation than using the bone substitute alone for maxillary atrophy. Histological analysis showed that rhBMP-7 was less effective than hydroxyapatite for sinus augmentation before implants [128]. A multicenter, randomized, prospective clinical trial showed that rhBMP-2 applied on an absorbable collagen sponge (ACS) is a reliable option for augmentation of maxillary sinus floor, achieving similar results to those of traditional autogenous bone grafts [129]. In an open-label trial, a composite graft proved to be as effective as an autogenous graft in regenerating bone in large maxillary defects, offering reduced morbidity, similar costs, and greater new bone formation. However, it was associated with increased edema and the absence of nonviable particles [130]. A systematic review found that rhBMP-2/ACS aids bone formation in augmentation of maxillary sinus for dental implant placement, with no significant variation in rhBMP-2 concentrations. However, autogenous bone grafts achieved significant bone height compared to rhBMP-2/ACS for sinus augmentation [131]. A meta-analysis revealed that rhBMP-2 enhanced bone height in alveolar ridge and maxillary sinus floor augmentations, but it was less effective than autografts or allografts in maxillary sinus floor augmentation [132].

12.3.2 Platelet-Derived Growth Factor

PDGF is a dimeric protein primarily found in platelets and other cells, which promotes interactions between mesenchymal cells. It stimulates the growth of fibroblasts and osteoblasts, acting as a potent mitogen to enhance their proliferation [133]. PDGF-AA, PDGF-AB, and PDGF-BB are essential for the development of anatomical structures and vasculogenesis [134]. Among them, PDGF-BB is particularly effective in stimulating periodontal ligament cells [135]. Recombinant human PDGF-BB (rhPDGF-BB) has been FDA-approved for the treatment of periodontal and long bone defects, as well as dermal wound healing [136].

12.3.2.1 Mechanism of Action

PDGF plays a crucial part in bone regeneration and wound healing by stimulating cell growth, angiogenesis, and macrophage activation [137, 138]. PDGF binds to α-PDGFR and β-PDGFR, leading to receptor activation and signaling through pathways like PI 3-kinase, PLC-γ, Src kinases, and Ras/MAPK. This activity promotes cellular functions like chemotaxis, growth, and anti-apoptosis [139]. PDGF attracts and proliferates cells, regulates extracellular matrix deposition, and activates osteoblasts, making it essential for effective bone grafting and accelerated wound healing [137, 138, 140].

12.3.2.2 Clinical Applications

RhPDGF has been studied in human trials for dental implant procedures, including sinus augmentation, ridge preservation, and horizontal bone augmentation [141–143]. However, clinical studies have primarily focused on its use for periodontal and peri-implant regeneration [144]. A phase I/II study on periodontal disease patients showed that rhPDGF-BB and rhIGF-I, when applied locally, were safe for treating osseous defects. High-dose treatment significantly enhanced bone regeneration, unlike low-dose treatment, which did not increase defect fill [145]. In a systematic review, rhPDGF-BB showed 40% more bone fill and about a 2-mm-higher bone growth rate than beta-tricalcium phosphate (β-TCP), demonstrating its effectiveness in periodontal regeneration [146]. A meta-analysis revealed that rhPDGF-BB significantly improved defect fill and CALs in the treatment of periodontal intrabony defects when compared to the control group. In contrast, recombinant human fibroblast growth factor-2 caused a significant linear defect fill [147]. A literature review highlighted that rhPDGF-BB significantly promoted CALs and bone regeneration in alveolar ridge augmentation before implant placement [148]. Furthermore, a systematic review found recombinant human fibroblast growth factor-2 to be both safe and effective for regenerating alveolar bone and soft tissues, particularly in combination with bone allografts, xenografts, or β-TCP for treating periodontal defects and gingival recession [149].

12.3.3 Transforming Growth Factor-Beta

TGF-β, a cytokine released by cells like macrophages, is key in regulating cell processes like growth, differentiation, and apoptosis by binding to specific receptors. The subfamily comprises three isoforms (TGF-β1–β3) with comparable activities and sequence homology [137, 150]. TGF-β facilitates the mesenchymal stem cells (MSC) differentiation into osteoblasts, which is essential for formation of bone. It also boosts bone regeneration by promoting cell proliferation, differentiation, bone matrix production, and angiogenesis, ultimately enhancing graft success [150]. Additionally, TGF-β modulates the inflammatory response and reduces the risk of excessive inflammation and fibrosis [151, 152]. Incorporating TGF-β into bone graft materials enhances bone regeneration, benefiting dental procedures such as implant placement and bone defect repair by accelerating healing and improving graft integration [127]. However, its use requires careful consideration of dosage, short half-life, and cost [153, 154].

12.3.3.1 Mechanism of Action

TGF-β controls the MSC differentiation into osteoblasts by both Smad-dependent and Smad-independent pathways [155, 156]. In the Smad-dependent pathway, TGF-β activates R-Smad phosphorylation upon binding, forming a complex with common-mediator Smad (Co-Smad) to regulate the target genes, such as Runx2, which is vital for osteoblast differentiation. Additionally, TGF-β stimulates Smad-independent pathways, like p38 mitogen-activated protein kinase (MAPK), to further promote osteogenic differentiation of MSCs by targeting Runx2. This process forms osteoblasts that mineralize the bone matrix, leading to new bone tissue formation [156, 157].

12.3.3.2 Clinical Applications

Human clinical studies on TGF-β use in jawbone grafting are presently limited. Preclinical models have demonstrated the significant impact of TGF-β on bone healing and regeneration, highlighting its potential clinical applications [158, 159]. However, most studies have focused on broader applications in craniofacial development and bone healing rather than on specific jawbone grafting procedures. Further studies are needed to explore TGF-β in bone regeneration for jawbone grafting, addressing the lack of clinical evidence on its efficacy and safety, highlighting the importance of improving outcomes [160]. Future research may optimize TGF-β for jawbone grafting, enhancing its therapeutic potential.

12.3.4 Enamel Matrix Derivatives

Enamel matrix derivatives (EMDs), composed mainly of amelogenin (90%) with enamelin and ameloblastin, are key biomaterials for periodontal regeneration [161]. These proteins, evolved from porcine tooth buds, are essential in forming periodontal attachment during tooth development [162, 163]. EMDs have been effective in promoting tissue recovery and reducing inflammation since their initial demonstration of efficacy, benefiting various cell types [161, 164]. Histological studies indicate that EMD promotes healing in periodontal tissues by stimulating the formation of periodontal ligament, acellular cementum, and alveolar bone in experimental defects [165–167]. Emdogain, derived from enamel matrix proteins (EMPs), is the only commercially available option for enhancing bone regeneration and periodontal healing [168].

12.3.4.1 Mechanism of Action

EMDs enhance jawbone grafting by mimicking natural tooth development processes. In brief, EMDs trigger the release of local growth factors and cytokines that contribute to the formation of an extracellular matrix, facilitating the attachment and differentiation of MSCs into osteoblasts, cementoblasts, and fibroblasts. EMDs create a scaffold for tissue regeneration, modulate inflammation by reducing pro-inflammatory cytokines, promote angiogenesis for nutrient delivery, and promote wound healing by stimulating epithelial cell proliferation and migration [169, 170]. Additionally, EMDs affect gene expression and trigger vital signaling pathways like BMP, TGF-β, VEGF, and PDGF, crucial for periodontal and bone regeneration [170, 171].

12.3.4.2 Clinical Applications

In the past two decades, EMD has significantly advanced the field of periodontal tissue engineering [161]. Clinical studies suggest that EMD, whether used alone or alongside other treatments, leads to improved clinical outcomes [172–176]. A systematic review showed EMD significantly improved CALs and pocket depths compared to placebo or control at 1 year. However, caution is needed due to high heterogeneity among trials [163]. The combination of bone grafts and EMD in periodontal regenerative surgery for intrabony defects leads to better outcomes in CAL gain and reduction of probing depth (PD), in comparison to using EMD alone as shown in one meta-analysis [177]. However, a comprehensive systematic review showed that using EMDs during alveolar ridge preservation post tooth extraction results in improved outcomes (i.e., increased new bone formation and reduced postoperative discomfort) [178]. Similarly, a meta-analysis suggested that combining EMD with autogenous bone graft for periodontal intrabony defects might not offer substantial benefits over using EMD alone in terms of clinical outcomes (CAL, PD, and gingival recession). Surgical protocol variations might have concealed the possible advantages of the combined treatment approach [179].

12.4 Conclusions

In conclusion, advancements in jawbone grafting techniques have significantly improved the outcomes of reconstructive procedures. Various graft materials, like autogenous, allogeneic, xenogeneic, and alloplastic grafts, offer tailored options to clinicians based on patient-specific needs. Supplementary techniques, such as platelet concentrates (PRP, PRF, and CGF) and other growth factors (BMPs, PDGF, TGF-β, and EMDs), have further enhanced bone regeneration and graft integration. These innovations have demonstrated potential in healing, improving graft stability, and accelerating recovery. Despite these advancements, there is a need to optimize these techniques, understand their mechanisms of action, and develop personalized treatment strategies. Future studies should optimize these techniques, clarify mechanisms of action, and develop personalized strategies to improve long-term outcomes. Further research on the therapeutic efficacy could provide valuable insights on these supplementary techniques, leading to better patient outcomes in dental and maxillofacial surgeries.

AI disclosure statement: The author acknowledges the use of AI-based tools for minor language editing or grammatical correction. However, all intellectual contributions, analyses, and conclusions presented in this chapter are entirely the author's own.

References

1. Miron, R.J., Optimized bone grafting. *Periodontol. 2000*, 94, 143–160, 2024.
2. Alyahya, A. and Swennen, G.R.J., Bone grafting in orthognathic surgery: A systematic review. *Int. J. Oral Maxillofac. Surg.*, 48, 3, 322–331, 2019.
3. Moussa, N.T. and Dym, H., Maxillofacial bone grafting materials. *Dent. Clin. North Am.*, 64, 2, 473–490, 2020.
4. Titsinides, S., Bone grafting as a method to regenerate jaw defects present and future. *J. Dent. Health Oral Disord. Ther.*, 5, 195, 2016.
5. Rothe, R., Hauser, S., Neuber, C., Laube, M., Schulze, S., Rammelt, S., Pietzsch, J., Adjuvant drug-assisted bone healing: Advances and challenges in drug delivery approaches. *Pharmaceutics*, 12, 5, 428, 2020.
6. Feigin, K. and Shope, B., Use of platelet-rich plasma and platelet-rich fibrin in dentistry and oral surgery: Introduction and review of the literature. *J. Vet. Dent.*, 36, 2, 109–123, 2019.
7. Feroz, S., Cathro, P., Ivanovski, S., Muhammad, N., Biomimetic bone grafts and substitutes: A review of recent advancements and applications. *Biomed. Eng. Adv.*, 6, 100107, 2023.
8. Aghaloo, T.L., Tencati, E., Hadaya, D., Biomimetic enhancement of bone graft reconstruction. *Oral Maxillofac. Surg. Clin. North Am.*, 31, 2, 193–205, 2019.

9. Mohan, S.P., Jaishangar, N., Devy, S., Narayanan, A., Cherian, D., Madhavan, S.S., Platelet-rich plasma and platelet-rich fibrin in periodontal regeneration: A review. *J. Pharm. Bioallied Sci.*, 11, S126–S130, 2019.
10. Mościcka, P. and Przylipiak, A., History of autologous platelet-rich plasma: A short review. *J. Cosmet. Dermatol.*, 20, 9, 2712–2714, 2021.
11. Qu, C., Luo, F., Hong, G., Wan, Q., Effects of platelet concentrates on implant stability and marginal bone loss: A systematic review and meta-analysis. *BMC Oral Health*, 21, 579, 2021.
12. Al-Hamed, F.S., Mahri, M., Al-Waeli, H., Torres, J., Badran, Z., Tamimi, F., Regenerative effect of platelet concentrates in oral and craniofacial regeneration. *Front. Cardiovasc. Med.*, 6, 126, 2019.
13. Noh, N.Z.M., Mohamed, N.A.H., Noor, E., Platelet concentrates effect on bone regeneration in dental surgery: A narrative review. *Dent. Rev.*, 2, 2, 100047, 2022.
14. Plachokova, A.S., Nikolidakis, D., Mulder, J., Jansen, J.A., Creugers, N.H.J., Effect of platelet-rich plasma on bone regeneration in dentistry: A systematic review. *Clin. Oral Investig.*, 19, 6, 539–545, 2008.
15. Bastami, F. and Khojasteh, A., Use of leukocyte-and platelet-rich fibrin for bone regeneration: A systematic review. *Regen. Reconstr. Restor.*, 1, 12, 47–68, 2016.
16. Hou, X., Yuan, J., Aisaiti, A., Liu, Y., Zhao, J., The effect of platelet - rich plasma on clinical outcomes of the surgical treatment of periodontal intrabony defects: A systematic review and meta–analysis. *BMC Oral Health*, 16, 1, 71–83, 2016.
17. Ortega-Mejia, H., Estrugo-Devesa, A., Saka-Herran, C., Ayuso-Montero, R., Lopez-Lopez, J., Velasco-Ortega, E., Platelet-rich plasma in maxillary sinus augmentation: Systematic review. *Materials (Basel)*, 13, 3, 1–23, 2020.
18. Andersen, C., Wragg, N.M., Shariatzadeh, M., Wilson, S.L., The use of platelet-rich plasma (PRP) for the management of non-union fractures. *Curr. Osteoporos. Rep.*, 19, 1–14, 2021.
19. Del Fabbro, M., Bortolin, M., Taschieri, S., Weinstein, R., Is platelet concentrate advantageous for the surgical treatment of periodontal diseases? A systematic review and meta-analysis. *J. Periodontol.*, 82, 8, 1101–1111, 2011.
20. Rock, L., Potential of platelet rich fibrin in regenerative periodontal therapy: Literature review. *Can. J. Dent. Hyg.*, 47, 1, 33–37, 2013.
21. Panda, S., Doraiswamy, J., Malaiappan, S., Varghese, S.S., Del Fabbro, M., Additive effect of autologous platelet concentrates in treatment of intrabony defects: A systematic review and meta-analysis. *J. Investig. Clin. Dent.*, 7, 1, 13–26, 2016.
22. Panda, S., Karanxha, L., Goker, F., Satpathy, A., Taschieri, S., Francetti, L., Das, A.C., Kumar, M., Panda, S., Fabbro, M.D., Autologous platelet concentrates in treatment of furcation defects –A systematic review and meta-analysis. *Int. J. Mol. Sci.*, 20, 6, 1347, 2019.

23. Troiano, G., Laino, L., Dioguardi, M., Giannatempo, G., Muzio, L.L., Mandibular class II furcation defects treatment: Effects of the addition of platelet concentrates to open flap. A systematic review and meta-analysis of RCT. *J. Periodontol.*, 87, 9, 1030–1038, 2016.
24. Miron, R.J., Zucchelli, G., Pikos, M.A., Salama, M., Lee, S., Guillemette, V., Fujioka-Kobayashi, M., Bishara, M., Zhang, Y., Wang, H.L., Chandad, F., Nacopoulos, C., Simonpieri, A., Aalam, A.A., Felice, P., Sammartino, G., Ghanaati, S., Hernandez, M.A., Choukroun, J., Use of platelet-rich fibrin in regenerative dentistry: a systematic review. *Clin. Oral Investig.*, 21, 6, 1913–1927, 2017.
25. Li, R., Liu, Y., Xu, T., Zhao, H., Hou, J., Wu, Y., Zhang, D., The additional effect of autologous platelet concentrates to coronally advanced flap in the treatment of gingival recessions: A systematic review and meta-analysis. *Biomed Res. Int.*, 2019, 1–14, 2019.
26. Rodriguez, I.A., Growney Kalaf, E.A., Bowlin, G.L., Sell, S.A., Platelet-rich plasma in bone regeneration: engineering the delivery for improved clinical efficacy. *Biomed Res. Int.*, 2014, 392398, 2014.
27. Dohan Ehrenfest, D.M., Andia, I., Zumstein, M.A., Zhang, C.Q., Pinto, N.R., Bielecki, T., Classification of platelet concentrates (platelet-rich plasma-PRP, platelet-rich fibrin-PRF) for topical and infiltrative use in orthopedic and sports medicine: current consensus, clinical implications and perspectives. *Muscles Ligaments Tendons J.*, 4, 1, 3–9, 2014.
28. Halepas, S., Chen, X.J., Koch, A., PRP in oral and maxillofacial surgery and Dental Implants, in: *Platelet Rich Plasma in Medicine*. Ferneini, E.M., Landesberg, R., Halepas, S. (eds), Springer, Cham, Switzerland, 2022.
29. Ramya, D., Krishna, P.S., Latha, H.A., Kommalapati, V., Applications of PRP in dental procedures. *RJPT*, 16, 1, 87–93, 2023.
30. Consolo, U., Zaffe, D., Bertoldi, C., Ceccherelli, G., Platelet-rich plasma activity on maxillary sinus floor augmentation by autologous bone. *Clin. Oral Implants Res.*, 18, 252–262, 2007.
31. Ilgenli, T., Dündar, N., Kal, B.I., Demineralized freeze-dried bone allograft and platelet-rich plasma vs platelet-rich plasma alone in infrabony defects: A clinical and radiographic evaluation. *Clin. Oral Investig.*, 11, 1, 51–59, 2007.
32. Aimetti, M., Romano, F., Dellavia, C., Paoli, S.D., Sinus grafting using autogenous bone and platelet-rich plasma: Histologic outcomes in humans. *Int. J. Periodontics Restorative Dent.*, 28, 585–591, 2008.
33. Schaaf, H., Streckbein, P., Lendeckel, S., Heidinger, K., Görtz, B., Bein, G., Boedeker, R.H., Schlegel, K.A., Howaldt, H.P., Topical use of platelet-rich plasma to influence bone volume in maxillary augmentation: A prospective randomized trial. *Vox Sang.*, 94, 64–69, 2008.
34. Schaaf, H., Streckbein, P., Lendeckel, S., Heidinger, K.S., Rehmann, P., Boedeker, R.H., Howaldt, H.P., Sinus lift augmentation using autogenous bone grafts and platelet-rich plasma: Radiographic results. *Oral Surg. Oral Med. Oral Pathol. Oral Radiol. Endod.*, 106, 673–678, 2008.

35. Bettega, G., Brun, J.P., Boutonnat, J., Cracowski, J.L., Quesada, J.L., Hegelhofer, H., Drillat, P., Richard, M.J., Autologous platelet concentrates for bone graft enhancement in sinus lift procedure. *Transfusion*, 49, 779–785, 2009.
36. Arora, N.S., Ramanayake, T., Ren, Y.F., Romanos, G.E., Platelet-rich plasma in sinus augmentation procedures: A systematic literature review: Part II. *Implant Dent.*, 19, 145–157, 2010.
37. Raghoebar, G.M., Schortinghuis, J., Liem, R.S.B., Ruben, J.L., Van Der Wal, J.E., Vissink, A., Does platelet-rich plasma promote remodeling of autologous bone grafts used for augmentation of the maxillary sinus floor? *Clin. Oral Implants Res.*, 16, 3, 349–356, 2005.
38. Jalaluddin, M., Mahesh, J., Mahesh, R., Jayanti, I., Faizuddin, M., Kripal, K., Nazeer, N., Effectiveness of platelet rich plasma and bone graft in the treatment of intrabony defects: A clinico-radiographic study. *Open Dent. J.*, 12, 133–154, 2018.
39. Attia, S., Narberhaus, C., Schaaf, H., Streckbein, P., Pons-Kühnemann, J., Schmitt, C., Neukam, F.W., Howaldt, H.P., Böttger, S., Long-term influence of platelet-rich plasma (PRP) on dental implants after maxillary augmentation: Retrospective clinical and radiological outcomes of a randomized controlled clinical trial. *J. Clin. Med.*, 9, 2, 355, 2020.
40. Arenaz-Búa, J., Luaces-Rey, R., Sironvalle-Soliva, S., Otero-Rico, A., Charro-Huerga, E., Patiño-Seijas, B., García-Rozado, A., Ferreras-Granados, J., Vázquez-Mahía, I., Lorenzo-Franco, F., Martín-Sastre, R., López-Cedrún, J.L., A comparative study of platelet-rich plasma, hydroxyapatite, demineralized bone matrix and autologous bone to promote bone regeneration after mandibular impacted third molar extraction. *Med. Oral Patol. Oral Cir. Bucal*, 15, 3, e483–e489, 2010.
41. Marx, R.E., Carlson, E.R., Eichstaedt, R.M., Schimmele, S.R., Strauss, J.E., Georgeff, K.R., Platelet-rich plasma: Growth factor enhancement for bone grafts. *Oral Surg. Oral Med. Oral Pathol. Oral Radiol. Endod.*, 85, 6, 638–46, 1998.
42. Sivakumar, I., Arunachalam, S., Mahmoud Buzayan, M., Sharan, J., Does the use of platelet-rich plasma in sinus augmentation improve the survival of dental implants? A systematic review and meta-analysis. *J. Oral Biol. Craniofac. Res.*, 13, 1, 57–66, 2023.
43. Dohan, D.M., Choukroun, J., Diss, A., Dohan, S.L., Dohan, A.J., Mouhyi, J., Gogly, B., Platelet-rich fibrin (PRF): A second-generation platelet concentrate. Part I: Technological concepts and evolution. *Oral Surg. Oral Med. Oral Pathol. Oral Radiol. Endod.*, 101, e37–e44, 2006.
44. Agrawal, M. and Agrawal, V., Platelet-rich fibrin and its applications in dentistry–A review article. *Natl. J. Med. Dent. Res.*, 2, 51–58, 2014.
45. Del Corso, M., Vervelle, A., Simonpieri, A., Current knowledge and perspectives for the use of platelet-rich plasma (PRP) and platelet-rich fibrin (PRF)

in oral and maxillofacial surgery part 1: Periodontal and dentoalveolar surgery. *Curr. Pharm. Biotechnol.*, 13, 7, 1207–1230, 2012.

46. Zhang, Y., Ruan, Z., Shen, M., Tan, L., Huang, W., Wang, L., Huang, Y., Clinical effect of platelet-rich fibrin on the preservation of the alveolar ridge following tooth extraction. *Exp. Ther. Med.*, 5, 2277–2286, 2018.
47. Wang, X., Zhang, Y., Choukroun, J., Ghanaati, S., Miron, R.J., Effects of an injectable platelet-rich fibrin on osteoblast behavior and bone tissue formation in comparison to platelet-rich plasma. *Platelets*, 9, 48–55, 2018.
48. Alrayyes, Y. and Al-Jasser, R., Regenerative potential of platelet rich fibrin (PRF) in socket preservation in comparison with conventional treatment modalities: A systematic review and meta-analysis. *Tissue Eng. Regen. Med.*, 19, 3, 463–475, 2022.
49. Liu, Y., Sun, X., Yu, J., Wang, J., Zhai, P., Chen, S., Liu, M., Zhou, Y., Platelet-rich fibrin as a bone graft material in oral and maxillofacial bone regeneration: Classification and summary for better application. *Biomed Res. Int.*, 2019, 3295756, 2019.
50. Pietruszka, P., Chruścicka, I., Duś-Ilnicka, I., Paradowska-Stolarz, A., PRP and PRF-Subgroups and Divisions When Used in Dentistry. *J. Pers. Med.*, 11, 10, 944, 2021.
51. Dohan, D.M., Choukroun, J., Diss, A., Dohan, S.L., Dohan, A.J., Mouhyi, J., Gogly, B., Platelet-rich fibrin (PRF): A second-generation platelet concentrate. Part II: Platelet-related biologic features. *Oral Surg. Oral Med. Oral Pathol. Oral Radiol. Endod.*, 101, e45–e50, 2006.
52. Tadepalli, A., Chekurthi, S., Kavassery Balasubramanian, S., Parthasarathy, H., Ponnaiyan, D., Comparative evaluation of clinical efficacy of leukocyte-rich platelet-rich fibrin with advanced platelet-rich fibrin in management of gingival recession defects: A randomized controlled trial. *Med. Princ. Pract.*, 31, 4, 376–383, 2022.
53. Qurban, H.A., Hamadallah, H.H., Madkhaly, M.A., Hakeem, M.M., Alqutaibi, A.Y., Leukocyte-platelet-rich fibrin in bone regeneration after periapical surgery: A 30-month follow-up clinical report. *Reports*, 7, 32, 2024.
54. Wang, Z., Mudalal, M., Sun, Y., Liu, Y., Wang, J., Wang, Y., Sun, X., Zhou, Y., The effects of leukocyte-platelet rich fibrin (L-PRF) on suppression of the expressions of the pro-inflammatory cytokines, and proliferation of Schwann cell, and neurotrophic factors. *Sci. Rep.*, 10, 2421, 2020.
55. Ghanaati, S., Booms, P., Orlowska, A., Kubesch, A., Lorenz, J., Rutkowski, J., Landes, C., Sader, R., Kirkpatrick, C., Choukroun, J., Advanced platelet-rich fibrin: A new concept for cell-based tissue engineering by means of inflammatory cells. *J. Oral Implantol.*, 40, 679–689, 2014.
56. Kobayashi, E., Flückiger, L., Fujioka-Kobayashi, M., Sawada, K., Sculean, A., Schaller, B., Miron, R.J., Comparative release of growth factors from PRP, PRF, and advanced-PRF. *Clin. Oral Investig.*, 20, 9, 2353–2360, 2016.

57. Chiara, M., Mariaelena, C., Alessandro, C., Davide, B., Lavinia, C., Paola, M.M., Barbara, L., Chiara, D.P., Flagiello, F., Pia, P.M., Influence of haematological parameters on size of the advanced platelet-rich fibrin+ (A-PRF+) in the horse. *Res. Vet. Sci.*, 177, 105367, 2024.
58. Walch, B., Kolk, A., Scheibl, D., Guarda, M., Maier, S.C., Denk, L., The effect of advanced platelet-rich fibrin plus (A-PRF+) on graft stability in dental implants and alveolar ridge augmentation procedures: A new low-speed standardized centrifugation protocol. *Dent. J.*, 12, 349, 2024.
59. Song, P., He, D., Ren, S., Fan, L., Sun, J., Platelet-rich fibrin in dentistry. *J. Appl. Biomater. Funct. Mater.*, 22, 2024. 10.1177/22808000241299588.
60. Pereira, V.B.S., Lago, C.A.P., Almeida, R.d.A.C., Barbirato, D.d.S., Vasconcelos, B.C.d.E., Biological and cellular properties of advanced platelet-rich fibrin (A-PRF) compared to other platelet concentrates: systematic review and meta-analysis. *Int. J. Mol. Sci.*, 25, 482, 2024.
61. Miron, R.J. and Choukroun, J., Platelet Rich Fibrin in: *Regenerative Dentistry: Biological Background and Clinical Indications*, John Wiley & Sons, Hoboken, NJ, USA, 2017.
62. Fujioka-Kobayashi, M., Schaller, B., Mourão, C.F.D.A.B., Zhang, Y., Sculean, A., Miron, R.J., Biological characterization of an injectable platelet-rich fibrin mixture consisting of autologous albumin gel and liquid platelet-rich fibrin (Alb-PRF). *Platelets*, 32, 74–81, 2021.
63. Farshidfar, N., Jafarpour, D., Firoozi, P., Sahmeddini, S., Hamedani, S., de Souza, R.F., Tayebi, L., The application of injectable platelet-rich fibrin in regenerative dentistry: A systematic scoping review of *in vitro* and *in vivo* studies. *Jpn. Dent. Sci. Rev.*, 58, 89–123, 2022.
64. Dohan Ehrenfest, D.M., Rasmusson, L., Albrektsson, T., Classification of platelet concentrates: from pure platelet-rich plasma (P-PRP) to leucocyte- and platelet-rich fibrin (L-PRF). *Trends Biotechnol.*, 27, 3, 158–167, 2009.
65. Atalay, B. and Doganay, O. The use of platelet-rich fibrin in bone grafting in: *Bone Grafting - Recent Advances with Special References to Cranio-Maxillofacial Surgery*, IntechOpen, London, UK, 2018.
66. Halepas, S., Chen, X.J., Koch, A. PRF in oral and maxillofacial surgery and dental implants, in: *Platelet Rich Plasma in Medicine*, pp. 81–93, Springer, Cham, Switzerland, 2022.
67. Thakkar, D.J., Deshpande, N.C., Dave, D.H., Narayankar, S.D., A comparative evaluation of extraction socket preservation with demineralized freeze-dried bone allograft alone and along with platelet-rich fibrin: A clinical and radiographic study. *Contemp. Clin. Dent.*, 7, 371–376, 2016.
68. Malhotra, A., Kapur, I., Das, D., Sharma, A., Gupta, M., Kumar, M., Comparative evaluation of bone regeneration with platelet-rich fibrin in mandibular third molar extraction socket: A randomized split-mouth study. *Natl. J. Maxillofac. Surg.*, 11, 2, 241–247, 2020.
69. Girish Kumar, N., Chaudhary, R., Kumar, I., Arora, S.S., Kumar, N., Singh, H., To assess the efficacy of socket plug technique using platelet rich fibrin

with or without the use of bone substitute in alveolar ridge preservation: A prospective randomised controlled study. *Oral Maxillofac. Surg.*, 22, 2, 135–142, 2018.
70. Clark, D., Rajendran, Y., Paydar, S., Ho, S., Cox, D., Ryder, M., Dollard, J., Kao, R.T., Advanced platelet-rich fibrin and freeze-dried bone allograft for ridge preservation: A randomized controlled clinical trial. *J. Periodontol.*, 89, 4, 379–387, 2018.
71. Kollati, P., Koneru, S., Dwarakanath, C.D., Gottumukkala, S.N., Effectiveness of naturally derived bovine hydroxyapatite (Cerabone™) combined with platelet-rich fibrin matrix in socket preservation: A randomized controlled clinical trial. *J. Indian Soc. Periodontol.*, 23, 145–151, 2019.
72. De Angelis, P., De Angelis, S., Passarelli, P.C., Liguori, M.G., Manicone, P.F., D'Addona, A., Hard and soft tissue evaluation of different socket preservation procedures using leukocyte and platelet-rich fibrin: A retrospective clinical and volumetric analysis. *J. Oral Maxillofac. Surg.*, 77, 9, 1807–1815, 2019.
73. Yewale, M., Bhat, S., Kamath, A., Tamrakar, A., Patil, V., Algal, A.S., Advanced platelet-rich fibrin plus and osseous bone graft for socket preservation and ridge augmentation – A randomized control clinical trial. *J. Oral Biol. Craniofac. Res.*, 11, 2, 225–233, 2021.
74. Li, A., Piao, H., Zhang, J., Cheng, Q., Piao, F., Cao, C., Yan, Y., Li, J., Jin, B., Clinical effect of platelet-rich fibrin combined with bio-gene artificial bone meal in bone defects after jaw cyst surgery. *Int. J. Gen. Med.*, 16, 5225–5234, 2023.
75. Azangookhiavi, H., Habibzadeh, S., Zahmatkesh, H., Mellati, E., Mosaddad, S.A., Dadpour, Y., The effect of platelet-rich fibrin (PRF) versus freeze-dried bone allograft (FDBA) used in alveolar ridge preservation on the peri-implant soft and hard tissues: A randomized clinical trial. *BMC Oral Health*, 24, 693, 2024.
76. Blinstein, B. and Bojarskas, S., Efficacy of autologous platelet rich fibrin in bone augmentation and bone regeneration at extraction socket. *Stomatologija*, 20, 4, 111–118, 2018.
77. Theodosaki, A.M., Filippoua, S., Kazantzidis, G., Doufexi, A.E., Effectiveness of platelet rich fibrin alone or in combination with bone grafts in the treatment of infrabony defects: Systematic review and metanalysis. *Health Sci. Rev.*, 5100066, 2022.
78. Neal, T.W., Sullivan, S.R., Cannon, S., Spresser, W., Schlieve, T., Platelet rich fibrin: A literature review of applications in oral and maxillofacial surgery. *J. Oral Maxillofac. Anesth.*, 3, 6, 2024.
79. Dong, K., Zhou, W.J., Liu, Z.H., Hou, P.J., The extract of concentrated growth factor enhances osteogenic activity of osteoblast through PI3K/AKT pathway and promotes bone regeneration *in vivo*. *Int. J. Implant Dent.*, 7, 70, 2021.
80. Khiste, S.V. and Tari, R.N., Platelet-rich fibrin as a biofuel for tissue regeneration. *Int. Sch. Res. Not.*, 2013, 1–6, 2013.

81. Chen, J. and Jiang, H., A comprehensive review of concentrated growth factors and their novel applications in facial reconstructive and regenerative medicine. *Aesthetic Plast. Surg.*, 44, 1047–57, 2020.
82. Mansour, P. and Kim, P., Use of concentrated growth factor (CGF) in implantology. *Australas. Dent. Pract.*, 162–168, 2010.
83. Nityasri, Aromal, S., Kumar, Y.P., Kalaivani, V., Pandian, R., Role of CGF (concentrated growth factor) in periodontal regeneration. *J. Dent. Health Oral Disord. Ther.*, 9, 5, 350–352, 2018.
84. Dai, Y., Han, X.H., Hu, L.H., Wu, H.W., Huang, S.Y., Lü, Y.P., Efficacy of concentrated growth factors combined with mineralized collagen on quality of life and bone reconstruction of guided bone regeneration. *Regen. Biomater.*, 7, 3, 313–320, 2020.
85. Kavitha, M., Shakthipriya, S., Arunaraj, D., Hemamalini, R., Velayudham, S., Bakthavatchalam, B., Comparative evaluation of platelet-rich fibrin and concentrated growth factor as scaffolds in regenerative endodontic procedure: A randomized controlled clinical trial. *J. Contemp. Dent. Pract.*, 23, 12, 1211–1217, 2022.
86. Borsani, E., Bonazza, V., Buffoli, B., Cocchi, M.A., Castrezzati, S., Scarì, G., Baldi, F., Pandini, S., Licenziati, S., Parolini, S., Rezzani, R., Rodella, L.F., Biological characterization and *in vitro* effects of human concentrated growth factor preparation: An innovative approach to tissue regeneration. *Biol. Med.*, 7, 5, 1–11, 2015.
87. Lei, L., Yu, Y., Han, J., Shi, D., Sun, W., Zhang, D., Quantification of growth factors in advanced platelet-rich fibrin and concentrated growth factors and their clinical efficiency as adjunctive to the GTR procedure in periodontal intrabony defects. *J. Periodontol.*, 91, 4, 462–472, 2020.
88. Rodella, L.F., Favero, G., Boninsegna, R., Buffoli, B., Labanca, M., Scarì, G., Sacco, L., Batani, T., Rezzani, R., Growth factors, CD34 positive cells, and fibrin network analysis in concentrated growth factors fraction. *Microsc. Res. Tech.*, 74, 8, 772–777, 2011.
89. Rochira, A., Siculella, L., Damiano, F., Palermo, A., Ferrante, F., Carluccio, M.A., Calabriso, N., Giannotti, L., Stanca, E., Concentrated growth factors (CGF) induce osteogenic differentiation in human bone marrow stem cells. *Biology (Basel)*, 9, 370, 2020.
90. Ma X., Ding L., Tang S., Li T., Pei J., Li Y. Effects of concentrated growth factors on proliferation and osteogenic differentiation in Beagle adipose-derived stem cells. *Zhong Nan Da Xue Xue Bao Yi Xue Ban*, 43, 1–6, 2018.
91. Sohn, D.S., Huang, B., Kim, J., Park, W.E., Park, C.C., Utilization of autologous concentrated growth factors (CGF) enriched bone graft matrix (sticky bone) and CGF-enriched fibrin membrane in implant dentistry. *J. Implant Adv. Clin. Dent.*, 7, 10, 2015.
92. Calabriso, N., Stanca, E., Rochira, A., Damiano, F., Giannotti, L., Di Chiara Stanca, B., Massaro, M., Scoditti, E., Demitri, C., Nitti, P., Palermo, A., Siculella, L., Carluccio, M.A., Angiogenic properties of concentrated

growth factors (CGFs): The role of soluble factors and cellular components. *Pharmaceutics*, 13, 5, 635, 2021.
93. Gökmenoğlu, C., Yavuz, M.C., Sadik, E., Kara, C., Treatment of different types of bone defects with concentrated growth factor: Four case reports. *Int. J. Oral Dent. Health*, 2, 2, 29, 2016.
94. Koyuncu, B.Ö., The use of concentrated growth factor in dentistry. *ASDS*, 2, 5, 81–93, 2018.
95. Lin, S., Li, X., Liu, H., Wu, F., Yang, L., Su, Y., Li, J., Duan, S.Y., Clinical applications of concentrated growth factors combined with bone substitutes for alveolar ridge preservation in maxillary molar area: A randomized controlled trial. *Int. J. Implant Dent.*, 7, 115, 2021.
96. Hemalata, M., Jayanthi, D., Vivekanand, L., Shafi, G.A., Keerti, V., Sandwich technique of socket preservation using concentrated growth factor and tricalcium phosphate and an immediate interim prosthesis with a natural tooth pontic: A case report. *Int. J. Adv. Health Sci.*, 2, 18–25, 2016.
97. Sohn, D.S., Moon, J.W., Moon, Y.S., Park, J.S., Jung, H.S., The use of concentrated growth factor (CGF) for sinus augmentation. *J. Oral Implantol.*, 38, 25–38, 2009.
98. Javid, K., Kurtzman, G.M., Nadi, M., Javid, H., Utilization of concentrated growth factor as a sole sinus augmentation material. *Int. J. Growth Factors Stem Cells Dent.*, 1, 95–100, 2018.
99. Lokwani, B.V., Gupta, D., Agrawal, R.S., Mehta, S., Nirmal, N.J., The use of concentrated growth factor in dental implantology: A systematic review. *J. Indian Prosthodont. Soc.*, 20, 1, 3–10, 2020.
100. Kim, J.M., Sohn, D.S., Bae, M.S., Moon, J.W., Lee, J.H., Park, I.S., Flapless transcrestal sinus augmentation using hydrodynamic piezoelectric internal sinus elevation with autologous concentrated growth factors alone. *Implant Dent.*, 23, 168–174, 2014.
101. Chen, Y., Cai, Z., Zheng, D., Lin, P., Cai, Y., Hong, S., Lai, Y., Wu, D., Inlay osteotome sinus floor elevation with concentrated growth factor application and simultaneous short implant placement in severely atrophic maxilla. *Sci. Rep.*, 6, 1–8, 2016.
102. Adali, E., Yüce, M.O., Günbay, T., Günbay, S., Does concentrated growth factor used with allografts in maxillary sinus lifting have adjunctive benefits? *J. Oral Maxillofac. Surg.*, 79, 1, 98–108, 2021.
103. Ntontoulos, V. and Dabarakis, N., The effect of denatured albumin with concentrated growth factors in minimally invasive sinus piezosurgery: Preliminary pilot study results. *Eur. J. Dent.*, 2023.
104. Kamal, A., Salman, B., Abdul Razak, N.H., Samsudin, A.R., A comparative clinical study between concentrated growth factor and low-level laser therapy in the management of dry socket. *Eur. J. Dent.*, 14, 4, 613–620, 2020.
105. Kamal, A., Salman, B., Abdul Razak, N.H., Al Qabbani, A., Samsudin, A.R., The efficacy of concentrated growth factor in the healing of alveolar osteitis: A clinical study. *Int. J. Dent.*, 2020, 1–9, 2020.

106. Yao, M., Hu, J., Jiang, L., Guo, R., Wang, X., Efficacy of concentrated growth factor combined with grafting materials *vs.* grafting materials alone for the treatment of periodontal intrabony defects: A systematic review and meta-analysis. *Ann. Transl. Med.*, 11, 4, 184, 2023.
107. Inchingolo, F., Georgakopoulos, P.G., Dipalma, G., Tsantis, S., Batani, T., Cheno, E., Georgakopoulos, I.P., Computer based textural evaluation of concentrated growth factors (CGF) in osseointegration of oral implants in dental panoramic radiography. *JIACD*, 9, 3, 20–29, 2017.
108. Manoj, S., Punit, J., Chethan, H., Nivya, J., A study to assess the bone formed around immediate postextraction implants grafted with concentrated growth factor in the mandibular posterior region. *J. Osseointegration*, 10, 121–129, 2018.
109. Shetty, M., Kalra, R., Hegde, C., Maxillary sinus augmentation with concentrated growth factors: Radiographic evaluation. *J. Osseointegration*, 10, 109–114, 2018.
110. Mortellaro, C. and Fabbro, M.D., Tissue engineering: Use of growth factors in bone regeneration, InTech, 2018, 10.5772/intechopen.69875.
111. Pilipchuk, S.P., Fretwurst, T., Yu, N., Larsson, L., Kavanagh, N.M., Asa'ad, F., Cheng, K.C.K., Lahann, J., Giannobile, W.V., Micropatterned scaffolds with immobilized growth factor genes regenerate bone and periodontal ligament-like tissues. *Adv. Healthc. Mater.*, 7, 22, e1800750, 2018.
112. Vaquette, C., Pilipchuk, S.P., Bartold, P.M., Hutmacher, D.W., Giannobile, W.V., Ivanovski, S., Tissue engineered constructs for periodontal regeneration: current status and future perspectives. *Adv. Healthc. Mater.*, 7, 21, e1800457, 2018.
113. Marian, D., Toro, G., D'Amico, G., Trotta, M.C., D'Amico, M., Petre, A., Lile, I., Hermenean, A., Fratila, A., Challenges and innovations in alveolar bone regeneration: A narrative review on materials, techniques, clinical outcomes, and future directions. *Medicina*, 61, 20, 2025.
114. On, S.W., Park, S.Y., Yi, S.M., Park, I.Y., Byun, S.H., Yang, B.E., Current status of recombinant human bone morphogenetic protein-2 (rhBMP-2) in maxillofacial surgery: Should it be continued? *Bioengineering (Basel)*, 10, 9, 1005, 2023.
115. El Bialy, I., Jiskoot, W., Reza Nejadnik, M., Formulation, delivery and stability of bone morphogenetic proteins for effective bone regeneration. *Pharm. Res.*, 34, 1152–1170, 2017.
116. Khojasteh, A., Behnia, H., Naghdi, N., Esmaeelinejad, M., Alikhassy, Z., Stevens, M., Effects of different growth factors and carriers on bone regeneration: A systematic review. *Oral Surg. Oral Med. Oral Pathol. Oral Radiol.*, 116, 6, e405–e423, 2013.
117. Al-Hezaimi, K., Nevins, M., Kim, S.W., Fateh, A., Kim, D.M., Efficacy of growth factor in promoting early osseointegration. *J. Oral Implantol.*, 40, 5, 543–548, 2014.

118. Ayoub, A., Roshan, C.P., Gillgrass, T., Naudi, K., Ray, A., The clinical application of rhBMP-7 for the reconstruction of alveolar cleft. *J. Plast. Reconstr. Aesthet. Surg.*, 69, 1, 101–117, 2016.
119. Park, S.Y., Kim, K.H., Kim, S., Lee, Y.M., Seol, Y.J., BMP-2 gene delivery-based bone regeneration in dentistry. *Pharmaceutics*, 11, 8, 393, 2019.
120. Gillman, C.E. and Jayasuriya, A.C., FDA-approved bone grafts and bone graft substitute devices in bone regeneration. *Mater. Sci. Eng. C. Mater. Biol. Appl.*, 130, 112466, 2021.
121. Zang, S., Xiao, C., He, M., Chen, B., Liu, B., Yi, S., Wang, L., Li, J., Shi, X., Bu, S., Jin, L., RGD and rhBMP-7 immobilized on zirconia scaffold with interweaved human dental pulp stem cells for promoting bone regeneration. *Mater. Des.*, 232, 112052, 2023.
122. Karataş, E., Karasulu, H.Y., Azizoğlu, G.A., Öcal, G.K., Armağan, G., Nizam, N., Özkaya, C.A., Tezel, H., Dental implants coated with BMP-2- and α-tocopherol-loaded nanofibers enhance osseointegration. *Int. J. Pharm.*, 125136, 2024.
123. Titsinides, S., Agrogiannis, G., Karatzas, T., Bone grafting materials in dentoalveolar reconstruction: A comprehensive review. *Jpn. Dent. Sci. Rev.*, 55, 1, 26–32, 2019.
124. Shah, P., Keppler, L., Rutkowski, J., Bone morphogenic protein: An elixir for bone grafting – a review. *J. Oral Implantol.*, 38, 6, 767–778, 2012.
125. Fan, L., Ren, Y., Emmert, S., Vučković, I., Stojanovic, S., Najman, S., Schnettler, R., Barbeck, M., Schenke-Layland, K., Xiong, X., The use of collagen-based materials in bone tissue engineering. *Int. J. Mol. Sci.*, 24, 4, 3744, 2023.
126. Szwed-Georgiou, A., Płociński, P., Kupikowska-Stobba, B., Urbaniak, M.M., Rusek-Wala, P., Szustakiewicz, K., Piszko, P., Krupa, A., Biernat, M., Gazińska, M., Kasprzak, M., Nawrotek, K., Mira, N.P., Rudnicka, K., Bioactive materials for bone regeneration: Biomolecules and delivery systems. *ACS Biomater. Sci. Eng.*, 9, 9, 5222–5254, 2023.
127. Nicolae, C.L., Pîrvulescu, D.C., Niculescu, A.G., Epistatu, D., Mihaiescu, D.E., Antohi, A.M., Grumezescu, A.M., Croitoru, G.A., An up-to-date review of materials science advances in bone grafting for oral and maxillofacial pathology. *Mater.*, 17, 4782, 2024.
128. Corinaldesi, G., Piersanti, L., Piattelli, A., Iezzi, G., Pieri, F., Marchetti, C., Augmentation of the floor of the maxillary sinus with recombinant human bone morphogenetic protein-7: A pilot radiological and histological study in humans. *Br. J. Oral Maxillofac. Surg.*, 51, 3, 247–252, 2013.
129. Triplett, R.G., Nevins, M., Marx, R.E., Spagnoli, D.B., Oates, T.W., Moy, P.K., Boyne, P.J., Pivotal, randomized, parallel evaluation of recombinant human bone morphogenetic protein-2/absorbable collagen sponge and autogenous bone graft for maxillary sinus floor augmentation. *J. Oral Maxillofac. Surg.*, 67, 9, 1947–1960, 2009.
130. Marx, R.E., Armentano, L., Olavarria, A., Samaniego, J., rhBMP-2/ACS grafts versus autogenous cancellous marrow grafts in large vertical defects of

the maxilla: An unsponsored randomized open-label clinical trial. *Int. J. Oral Maxillofac. Implants*, 28, 5, e243–e251, 2013.
131. Freitas, R.M., Spin-Neto, R., Marcantonio Junior, E., Pereira, L.A., Wikesjö, U.M., Susin, C., Alveolar ridge and maxillary sinus augmentation using rhBMP-2: A systematic review. *Clin. Implant Dent. Relat. Res.*, 17, Suppl 1, e192–c201, 2015.
132. Kelly, M.P., Vaughn, O.L., Anderson, P.A., Systematic review and meta-analysis of recombinant human bone morphogenetic protein-2 in localized alveolar ridge and maxillary sinus augmentation. *J. Oral Maxillofac. Surg.*, 74, 5, 928–939, 2016.
133. Galarraga-Vinueza, M.E., Barootchi, S., Nevins, M.L., Nevins, M., Miron, R.J., Tavelli, L., Twenty-five years of recombinant human growth factors rhP-DGF-BB and rhBMP-2 in oral hard and soft tissue regeneration. *Periodontol. 2000*, 94, 1, 483–509, 2024.
134. Andrae, J., Gallini, R., Betsholtz, C., Role of platelet-derived growth factors in physiology and medicine. *Genes Dev.*, 22, 10, 1276–1312, 2008.
135. Ghassib, I.H., Saleh, M.H.A., Wang, H.L., Human platelet-derived growth factor-BB (rhPDGF-BB) with collagen matrix for sinus elevation without using a bone graft. *Clin. Adv. Periodontics*, 14, 4, 237–243, 2024.
136. Tavelli, L., Ravidà, A., Barootchi, S., Chambrone, L., Giannobile, W.V., Recombinant human platelet-derived growth factor: A systematic review of clinical findings in oral regenerative procedures. *JDR. Clin. Trans. Res.*, 6, 2, 161–173, 2021.
137. Kaigler, D., Avila, G., Wisner-Lynch, L., Chambrone, L., Giannobile, W.V., Platelet-derived growth factor applications in periodontal and peri-implant bone regeneration. *Expert Opin. Biol. Ther.*, 11, 3, 375–385, 2011.
138. Wang, H., Qi, L.L., Shema, C., Jiang, K.Y., Ren, P., Wang, H., Wang, L., Advances in the role and mechanism of fibroblasts in fracture healing. *Front. Endocrinol. (Lausanne)*, 15, 1350958, 2024.
139. Shah, P., Keppler, L., Rutkowski, J., A review of platelet derived growth factor playing pivotal role in bone regeneration. *J. Oral Implantol.*, 40, 3, 330–340, 2014.
140. Nugraha, M.A., Mulyawan, I., Jayakusuma, A.A., Osteoinductive capacity of platelet-rich fibrin vs biodentine for mandible fracture. *Majalah Biomorfologi–Biomorphol. J.*, 34, 2, 134–142, 2024.
141. Simion, M., Rocchietta, I., Dellavia, C., Three-dimensional ridge augmentation with xenograft and recombinant human platelet-derived growth factor-BB in humans: Report of two cases. *Int. J. Periodontics Restorative Dent.*, 27, 2, 109–115, 2007.
142. Nevins, M., Garber, D., Hanratty, J.J., McAllister, B.S., Nevins, M.L., Salama, M., Schupbach, P., Wallace, S., Bernstein, S.M., Kim, D.M., Human histologic evaluation of anorganic bovine bone mineral combined with recombinant human platelet-derived growth factor BB in maxillary sinus augmentation: case series study. *Int. J. Periodontics Restorative Dent.*, 29, 6, 583–591, 2009.

143. Nevins, M.L., Camelo, M., Schupbach, P., Kim, D.M., Camelo, J.M., Nevins, M., Human histologic evaluation of mineralized collagen bone substitute and recombinant platelet-derived growth factor-BB to create bone for implant placement in extraction socket defects at 4 and 6 months: A case series. *Int. J. Periodontics Restorative Dent.*, 29, 2, 129–139, 2009.
144. McAllister, B.S. and Haghighat, K., Bone augmentation techniques. *J. Periodontol.*, 78, 3, 377–396, 2007.
145. Howell, T.H., Fiorellini, J.P., Paquette, D.W., Offenbacher, S., Giannobile, W.V., Lynch, S.E., A phase I/II clinical trial to evaluate a combination of recombinant human platelet-derived growth factor-BB and recombinant human insulin-like growth factor-I in patients with periodontal disease. *J. Periodontol.*, 68, 12, 1186–1193, 1997.
146. Darby, I.B. and Morris, K.H., A systematic review of the use of growth factors in human periodontal regeneration. *J. Periodontol.*, 84, 4, 465–476, 2013.
147. Khoshkam, V., Chan, H.L., Lin, G.H., Mailoa, J., Giannobile, W.V., Wang, H.L., Oh, T.J., Outcomes of regenerative treatment with rhPDGF-BB and rhFGF-2 for periodontal intra-bony defects: A systematic review and meta-analysis. *J. Clin. Periodontol.*, 42, 3, 272–280, 2015.
148. Scheines, C., Hokett, S.D., Katancik, J.A., Recombinant human platelet-derived growth factor-BB in human alveolar ridge augmentation: A review of the literature. *Int. J. Oral Maxillofac. Implants*, 33, 5, 1047–1056, 2018.
149. Nevins, M., Giannobile, W.V., McGuire, M.K., Kao, R.T., Mellonig, J.T., Hinrichs, J.E., McAllister, B.S., Murphy, K., Burgess, A.M., McClain, P.K., Nevins, M.L. Platelet-derived growth factor stimulates bone fill and rate of attachment level gain: results of a large multicenter randomized controlled trial. *J. Periodontol.*, 76, 12, 2205–2215, 2005.
150. Gao, P., Liu, C., Dong, H., Li, Q., Chen, Y., TGF-β promotes the proliferation and osteogenic differentiation of dental pulp stem cells a systematic review and meta-analysis. *Eur. J. Med. Res.*, 28, 261, 2023.
151. Sanjabi, S., Oh, S.A., Li, M.O., Regulation of the immune response by TGF-β: From conception to autoimmunity and infection. *Cold Spring Harb. Perspect. Biol.*, 9, 6, a022236, 2017.
152. Tie, Y., Tang, F., Peng, D., Zhang, Y., Shi, H., TGF-beta signal transduction: biology, function and therapy for diseases. *Mol. Biomed.*, 3, 45, 2022.
153. Danielpour, D., Advances and challenges in targeting TGF-β isoforms for therapeutic intervention of cancer: A mechanism-based perspective. *Pharmaceuticals (Basel)*, 17, 533, 2024.
154. Wei, E., Hu, M., Wu, L., Pan, X., Zhu, Q., Liu, H., Liu, Y., TGF-β signaling regulates differentiation of MSCs in bone metabolism: disputes among viewpoints. *Stem Cell Res. Ther.*, 15, 156, 2024.
155. Zou, M.L., Chen, Z.H., Teng, Y.Y., Liu, S.Y., Jia, Y., Zhang, K.W., Sun, Z.L., Wu, J.J., Yuan, Z.D., Feng, Y., Li, X., Xu, R.S., Yuan, F.L., The Smad dependent TGF-β and BMP signaling pathway in bone remodeling and therapies. *Front. Mol. Biosci.*, 8, 593310, 2021.

156. Wu, M., Wu, S., Chen, W., Li, Y.P., The roles and regulatory mechanisms of TGF-β and BMP signaling in bone and cartilage development, homeostasis and disease. *Cell Res.*, 34, 101–123, 2024.
157. Chen, G., Deng, C., Li, Y.P., TGF-β and BMP signaling in osteoblast differentiation and bone formation. *Int. J. Biol. Sci.*, 8, 2, 272–288, 2012.
158. Shi, A., Heinayati, A., Bao, D., Liu, H., Ding, X., Tong, X., Wang, L., Wang, B., Qin, H., Small molecule inhibitor of TGF-β signaling enables robust osteogenesis of autologous GMSCs to successfully repair minipig severe maxillofacial bone defects. *Stem Cell Res. Ther.*, 10, 172, 2019.
159. Houchen, C.J., Ghanem, S., Kaartinen, V., Bumann, E.E., TGF-β signaling in the cranial neural crest affects late-stage mandibular bone resorption and length. *Front. Physiol.*, 15, 1435594, 2024.
160. Asparuhova, M.B., Riedwyl, D., Aizawa, R., Raabe, C., Couso-Queiruga, E., Chappuis, V., Local concentrations of TGF-β1 and IGF-1 appear determinant in regulating bone regeneration in human postextraction tooth sockets. *Int. J. Mol. Sci.*, 24, 8239, 2023.
161. Miron, R.J., Sculean, A., Cochran, D.L., Froum, S., Zucchelli, G., Nemcovsky, C., Donos, N., Lyngstadaas, S.P., Deschner, J., Dard, M., Stavropoulos, A., Zhang, Y., Trombelli, L., Kasaj, A., Shirakata, Y., Cortellini, P., Tonetti, M., Rasperini, G., Jepsen, S., Bosshardt, D.D., Twenty years of enamel matrix derivative: the past, the present and the future. *J. Clin. Periodontol.*, 43, 8, 668–683, 2016.
162. Brookes, S.J., Robinson, C., Kirkham, J., Bonass, W.A., Biochemistry and molecular biology of amelogenin proteins of developing dental enamel. *Arch. Oral Biol.*, 40, 1, 1–14, 1995.
163. Esposito, M., Grusovin, M.G., Papanikolaou, N., Coulthard, P., Worthington, H.V., Enamel matrix derivative (Emdogain(R)) for periodontal tissue regeneration in intrabony defects. *Cochrane Database Syst. Rev.*, 2009, 4, CD003875, 2009.
164. Heijl, L., Heden, G., Svärdström, G., Ostgren, A., Enamel matrix derivative (EMDOGAIN) in the treatment of intrabony periodontal defects. *J. Clin. Periodontol.*, 24, 9 Pt 2, 705–714, 1997.
165. Heijl, L., Periodontal regeneration with enamel matrix derivative in one human experimental defect. A case report. *J. Clin. Periodontol.*, 24, 9 Pt 2, 693–696, 1997.
166. Yukna, R.A. and Mellonig, J.T., Histologic evaluation of periodontal healing in humans following regenerative therapy with enamel matrix derivative. A 10-case series. *J. Periodontol.*, 71, 5, 752–759, 2000.
167. Cochran, D.L., King, G.N., Schoolfield, J., Velasquez-Plata, D., Mellonig, J.T., Jones, A., The effect of enamel matrix proteins on periodontal regeneration as determined by histological analyses. *J. Periodontol.*, 74, 7, 1043–1055, 2003.
168. Mumulidu, A., Hildebrand, B., Fabi, B., Hammarström, L., Cochran, D.L., Dard, M., Lemoult, S., Purification and analysis of a 5kDa component of

enamel matrix derivative. *J. Chromatogr. B. Analyt. Technol. Biomed. Life Sci.*, 857, 2, 210–218, 2007.
169. Hammarström, L., Enamel matrix, cementum development and regeneration. *J. Clin. Periodontol.*, 24, 658–668, 1997.
170. Lyngstadaas, S.P., Wohlfahrt, J.C., Brookes, S.J., Paine, M.L., Snead, M.L., Reseland, J.E., Enamel matrix proteins; old molecules for new applications. *Orthod. Craniofac. Res.*, 12, 3, 243–253, 2009.
171. Wyganowska-Świątkowska, M., Urbaniak, P., Nohawica, M.M., Kotwicka, M., Jankun, J., Enamel matrix proteins exhibit growth factor activity: A review of evidence at the cellular and molecular levels. *Exp. Ther. Med.*, 9, 6, 2025–2033, 2015.
172. Jepsen, S., Topoll, H., Rengers, H., Heinz, B., Teich, M., Hoffmann, T., Al-Machot, E., Meyle, J., Jervøe-Storm, P.M., Clinical outcomes after treatment of intra-bony defects with an EMD/synthetic bone graft or EMD alone: A multicentre randomized-controlled clinical trial. *J. Clin. Periodontol.*, 35, 5, 420–428, 2008.
173. Gupta, S.J., Jhingran, R., Gupta, V., Bains, V.K., Madan, R., Rizvi, I., Efficacy of platelet-rich fibrin vs. enamel matrix derivative in the treatment of periodontal intrabony defects: A clinical and cone beam computed tomography study. *J. Int. Acad. Periodontol.*, 16, 3, 86–96, 2014.
174. Lee, J.H., Kim, D.H., Jeong, S.N., Comparative assessment of anterior maxillary alveolar ridge preservation with and without ad-junctive use of enamel matrix derivative: A randomized clinical trial. *Clin. Oral Implants Res.*, 31, 1–9, 2020.
175. Lee, J.H. and Jeong, S.N., Effect of enamel matrix derivative on alveolar ridge preservation in the posterior maxilla: A randomized controlled clinical trial. *Clin. Implant Dent. Relat. Res.*, 22, 622–630, 2020.
176. Mercado, F., Vaquette, C., Hamlet, S., Ivanovski, S., Enamel matrix derivative promotes new bone formation in xenograft assisted maxillary anterior ridge preservation – A randomized controlled clinical trial. *Clin. Oral Implants Res.*, 32, 732–744, 2021.
177. Matarasso, M., Iorio-Siciliano, V., Blasi, A., Ramaglia, L., Salvi, G.E., Sculean, A., Enamel matrix derivative and bone grafts for periodontal regeneration of intrabony defects. A systematic review and meta-analysis. *Clin. Oral Investig.*, 19, 7, 1581–1593, 2015.
178. Fakheran, O., Fischer, K.R., Schmidlin, P.R., Enamel matrix derivatives as an adjunct to alveolar ridge preservation – A systematic review. *Dent. J.*, 11, 100, 2023.
179. Annunziata, M., Piccirillo, A., Perillo, F., Cecoro, G., Nastri, L., Guida, L., Enamel matrix derivative and autogenous bone graft for periodontal regeneration of intrabony defects in humans: A systematic review and meta-analysis. *Materials (Basel)*, 12, 16, 2634, 2009.

13

Histological Assessment of Bone Grafts and Substitute Materials Used in Bone Regeneration

Sundar Ramalingam[1]*, Chalini Sundar[2] and Randa A. Alfotawi[3]

[1]*Department of Oral and Maxillofacial Surgery, College of Dentistry, King Saud University and Dental University Hospital, King Saud University Medical City, Riyadh, Saudi Arabia*
[2]*Saudi Dental Society, College of Dentistry, King Saud University, Riyadh, Saudi Arabia*
[3]*Department of Oral and Maxillofacial Surgery, College of Dentistry, King Saud University, Riyadh, Saudi Arabia*

Abstract

Bone regeneration is a cornerstone of oral and maxillofacial surgery, orthopedics, and implantology. The increasing use of bone grafts and bone substitute materials, with or without biological adjuncts such as mesenchymal stem cells (MSCs), bone morphogenetic proteins (BMPs), and growth factors, necessitates a comprehensive understanding of the biological events that control bone healing and integration. Histological assessment of bone regeneration and healing provides critical insight into these processes, allowing clinicians and researchers to assess the quality of new bone formation, scaffold resorption, vascularization, cellular infiltration, and inflammatory response. This chapter aims to serve as a practical and scientific reference for evaluating histological outcomes in bone regenerative procedures that utilize various bone grafts and substitute materials.

***Keywords*:** Histological assessment, histology, bone regeneration, bone defect healing, bone grafts, bone substitutes, adjuncts for bone regeneration

**Corresponding author:* smunusamy@ksu.edu.sa

Randa A. Alfotawi (ed.) Oro-Facial Bone Grafts and Biomaterials, (277–316) © 2026 Scrivener Publishing LLC

13.1 Introduction

Bone regeneration is a critical aspect of orthopedic, craniofacial, dental, and reconstructive surgery, particularly in cases of trauma, tumor resection, congenital defects, and degenerative diseases [1, 2]. The assessment of bone grafts and bone substitute materials is fundamental to advancing regenerative medicine. Among various evaluation methods, histological analysis remains the gold standard for understanding the biological performance of these materials at the tissue level [3]. Histology provides essential insights into cellular behavior, vascularization, host–graft interactions, and the quality and quantity of newly formed bone [4].

The advent of tissue engineering and regenerative techniques, including the incorporation of mesenchymal stem cells (MSCs), bone morphogenetic proteins (BMPs), and other growth factors, has necessitated more refined and comprehensive histological evaluations [5, 6]. These adjuncts influence cellular signaling pathways and extracellular matrix deposition, which are best characterized using microscopic tissue analysis [4, 7]. The integration of graft materials into host bone involves a complex sequence of events, including inflammation, osteoconduction, osteoinduction, and remodeling, all of which are best observed through histological methods [3, 8, 9].

Despite the availability of advanced imaging modalities like micro-computed tomography (μCT) and magnetic resonance imaging (MRI), these techniques cannot substitute for the cellular-level resolution and qualitative insights that histological evaluation provides [10–12]. Thus, histological assessment continues to be indispensable in preclinical and clinical studies of bone grafts and substitutes.

This chapter highlights the significance of histological assessment in correlating clinical and radiographic findings with microscopic evidence. It briefly describes about specimen processing and preparation techniques, key staining methods, and commonly used microscopy techniques. Furthermore, it addresses the implications of histological findings for clinical decision-making, the performance of various graft materials, and the use of biological adjuncts to enhance regeneration.

The main objectives of this chapter are to help the reader understand the significance of histological assessment in evaluating bone grafts and substitutes, apply appropriate preparation and staining techniques for bone analysis, select suitable microscopy methods for bone regeneration studies, and interpret findings related to osteogenesis, scaffold integration, vascularization, and remodeling. It also covers the effects of biological adjuncts like MSCs, BMPs, and growth factors, as well as current limitations and future directions in histological analysis and quantitative histomorphometry in bone regenerative research.

13.2 Histological Techniques in Bone Regeneration Research

13.2.1 Decalcified and Undecalcified Specimen Processing

The choice between decalcified and undecalcified histological processing depends on the specific objectives of the study. Decalcification is commonly employed to facilitate the sectioning of mineralized tissue using paraffin embedding [13]. It involves removing calcium deposits from the bone matrix using chelating agents like ethylenediaminetetraacetic acid (EDTA) or acidic solutions such as formic or nitric acid [14, 15]. While this process allows for routine staining and immunohistochemistry, it may compromise structural integrity and leach out some proteins and cellular components [13].

Undecalcified histology, on the other hand, retains the mineral content of the bone and is typically used when assessing the quality and quantity of mineralized tissue or implant integration. These specimens are embedded in poly-methyl-methacrylate (PMMA) or other plastic resins and require specialized microtomes for sectioning [16]. The challenge of undecalcified processing lies in the technical demands and time-consuming nature of sample preparation, but it offers superior preservation of the bone–implant interface and is invaluable for quantitative histology and fluorescent labeling studies [16].

13.2.2 Staining Techniques in Histological Assessment of Bone Regeneration

Histological staining is a cornerstone of evaluating bone grafts and bone substitute materials in both preclinical and clinical research. It allows for detailed visualization of cellular and extracellular structures, aiding in the assessment of new bone formation, scaffold integration, inflammatory response, and vascularization [17]. One of the most commonly employed staining techniques is hematoxylin and eosin (H&E) staining, which serves as the foundational method for general tissue morphology. Hematoxylin stains nuclei blue-purple, while eosin stains cytoplasmic and extracellular components in shades of pink. H&E is particularly useful for identifying the general architecture of regenerated bone, the presence of inflammatory infiltrates, and cellular responses to biomaterials [3].

For the assessment of collagen deposition and fibrous tissue maturation, Masson's trichrome staining is frequently utilized. This trichrome method distinctly stains collagen fibers in blue or green, muscle and cytoplasm in red, and nuclei in black. It is particularly effective for distinguishing between newly formed osteoid, fibrous encapsulation, and mature lamellar bone. This technique is highly valuable in studies evaluating the osteoconductivity and fibrogenic response of graft materials, especially in the context of scaffold biocompatibility and host integration [18].

Another significant stain in bone histology is Van Gieson's stain, often used in conjunction with picric acid, which stains collagen red and other tissues yellow. This stain provides excellent contrast for visualizing the deposition and orientation of collagen fibers, thereby aiding in the differentiation of mature versus immature bone. It is particularly useful in comparative analyses of different graft materials and their ability to support organized bone matrix formation [19].

In addition to these traditional stains, Goldner's trichrome is often applied to undecalcified, resin-embedded bone specimens. It offers a more nuanced view of mineralized versus unmineralized bone, staining mineralized bone green, osteoid red, and cell nuclei black. This stain is essential in dynamic histomorphometric studies where the quantification of mineral apposition rates and bone formation parameters is required [18]. Toluidine blue is another metachromatic stain widely employed in resin-embedded sections, particularly useful for identifying osteoblasts, osteoclasts, and cartilage remnants. Its high affinity for acidic tissue components makes it ideal for highlighting proteoglycan-rich areas, making it useful in osteochondral tissue engineering studies [20].

For mineral-specific visualization, Von Kossa and Alizarin Red S stains are indispensable. Von Kossa stain uses silver nitrate to detect phosphate and carbonate in calcium deposits, turning mineralized regions black [15, 21]. This method is particularly effective for evaluating the degree and distribution of mineralization in bone graft materials. Alizarin Red S, on the other hand, binds directly to calcium ions, staining mineralized tissues in red or orange hues. It is highly suitable for both *in vivo* and *in vitro* studies assessing osteogenic potential and mineral deposition of scaffolds, especially when mesenchymal stem cells or osteoinductive agents like bone morphogenetic proteins (BMPs) are involved [22].

Immunohistochemistry (IHC) and immunofluorescence (IF) represent more advanced staining modalities that use antigen–antibody reactions to detect specific bone-related proteins such as osteocalcin, osteopontin, RUNX2, and vascular markers like CD31. These techniques enable precise localization of cellular phenotypes and are critical for understanding the molecular mechanisms underlying bone regeneration. When bone grafts are loaded with adjuncts like MSCs or BMPs, IHC and IF allow researchers to track the differentiation status of implanted cells and the bioactivity of signaling molecules [5, 18].

Furthermore, tartrate-resistant acid phosphatase (TRAP) staining is employed to identify osteoclasts and assess bone resorption. This is particularly relevant in studies where bone remodeling and graft turnover are being analyzed. TRAP-positive multinucleated cells at the graft interface indicate active resorption, which is a crucial component of natural bone healing and remodeling dynamics [23].

The integration of these staining techniques offers a comprehensive histological toolkit that facilitates qualitative and quantitative evaluation of bone tissue regeneration. Their combined use is often tailored to the specific aims of each study, whether focusing on matrix deposition, mineralization, cellular infiltration, vascularization, or inflammatory responses. The continual advancement of histological staining methods, including multiplexed staining and digital pathology, further enhances the depth and precision of bone graft evaluation.

13.2.3 Quantitative Histology

Quantitative histomorphometry involves measuring specific parameters of bone formation and remodeling, such as bone volume/tissue volume (BV/TV), osteoid thickness, and mineral apposition rate. Stereological approaches and image analysis software now allow for objective, reproducible quantification of histological sections [24–26]. Dynamic histomorphometry, using fluorescent dyes such as Calcein and Alizarin Red, enables time-resolved measurement of bone deposition rates. This is especially useful in animal models where sequential labeling is possible [27]. Furthermore, advanced image processing and machine learning are being increasingly incorporated into histological analysis, promising enhanced accuracy and high-throughput capabilities.

13.3 Microscopy Techniques for Histological Assessment of Bone Grafts

The microscopic evaluation of bone grafts and substitute materials plays a pivotal role in understanding the integration, remodeling, and cellular responses within regenerated bone tissue. The choice of microscopy technique directly influences the type and quality of data obtained [28]. Depending on the research objectives ranging from assessing mineralization, cellular infiltration, vascularization, and scaffold degradation to osseointegration, different microscopy methods are used, either independently or in combination (Table 13.1) [29]. This report outlines the primary microscopy techniques used in bone histology, their indications, and their relevance in both preclinical and clinical research.

Table 13.1 Brief overview of the commonly employed microscopy techniques for histological assessment of bone grafts in osseous regeneration and healing, along with their indications, advantages, and limitations [18, 20, 28–33].

Technique	Description	Indications	Advantages	Limitations
Light Microscopy	Utilizes visible light and stains (e.g., H&E, Masson's trichrome, Van Gieson's) to visualize cellular and extracellular structures in decalcified or undecalcified sections.	- Routine assessment of graft–host interface - Detection of inflammation, angiogenesis, fibrosis - Morphological evaluation of bone regeneration	- Widely available and cost-effective - Compatible with image analysis software - Suitable for routine diagnostic histology	- Limited resolution - Cannot reveal ultrastructural or molecular details
Polarized Light Microscopy	Employs polarized light to detect birefringent materials like collagen and mineral crystals, enhancing visualization of bone microstructure.	- Analysis of collagen fiber orientation - Differentiation of woven vs. lamellar bone - Mineral orientation assessment in undecalcified bone	- Provides unique insights into matrix organization - Enhances quality control of grafts	- Interpretation requires expertise - Primarily qualitative and adjunctive
Fluorescence Microscopy	Uses fluorochrome-labeled molecules (e.g., calcein, alizarin, tetracycline) to track dynamic bone processes or specific cellular components.	- Bone formation rate and mineral apposition - Labeling of osteoblasts/osteoclasts - Protein/mRNA detection *via* immunofluorescence or fluorescence *in situ* hybridization (FISH)	- High specificity for biological targets - Enables dynamic histomorphometry - Ideal for assessing mesenchymal stem cell (MSC) behavior or signaling molecules	- Fluorophore degradation and tissue auto-fluorescence - Requires specialized equipment
Confocal Laser Scanning Microscopy	Utilizes a laser beam and spatial pinhole to generate high-resolution, optical section images, enabling 3D reconstruction.	- Cell–scaffold interactions - 3D imaging of vascularization - Subcellular localization of proteins	- Excellent depth resolution - Enables live-cell imaging - Compatible with thick or complex tissue samples	- High cost and complex operation - Labor-intensive sample preparation

(*Continued*)

Table 13.1 Brief overview of the commonly employed microscopy techniques for histological assessment of bone grafts in osseous regeneration and healing, along with their indications, advantages, and limitations [18, 20, 28–33]. (*Continued*)

Technique	Description	Indications	Advantages	Limitations
Scanning Electron Microscopy	Provides high-resolution 3D imaging by scanning specimen surfaces with an electron beam. Ideal for mineralized tissues and biomaterials.	- Evaluation of scaffold surface morphology - Bone–material integration analysis - Microstructure and porosity assessment	- Superb surface detail and magnification - Effective for bone substitute characterization	- Requires conductive coating (e.g., gold sputtering) - Not suitable for hydrated or live specimens
Transmission Electron Microscopy	Transmits electrons through ultra-thin sections to analyze internal cell structures and nanostructures at high magnification.	- Subcellular evaluation of osteoblasts/osteoclasts - Bone matrix ultrastructure analysis - Bone morphogenetic proteins (BMPs) and nanoparticle–cell interaction studies	- Exceptional resolution (nm scale) - Reveals organelle-level changes (e.g., autophagy, apoptosis)	- Technically demanding - Narrow field of view - Time-consuming preparation

The histological assessment of bone grafts and substitute materials requires a multi-modal microscopy approach tailored to specific research or clinical questions. Light and polarized light microscopy remain essential for general morphology and collagen organization. Fluorescence-based methods allow for dynamic and molecular analyses, while electron microscopy provides ultrastructural details crucial for advanced material characterization. The integration of confocal, electron microcopy techniques, and emerging digital and AI (Artifical Intelligence)-driven platforms is set to enhance the precision and throughput of bone histology in the future [30].

13.4 General Histological Characteristics of Different Bone Graft Materials

Bone grafting is a pivotal technique in regenerative medicine, aiming to restore bone defects resulting from trauma, disease, or surgical interventions. The selection of an appropriate graft material is crucial, as it influences the healing process, integration, and long-term functionality [18]. Histological evaluations provide insights into the biological behavior of these materials, including their osteoconductivity, osteoinductivity, resorption rates, and integration with host tissue [4]. This section delves into the histological characteristics of various bone graft materials, encompassing synthetic substitutes, allografts, autografts, xenografts, and alternative grafting tissues. In order to delineate differences in bone healing between grafted and non-grafted defects, Figure 13.1 shows representative histological images of impaired bone healing in a non-grafted defect. On the contrary, even placement of a simple resorbable scaffold like collagen sponge enhances bone regeneration within defects, as shown in Figure 13.2.

13.4.1 Synthetic Bone Substitutes

13.4.1.1 Beta-Tricalcium Phosphate (β-TCP)

Beta-tricalcium phosphate (β-TCP) is a synthetic, bioceramic material recognized for its osteoconductive properties and resorbability. Histologically, β-TCP exhibits prominent bone formation, particularly at the periphery of the grafted area. Osteoclast-like giant cells are often observed surrounding the material, indicating active resorption and remodeling. Over time, β-TCP is replaced by newly formed bone, demonstrating its biodegradable nature and compatibility with human bone tissue [3, 6, 34]. Representative histological images of bone defect healing and regeneration when grafted with β-TCP are shown in Figures 13.3, 13.4 and 13.5.

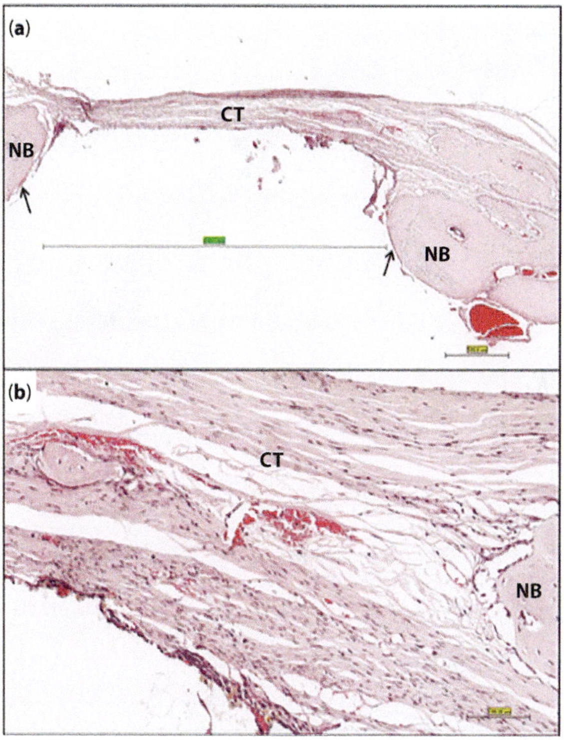

Figure 13.1 Representative photomicrographs of bone defect healing in a non-grafted defect, after 6 weeks (decalcified, HE staining). (a) At lower magnification (x4), there is no new bone formed within the defect, and the native bone (NB) on the defect edges (black arrows) is bridged by a fibrous connective tissue (CT) layer. (b) At higher magnification (x10), the CT is highly cellular and is seen interspersed with areas of homogeneous acellular acidophilic material indicative of collagen fibers, and the presence of a dense inflammatory infiltrate in the inferior portions indicative of prolonged inflammation, even after 6 weeks of healing.

In a study assessing large human bone defects implanted with β-TCP, ongoing bone remodeling was observed even 208 weeks post-implantation. Multinuclear giant cells were noted phagocytosing the biomaterial, and osteoclasts showed intense tartrate-resistant acid phosphatase (TRAP) positivity, indicating active resorption and remodeling processes [35].

13.4.1.2 Biphasic Calcium Phosphate (BCP)

Biphasic calcium phosphate (BCP) combines hydroxyapatite (HA) and β-TCP, aiming to balance the stability of HA with the resorbability of

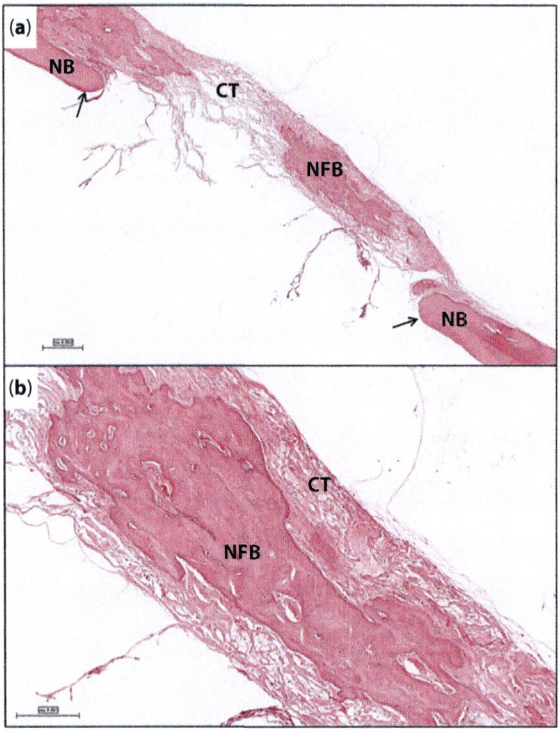

Figure 13.2 Representative photomicrographs of bone defect regeneration in a defect grafted only with collagen sponge, after 6 weeks of healing (decalcified, HE staining). (a) At lower magnification (x4), the native bone (NB) in the defect edges (black arrows) is seen bridged by a layer of connective tissue (CT) with islands of newly formed bone (NFB). (b) At higher magnification (x10), the NFB presents with irregular lamellae having multiple osteocytes and evidence of neovascularization indicative of immature osteoid that is undergoing mineralization, and the NFB is enveloped both superiorly and inferiorly by dense fibrous CT with interspersed areas of high cellularity and collagen fibers (homogeneous acellular acidophilic material).

β-TCP. Histological assessments reveal that BCP supports bone regeneration, with new bone formation observed around the material particles, as shown in Figure 13.6. The proportion of HA to β-TCP influences the resorption rate and the extent of new bone formation, allowing for tailored applications based on clinical needs [36, 37].

In a comparative study, BCP demonstrated the ability to differentiate bone marrow stromal cells toward the osteoblast lineage and promoted ectopic bone formation *in vivo*, confirming its osteoinductive potential [38].

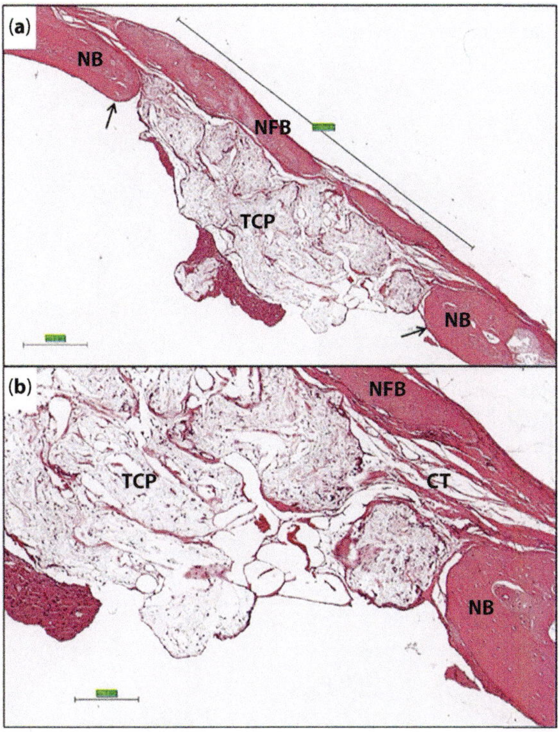

Figure 13.3 Representative photomicrographs of bone defect regeneration in a defect grafted with beta tricalcium phosphate (beta-TCP—alloplastic bone substitute) after 6 weeks of healing (decalcified, HE staining). (a) At lower magnification (x4), there is a layer of newly formed bone (NFB) extending between the edges of the defect (black arrows), and inferior to it is a thick layer of granular crystalline material indicative of beta-TCP particles (TCP). The layer of NFB is separated from the native bone (NB) by connective tissue. (b) At higher magnification (x10), the NFB layer is thin, has irregular lamellae unlike NB, and has osteoblasts in the osteoid. The CT layer separates the NFB from NB and the TCP particles.

13.4.2 Allografts

Allografts, derived from human donors, are utilized as bone substitutes due to their availability and structural similarity to autogenous bone [25]. Histological evaluations of allografts show varying degrees of integration and remodeling. Some studies report the presence of necrotic bone at earlier stages, which is gradually replaced by new bone over extended periods [38]. The incorporation of allografts is influenced by factors such as processing methods and the recipient's biological environment [25].

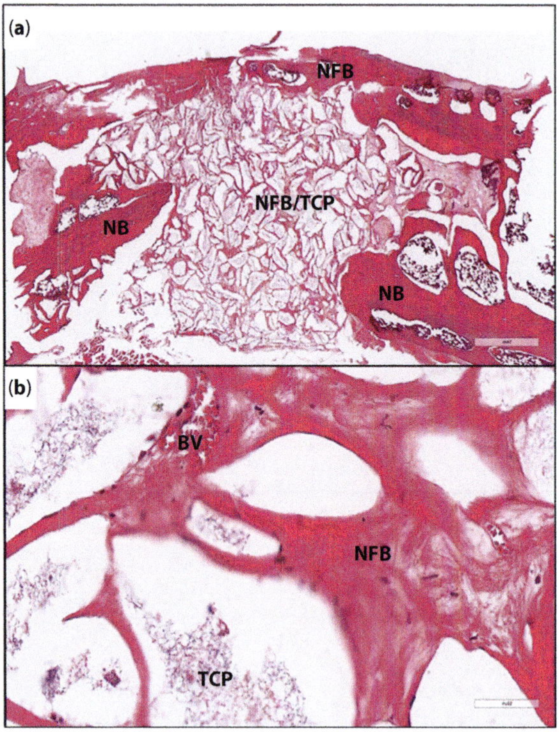

Figure 13.4 Representative photomicrographs of bone defect regeneration in a defect grafted with beta tricalcium phosphate (beta-TCP—alloplastic bone substitute) after 6 weeks of healing (decalcified, HE staining). (a) At lower magnification (x4), the segmental bone defect is seen bridged by a layer of newly formed bone (NFB) along with beta-TCP particles surrounded by newly forming bone and connective tissue. (b) At very high magnification (x40), the granular, crystalline, and amorphous beta-TCP particles are seen surrounded by new bone osteoid with an irregular lamellar pattern, trapped osteoblasts, and neovascularization (BV).

Demineralized freeze-dried bone allograft (DFDBA) is a specific type of allograft known for its osteoinductive properties. Histological studies have shown that DFDBA can induce new bone formation, making it a valuable material in periodontal and oral surgeries [25, 38]. Bone defect regeneration after grafting with allograft bone is shown in Figure 13.7.

13.4.3 Autografts

Autografts, harvested from the patient's own body, are considered the gold standard in bone grafting due to their osteogenic, osteoinductive, and osteoconductive properties [11]. Histologically, autografts demonstrate

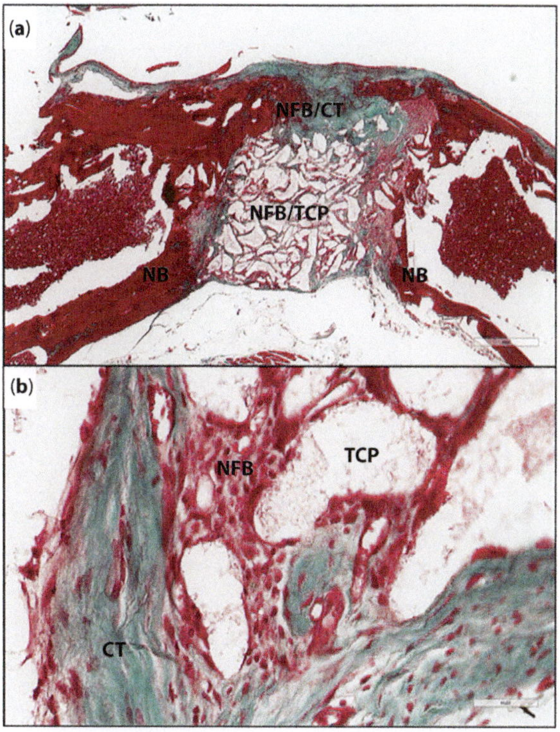

Figure 13.5 Representative photomicrographs of bone defect regeneration in a defect grafted with beta tricalcium phosphate (beta-TCP—alloplastic bone substitute) similar to the one shown in Figure 13.11, after 6 weeks of healing (decalcified, MT staining). (a) At lower magnification (x4), while the new bone bridging the superior edges of the segmental defect has mixed osseous and fibrous connective tissue areas (NFB/CT), the native bone (NB) in the inferior edges of the defect is predominantly bridged by beta-TCP and connective tissue. (b) At very high magnification (x40), the residual mineral content of the beta-TCP particles is visible (light red stain) and differentiated from the higher mineral content of new bone osteoid surrounding the TCP (NFB—dark red stain). The NFB is replete with osteoblasts and has interspersed areas of CT, which indicates resorption of TCP particles and new bone deposition.

viable osteocytes within the grafted bone, indicating successful integration and vitality, as shown in Figures 13.8 and 13.9. The presence of living bone cells facilitates remodeling and incorporation into the host site, leading to effective bone regeneration [38, 39].

However, the use of autografts is limited by donor site morbidity and the quantity of available bone. Despite these limitations, autografts remain a preferred choice in many clinical scenarios due to their superior regenerative capabilities [6].

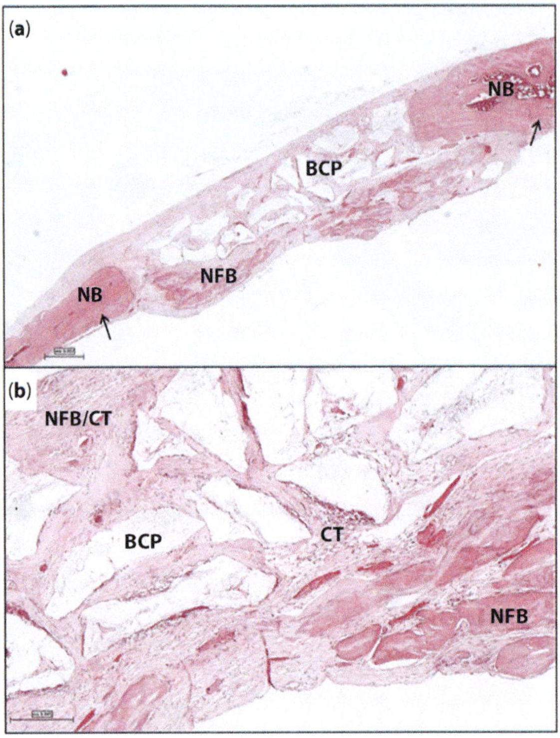

Figure 13.6 Representative photomicrographs of bone defect regeneration in a defect grafted with biphasic calcium phosphate (BCP—alloplastic bone substitute) after 6 weeks of healing (decalcified, HE staining). (a) At lower magnification (x4), the bone defect is seen bridged by a layer of particles (BCP) of amorphous crystalline material along with connective tissue and a layer of newly formed (NFB) in the inferior part of the healing defect. The NFB is seen separated from the native bone (NB) in the edges of the defect (black arrows) by fibrous connective tissue. (b) At higher magnification (x10), the healing defect site is filled with abundant BCP, which appears as a granular crystalline material, and is surrounded by abundant connective tissue (CT) and areas of NFB, indicating new bone formation through creeping substitution. The NFB, although less in quantity, is seen with irregular lamellae and osteoblasts.

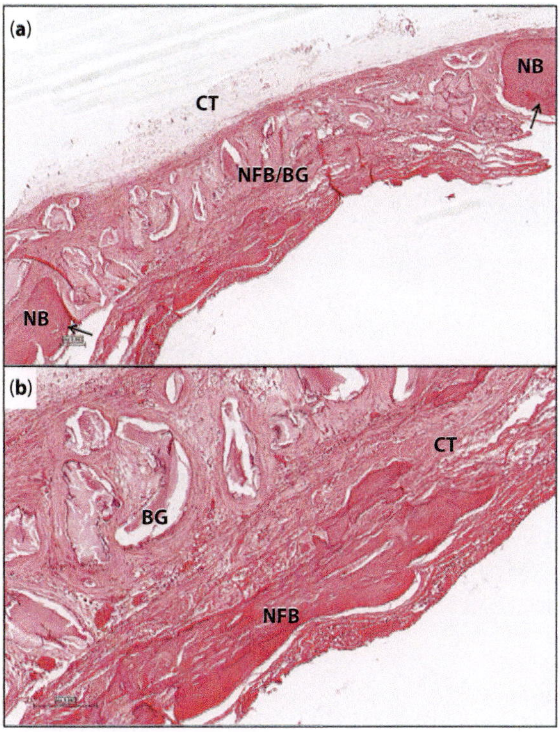

Figure 13.7 Representative photomicrographs of bone defect regeneration in a defect grafted with demineralized allograft bone, after 6 weeks of healing (decalcified, HE staining). (a) At lower magnification (x4), a bridge of newly formed bone (NFB) with connective tissue (CT) is seen extending between the native bone (NB) in the edges of the defect (black arrows). Additionally, multiple fragments of homogeneous acellular material resembling dead bone are seen indicative of demineralized bone allograft particles (BG) in differing stages of resorption. (b) At higher magnification (x10), a thick sheet of NFB with irregular lamellae, multiple osteoblasts, and blood vessels is seen in the inferior aspect of the healing bone defect. The BG particles are seen surrounded by areas of immature osteoid formation and is seen separated from the sheets of NFB by sparse layers of fibrous CT.

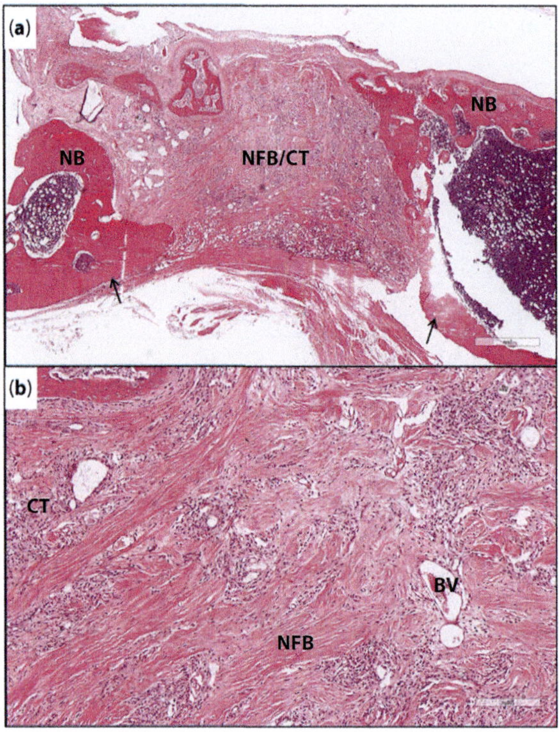

Figure 13.8 Representative photomicrographs of bone defect regeneration in a defect grafted with autologous bone, after 6 weeks of healing (decalcified, HE staining). (a) At lower magnification (x4), a thick sheet of newly formed bone (NFB) and connective tissue (CT) is seen extending from the native bone (NB) margins on either side of the edges of the defect (black arrows). (b) At higher magnification (x10), NFB with irregular lamellae, multiple osteoblasts, and blood vessels is seen all through the healing defect and is seen oriented in a random fashion, indicating multiple foci of new bone formation due to the combined osteoinductive, osteoconductive, and osteogenic potential of autologous bone graft. Although CT is seen in between the immature osteoid, it is not abundant, has less cellularity, and possesses more collagen fibers, signifying resorption of the autograft bone for deposition of new osteoid within the healing bone defect.

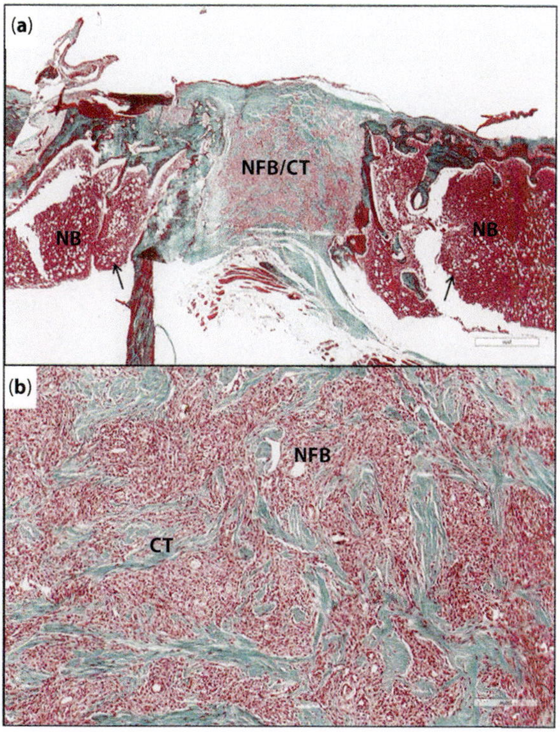

Figure 13.9 Representative photomicrographs of bone defect regeneration in the autologous bone grafted defect shown in Figure 13.4 (decalcified, MT staining). (a) At lower magnification (x4), a thick sheet of newly formed bone (NFB, red color) with interspersed connective tissue (CT, green color) is seen bridging the edges of the defect (black arrows) along with abundant CT surrounding the healing bone defect. (b) At higher magnification (x10), NFB with irregular lamellae, high cellularity, and abundant blood vessels is seen in the bone regeneration site, and the presence of sparse CT, which is predominantly collagenous than cellular, is discernible throughout the healing bone defect.

13.4.4 Xenografts

13.4.4.1 Bovine Bone

Bovine-derived bone grafts are widely used due to their structural similarity to human bone. Histological studies reveal that bovine bone grafts exhibit osteoconductive properties, supporting new bone formation around the graft particles, as shown in Figure 13.10. However, the resorption rate is relatively slow, and residual graft material may persist over extended periods. The integration of bovine bone grafts is generally favorable, with minimal inflammatory responses observed [5, 40, 41].

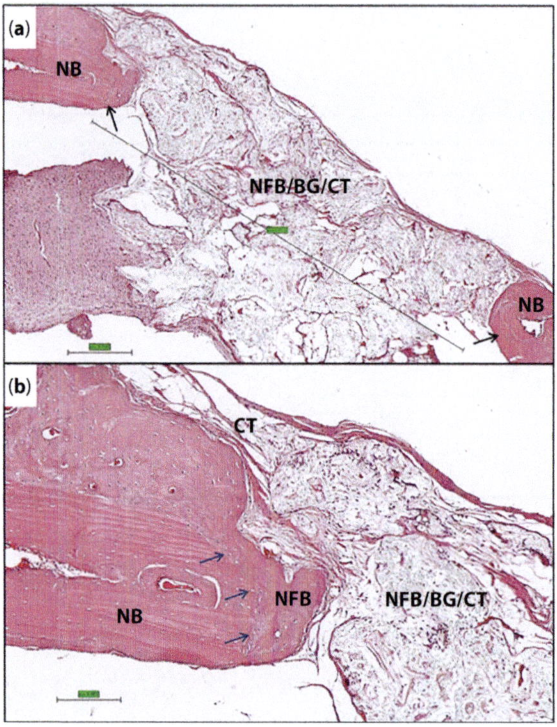

Figure 13.10 Representative photomicrographs of bone defect regeneration in a defect grafted with deproteinized bovine bone graft after 6 weeks of healing (decalcified, HE staining). (a) At lower magnification (x4), there is a layer of newly formed bone (NBF), remnant bone graft (BG), and connective tissue (CT) bridging the native bone (NB) between the edges of the defect (black arrows). The differentiation between NB and NFB is not clearly seen. (b) At higher magnification (x10), a clear line of separation between NB and NFB is appreciable (blue arrows), and it delineates the regularly lamellated NB and irregularly lamellated NFB. Mineralized bone osteoid without osteoblasts resembling dead bone is seen in the mid-portion of the defect and indicates the remnant BG particles, which are surrounded by NFB with interspersed CT.

13.4.4.2 Equine Bone

Equine-derived bone grafts are another xenogenic option, offering biocompatibility and structural support. Histological evaluations indicate that equine bone grafts can support new bone formation; however, the extent of integration and remodeling may vary. Some studies report the presence of connective tissue within the grafted area, suggesting a slower or less complete integration process compared to other graft materials [6, 11, 42].

Figures 13.11 and 13.12, show representative histological images of bone defect healing and regeneration after using equine bone graft.

In a comparative study, collagenated cancellous equine bone blocks used as inlay grafts demonstrated a higher percentage of new bone formation compared to onlay grafts, highlighting the influence of graft placement on regenerative outcomes [43].

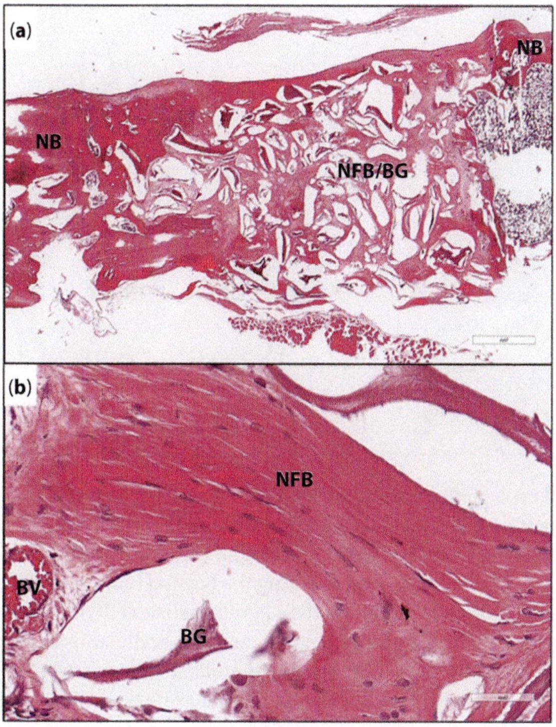

Figure 13.11 Representative photomicrographs of bone defect regeneration in a defect grafted with deproteinized equine bone graft after 6 weeks of healing (decalcified, HE staining). (a) At lower magnification (x4), the segmental bone defect is predominantly filled with a layer of newly formed bone (NFB) and remnant bone graft particles (BG). On the superior portion of the defect, a thin layer of NFB is seen bridging the native bone (NB) between the two edges of the defect. (b) At higher magnification (x40), the NFB is seen as a thick sheet of mineralized osteoid with irregular lamellae, plenty of osteoblasts, and blood vessels (BV), and is seen surrounding the dead bone chips of BG particles.

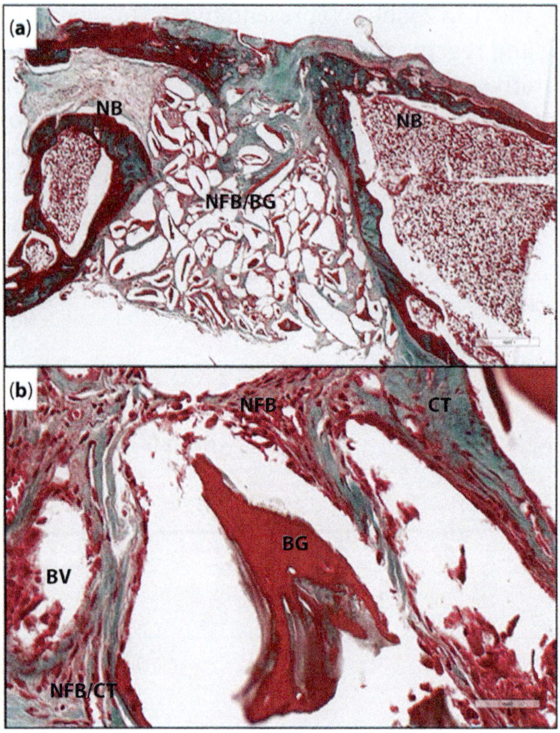

Figure 13.12 Representative photomicrographs of bone defect regeneration in a defect grafted with deproteinized equine bone graft similar to the one shown in Figure 13.16, after 6 weeks of healing (decalcified, MT staining). (a) At lower magnification (x4), connective tissue (green color) is seen invading the healing bone defect filled with newly formed bone (NFB, red color) and bone graft particles (BG). (b) At very high magnification (x40), the BG particle is clearly seen as an acellular osteoid or chip of dead bone and is surrounded by NFB with osteoblasts and blood vessels (BV). Even the NFB surrounding the BG particles has considerable amount of intervening connective tissue (CT), indicating continuous healing process in the absence of inflammation.

13.4.5 Alternative Grafting Tissues

13.4.5.1 Fat Grafts

Adipose tissue grafts have been explored for bone regeneration due to the presence of adipose-derived stem cells (ADSCs) [44]. Histological analyses demonstrate that fragmented adipose tissue can contribute to bone healing in critical-size defects, as shown in Figure 13.13. The presence of ADSCs within the graft may facilitate osteogenic differentiation and vascularization, promoting bone regeneration [45].

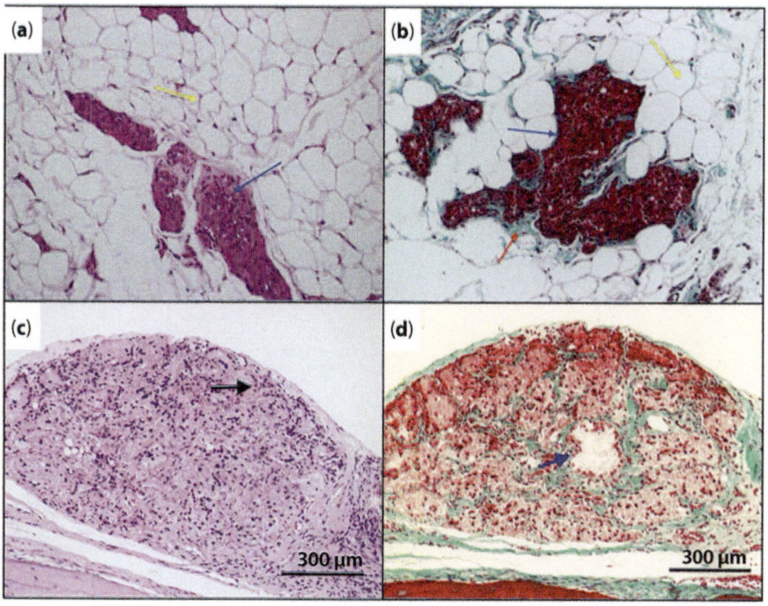

Figure 13.13 Representative photomicrographs of bone defect regeneration in a defect grafted with fat graft. The top photomicrographs showing decalcified sections stained with H&E (a) and Masson's trichrome (b). An island of immature cellular bone (blue arrow) is observed inside the remnant of fat tissue (yellow arrow). The immature bone is seen surrounded by cellular fibrous tissue, and the periosteum appears green (red arrow), 10x magnification. The bottom photomicrographs showing decalcified sections stained with H&E (c) and Masson's trichrome (d). Different cell populations are evident in the section. The connective tissue that replaced the fat tissue is seen as a highly cellular rim around bone (blue arrow), and osteoblasts and pre-osteoblasts (black arrow) are seen arranged around mineralized tissue in a ring-like structure, 5x magnification.

13.4.5.2 Skeletal Muscle Grafts

Skeletal muscle grafts, particularly decellularized skeletal muscle (DSM), have been investigated for their potential in bone regeneration [46]. Histological assessments reveal that DSM can support neovascularization and the infiltration of osteoprogenitor cells, contributing to bone healing in critical-size defects, as shown in Figure 13.14. The structural matrix of DSM provides a conducive environment for cell attachment and proliferation, aiding in the regenerative process [47].

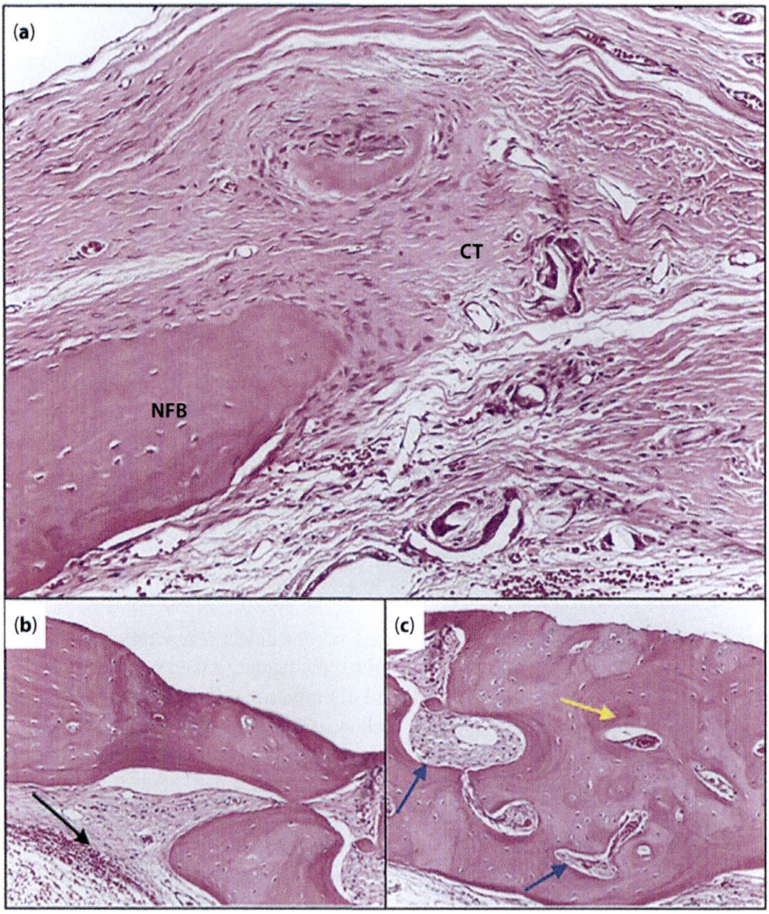

Figure 13.14 Representative photomicrographs of bone defect regeneration in a defect grafted with decellularized skeletal muscle (DSM), showing decalcified sections stained with H&E. The top photomicrograph shows (a) remnants of connective tissue with neovascularization (CT) along with cell population of osteoblasts and pre-osteoblasts, especially in woven bone (NFB). There is evidence of metaplastic changes in fibroblasts or myoblasts, 10x magnification. The bottom photomicrographs show (b) areas of bone bridging the defect surrounded by highly vascular, periosteum like connective tissue (black arrow). The regenerated bone shows high evidence of remodeling, with mixed lamellar and woven bone, 5x magnification. (c) Newly formed bone with multiple marrow spaces (blue arrows) and blood vessel (yellow arrow), is mixed with mature lamellar bone, cartilage-like structure, and woven bone, 5x magnification.

13.5 Adjunctive Biological Agents to Enhance Bone Regeneration

Bone grafting alone may not always provide optimal regenerative outcomes, especially in compromised or critical-sized defects [48]. To improve the osteogenic potential and clinical efficacy of grafts, adjunctive biological agents such as bone morphogenetic proteins (BMPs), platelet-derived growth factor (PDGF), and bone marrow-derived mesenchymal stem cells (BMSCs) have been widely investigated [49]. These adjuncts work through different mechanisms, including but not limited to osteoinduction, chemotaxis, angiogenesis, and cellular proliferation, to augment the biological environment for bone repair [49].

13.5.1 Bone Morphogenetic Proteins (BMPs)

Bone morphogenetic proteins are members of the transforming growth factor-beta (TGF-β) superfamily and are potent osteoinductive agents. Among them, BMP-2 and BMP-7 have been extensively studied and approved for clinical use in spinal fusion and long bone non-unions [36, 50]. BMPs promote the differentiation of mesenchymal stem cells into osteoblasts, upregulate the expression of osteogenic genes (e.g., Runx2, ALP, and osteocalcin), and enhance endochondral ossification.

When incorporated into scaffolds like collagen sponges, hydroxyapatite, or β-TCP, BMPs significantly accelerate new bone formation and improve graft integration [10, 51]. Histologically, BMP-treated grafts show earlier and more abundant bone deposition, increased osteoblast activity, and mature lamellar bone compared to untreated controls. However, supra-physiologic doses can lead to complications such as ectopic bone formation and inflammation, warranting controlled release systems and proper dosing protocols [49, 52]. Representative histological images of different scaffolds grafted with adjunct BMP are shown in Figures 13.15 (Collagen sponge + BMP) and 13.16 (BCP + BMP).

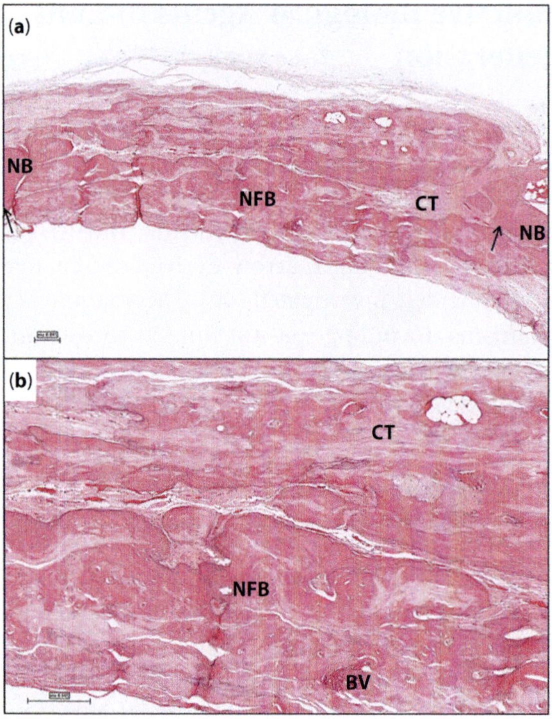

Figure 13.15 Representative photomicrographs of bone defect regeneration in a defect grafted with collagen sponge and adjunct recombinant human bone morphogenetic protein (rhBMP-2), after 6 weeks of healing (Decalcified, HE staining). (a) At lower magnification (x4), a thick sheet of newly formed bone (NFB) with intervening connective tissue (CT) is seen bridging the edges of the defect (black arrows), and the NFB is clearly discernible from the native bone (NB) by its irregular lamellae. (b) At higher magnification (x10), the immature osteoid of the NFB is seen with plenty of osteoblasts and abundant blood vessels, and there is interspersed fibrous CT within the NFB osteoid that is visibly lesser in quantity attributable to the osteoinductive potential of rhBMP-2.

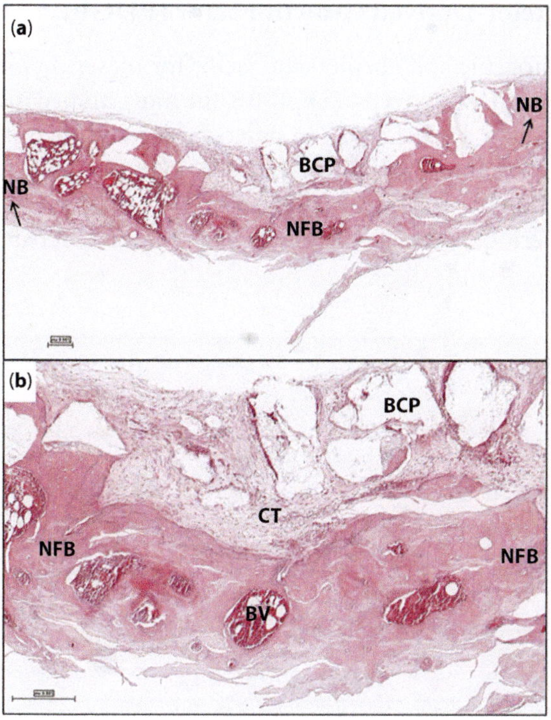

Figure 13.16 Representative photomicrographs of bone defect regeneration in a defect grafted with biphasic calcium phosphate (BCP—alloplastic bone substitute) with adjunct recombinant human bone morphogenetic protein (rhBMP-2) after 6 weeks of healing (decalcified, HE staining). (a) At lower magnification (x4), there is abundant newly formed bone (NFB) bridging the defect and the amount of remnant BCP particles is considerably less, and these particles are surrounded by areas of fibrous connective tissue. (b) At higher magnification (x10), the NFB is not only abundant in quantity with osteoblasts and blood vessels but also appears with areas of regular and irregular lamellae indicative of advanced stages of new bone formation and osteoid maturation. The BCP particles appearing as granular crystalline material are sparse and are surrounded by fibrous CT and NFB, suggesting active resorption and new bone deposition in the resorbed areas.

13.5.2 Platelet-Derived Growth Factor (PDGF)

PDGF is a mitogenic and chemotactic factor for mesenchymal cells, fibroblasts, and smooth muscle cells. PDGF-BB, the most studied isoform in bone regeneration, plays a crucial role in angiogenesis and recruitment of progenitor cells to the injury site [40, 53]. Based on *in vivo* and clinical studies, recombinant human PDGF-BB (rhPDGF-BB) has been used with β-TCP matrices for periodontal regeneration and alveolar bone repair [6, 12, 54].

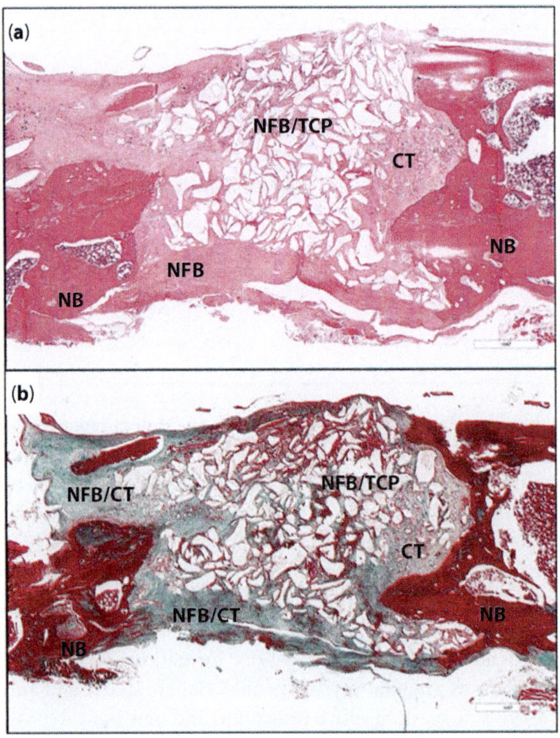

Figure 13.17 Representative photomicrographs of bone defect regeneration in a defect grafted with beta tricalcium phosphate (beta-TCP—alloplastic bone substitute) and adjunct platelet derived growth factor (PDGF) after 6 weeks of healing. (a) At lower magnification (x4, decalcified, HE staining), a dense sheet of newly formed bone (NFB) with intervening connective tissue (CT) and remaining TCP particles is seen connecting the edges (NB) of the segmental bone defect. (b) The same histological section, at lower magnification (x4, decalcified, MT staining), shows the differentiation between new bone osteoid (red color) and connective tissue (green color). Most of the new bone bridging the defect is seen mixed with fibrous CT, and the remnant beta-TCP particles are all seen surrounded by mineralized osteoid, indicating resorption of the bone substitute material and replacement by NFB.

PDGF enhances soft tissue healing and accelerates early-stage bone regeneration by stimulating vascular ingrowth, which is essential for nutrient and oxygen delivery in bone healing [55, 56]. Histological evaluations of PDGF-enhanced grafts show improved vascularization, early connective tissue matrix organization, and moderate enhancement in mineralized tissue formation. PDGF is especially beneficial in compromised healing environments such as diabetic or irradiated bone [54–56]. Bone defect regeneration following the use of adjunct PDGF with different graft materials is shown in Figures 13.17 (TCP + PDGF), 13.18 (Bovine xenograft + PDGF) and 13.19 (Equine xenograft + PDGF).

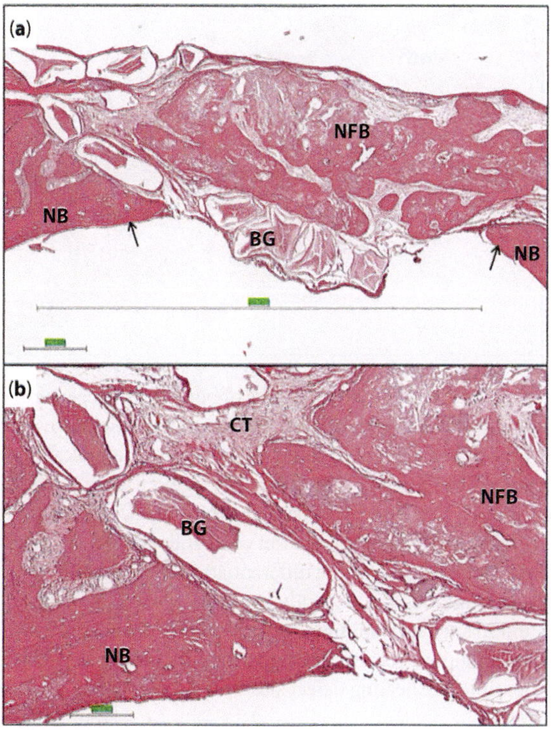

Figure 13.18 Representative photomicrographs of bone defect regeneration in a defect grafted with deproteinized bovine bone graft and adjunct platelet derived growth factor (PDGF) after 6 weeks of healing (decalcified, HE staining). (a) At lower magnification (x4), the layer of newly formed bone (NFB) and connective tissue (CT) along with bone graft particles (BG) is thick and extends for the complete thickness of the defect, between the native bone (NB) in the edges of the defect (black arrows). Abundant NFB within the defect is clearly seen even in lower magnification. (b) At higher magnification (x10), the BG particles, appearing as dead bone chips with no osteoblasts, are seen surrounded by a layer of NFB and CT. The NFB in the mid-portion of the defect is seen as irregularly lamellated osteoid with abundant osteoblasts and evidence of neovascularization.

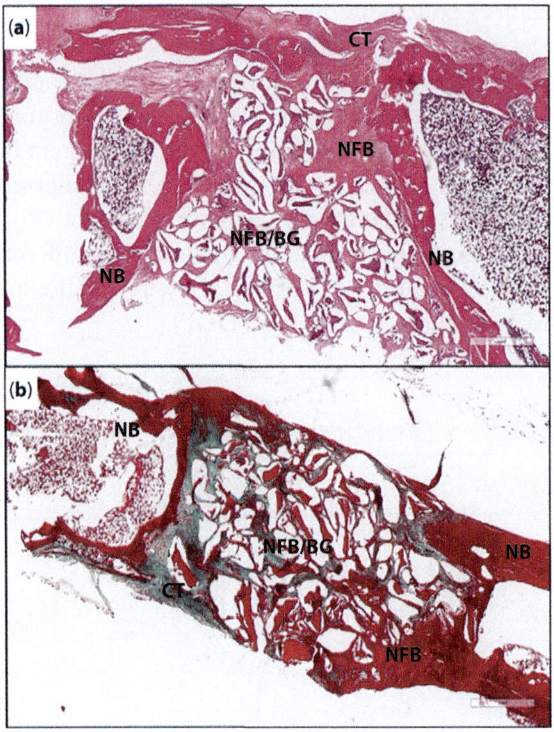

Figure 13.19 Representative photomicrographs of bone defect regeneration in a defect grafted with deproteinized equine bone graft and adjunct platelet derived growth factor (PDGF) after 6 weeks of healing. (a) At lower magnification (x4, decalcified, HE staining), a thick sheet of newly formed bone (NFB) surrounding bone graft particles (BG) along with connective tissue (CT) is seen between the native bone (NB), within the healing segmental bone defect. (b) Histological section of a similar defect, at lower magnification (x4, decalcified, MT staining), shows the differentiation between NFB (red color) and CT (green color). The amount of CT is evidently less than the NFB, both in areas away from the BG particles and in sites surrounding BG particles. This could be indicative of the osteogenic and osteoinductive role of PDGF that enables greater new bone formation and reduces CT invasion into the healing defect site.

13.5.3 Bone Marrow-Derived Mesenchymal Stem Cells (BMSCs)

BMSCs are multipotent progenitor cells capable of differentiating into osteoblasts, chondrocytes, and adipocytes. When used in conjunction with scaffolds, BMSCs provide both cellular and trophic support for bone regeneration [57, 58]. Figures 13.20 (Allograft + BMSC) and 13.21 (DSM + BMSC) show histological images of bone regeneration in defects while using BMSCs as adjuncts to graft materials. BMSCs can be harvested autologously from the iliac crest or tibial plateau and seeded onto various biomaterials including allografts, β-TCP, and collagen matrices. They enhance osteogenesis through direct differentiation and paracrine signaling, promoting angiogenesis and modulating the immune response [38, 59]. Histologically, constructs containing BMSCs show robust early osteoid formation, increased osteoblast population, and vascular infiltration. Moreover, BMSCs have been shown to synergize with BMPs or PDGF, enhancing the regenerative effect in both preclinical and clinical models [50, 56].

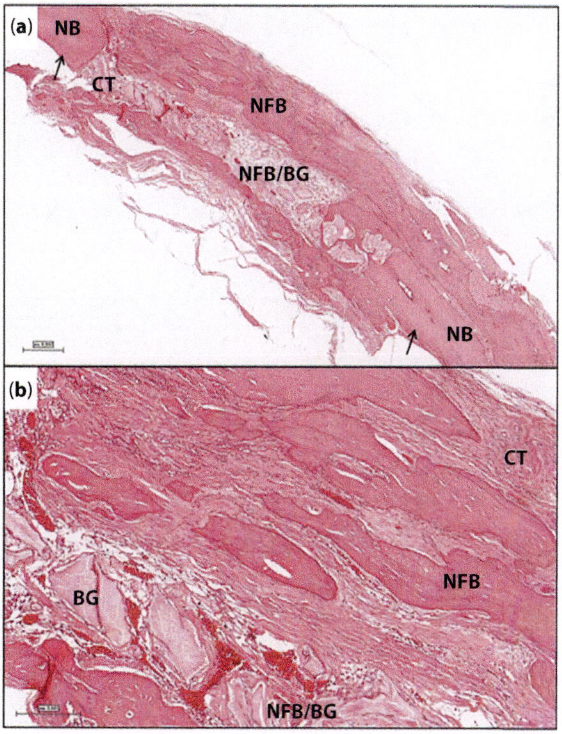

Figure 13.20 Representative photomicrographs of bone defect regeneration in a defect grafted with demineralized allograft bone and adjunct bone-marrow mesenchymal stem cells (BMSCs) after 6 weeks of healing (decalcified, HE staining). (a) At lower magnification (x4), the bone defect is filled by abundant newly formed bone (NFB) extending from the edges of the defects (black arrows). The delineation between the native bone (NB) and NFB is clearly discernible by the regular lamellar pattern of NB and irregular lamellae in NFB osteoid. Additionally, areas of NFB and remnant allograft bone (BG) particles are seen within the defect. (b) At higher magnification (x10), the NFB is visibly abundant within the healing defect site and is separated by fibrous connective tissue (CT), which also separated the NFB from the resorbing BG particles. The sparse areas of CT and new bone formation surrounding BG particles are indicative of active osseous healing probably attributable to the osteogenic potential of adjunct BMSCs.

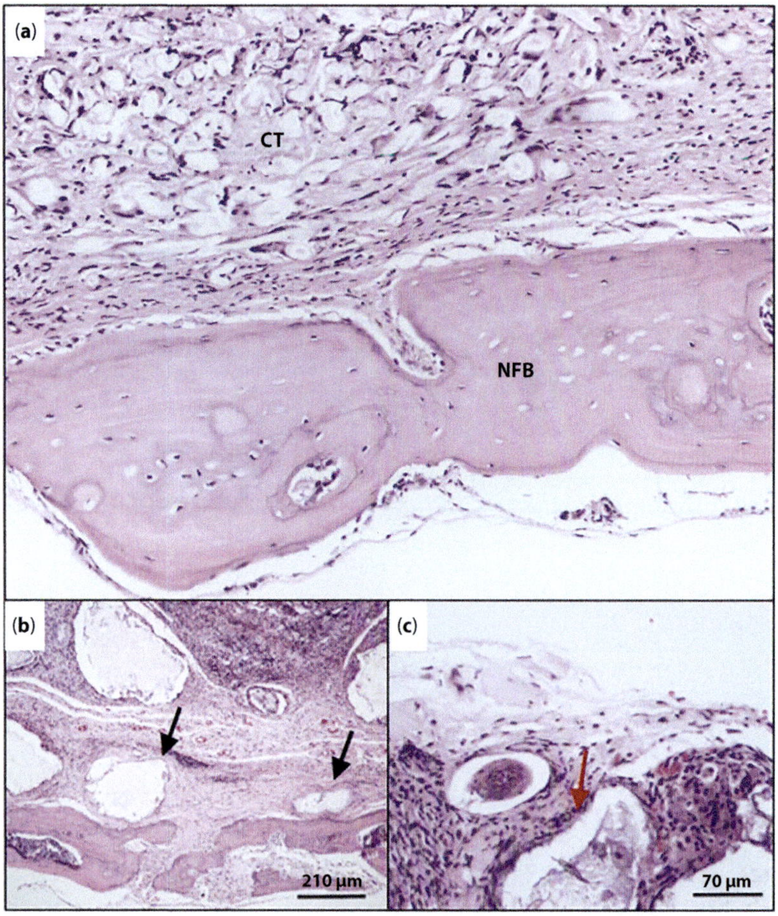

Figure 13.21 Representative photomicrographs of bone defect regeneration in a defect grafted with decellularized skeletal muscle (DSM), silica calcium phosphate composite (SCPC) and bone marrow mesenchymal stem cells (BMSCs), showing decalcified sections stained with H&E. The top photomicrograph shows (a) areas of bone growth (NFB) within the corticoid defect as well as the onlay graft. New woven bone bridges the defect and grows upward. Islands of mature bone can be seen surrounded by high cellular activity and immature bone and loose connective tissue (CT), 10x magnification. The bottom photomicrographs showing (b) tissue remnants of DSM with osteoblasts and pre-osteoblast cells (black arrows), 5x magnification; (c) The collagenous matrix becomes highly vascular and the presence of immature bone osteoid is noticed (red arrow), 5x magnification.

13.5.4 Vitamin D

Vitamin D has been shown to enhance the osteogenic differentiation of mesenchymal stem cells and osteoblasts *in vitro* [49]. This enhancement is evidenced by the increased expression of osteogenic markers such as alkaline phosphatase (ALP), osteocalcin (OCN), and osteopontin (OPN). These findings suggest that vitamin D plays a crucial role in promoting the expression of bone matrix proteins and facilitating cellular maturation, both of which are essential for bone formation [48]. *In vivo* studies have demonstrated that vitamin D, whether administered systemically or locally, significantly improves bone regeneration in osseous defects and increases bone-to-implant contact (BIC) during osseointegration [60, 61]. When combined with bone substitute materials and bone regenerative scaffolds, vitamin D promotes early bone formation and mineralization [48]. Notably, systemic administration is often more effective than local administration, particularly in cases of systemic illnesses such as diabetes, osteoporosis, or chronic kidney disease [62]. These findings highlight vitamin D's potential as a safe, cost-effective, and non-invasive adjunct to conventional bone grafting and tissue engineering techniques.

13.5.5 Synergistic Effects and Future Directions

The integration of these adjuncts into composite graft systems has opened new frontiers in regenerative medicine. Combinatorial approaches—such as BMSCs with BMP-2, or PDGF with β-TCP—show synergistic effects that outperform any single-agent use. Controlled delivery systems using nanoparticles, hydrogels, or 3D-printed scaffolds allow for spatial and temporal regulation of growth factor release, optimizing cellular responses. Emerging techniques such as gene-activated matrices, exosome-based delivery, and scaffold bio-functionalization continue to evolve, potentially offering next-generation bone graft substitutes with enhanced efficacy and safety profiles [49, 61].

13.6 Clinical Significance and Future Research Directions

13.6.1 Clinical Significance

The histological assessment of bone grafts has direct clinical relevance. Autografts remain the gold standard due to their osteogenic, osteoconductive, and osteoinductive properties; however, their limited availability and donor site morbidity have led to the widespread use of allografts, xenografts, and synthetic substitutes [2]. Histology helps to differentiate between viable and necrotic bone, assess the degree of vascularization, and monitor host response, including immune reactions and fibrous encapsulation. When adjuncts like MSCs or BMPs are used, histology becomes essential for verifying their bioactivity. MSCs contribute to bone formation through both differentiation and paracrine signaling [44, 49]. BMPs, particularly BMP-2 and BMP-7, are potent osteoinductive agents that modulate gene expression in progenitor cells [51, 52]. Histological techniques help validate these effects by showing increased osteoid formation, reduced inflammatory infiltrate, and improved integration with host bone [10, 51]. In dentistry and maxillofacial surgery, histology guides material selection and procedural planning. For example, socket preservation, sinus lift procedures, and alveolar ridge augmentation all benefit from preclinical histological data to predict clinical outcomes.

13.6.2 Future Research Directions

With advances in biomaterials and biotechnology, the horizon of bone regeneration is expanding [48]. Bioactive scaffolds incorporating peptides, growth factors, and nanoparticles are under investigation for their synergistic effects on osteogenesis and angiogenesis [49]. Histology remains crucial in evaluating these materials, not just qualitatively but also quantitatively through high-resolution imaging and computational morphometry. Tissue-engineered constructs seeded with stem cells or genetically modified cells are becoming increasingly complex, and future histological studies must adapt to assess cell fate, matrix deposition, and vascular integration in detail [18]. Emerging techniques like multiplex immunohistochemistry, confocal microscopy, and spatial transcriptomics may revolutionize the granularity with which histological assessment is conducted [63].

Moreover, translating histological data from animal models to human applications poses challenges due to interspecies differences in bone remodeling dynamics. Thus, developing standardized protocols for histological processing and interpretation is a priority for reproducibility and clinical relevance [33]. Finally, integration with digital pathology and artificial intelligence (AI) holds promise for the future. AI-based histological image analysis could automate pattern recognition, reduce observer variability, and uncover previously unrecognized biomarkers of successful bone regeneration [64].

13.7 Conclusion

Histological assessment remains a cornerstone in the evaluation of bone grafts and substitutes. By providing detailed insight into the tissue-level events of bone healing, histology complements other imaging and biochemical assays and plays an indispensable role in both experimental and clinical contexts. The integration of adjuncts such as MSCs, BMPs, and growth factors further highlights the necessity for meticulous tissue evaluation. As regenerative medicine continues to evolve, histological techniques must also advance, embracing new technologies and interdisciplinary approaches to enhance our understanding of bone biology and improve patient outcomes.

AI disclosure statment: The author confirms that no artificial intelligence (AI)-generated content or AI-assisted writing tools were used in the preparation of this chapter (including summaries and the abstract). All text, analysis, and conclusions are the result of the author's original work.

References

1. Starch-Jensen, T., Schou, S., Terheyden, H., Bruun, N.H., Aludden, H., Bone regeneration after maxillary sinus floor augmentation with different ratios of autogenous bone and deproteinized bovine bone mineral an *in vivo* experimental study. *Clin. Oral Implants Res.*, 34, 12, 1406–16, 2023. Epub 2023/09/28.
2. Choi, J.W., Park, J.Y., Cha, J.K., Hieu, P.D., Jung, H.D., Kim, C.S., Alveolar Ridge Regeneration With Open Versus Closed Healing in Damaged Extraction Sockets: A Preclinical *In Vivo* Study. *Clin. Oral Implants Res.*, 36, 2, 220–7, 2025. Epub 2024/10/28.
3. Ramalingam, S., Al-Rasheed, A., ArRejaie, A., Nooh, N., Al-Kindi, M., Al-Hezaimi, K., Guided bone regeneration in standardized calvarial defects using beta-tricalcium phosphate and collagen membrane: a real-time *in vivo* micro-computed tomographic experiment in rats. *Odontology*, 104, 2, 199–210, 2016. Epub 2015/07/15.
4. Tumedei, M., Mijiritsky, E., Mourão, C.F., Piattelli, A., Degidi, M., Mangano, C., *et al.*, Histological and Biological Response to Different Types of Biomaterials: A Narrative Single Research Center Experience over Three Decades. *Int. J. Environ. Res. Public Health*, 19, 13, 2022. Epub 2022/07/10.
5. de Freitas Silva, L., de Carvalho Reis, E.N.R., Barbara, T.A., Bonardi, J.P., Garcia, I.R.J., de Carvalho, P.S.P., *et al.*, Assessment of bone repair in critical-size defect in the calvarium of rats after the implantation of tricalcium

phosphate beta (β-TCP). *Acta Histochem.*, 119, 6, 624–31, 2017. Epub 2017/07/25.

6. Alkindi, M., Ramalingam, S., Alghamdi, O., Alomran, O.M., Binsalah, M.A., Badwelan, M., Guided bone regeneration with osteoconductive grafts and PDGF: A tissue engineering option for segmental bone defect reconstruction. *J. Appl. Biomater. Funct. Mater.*, 19, 2280800020987405, 2021. Epub 2021/02/06.
7. Cömert Kılıç, S., Güngörmüş, M., Parlak, S.N., Histologic and histomorphometric assessment of sinus-floor augmentation with beta-tricalcium phosphate alone or in combination with pure-platelet-rich plasma or platelet-rich fibrin: A randomized clinical trial. *Clin. Implant Dentistry Related Res.*, 19, 5, 959–67, 2017. Epub 2017/07/27.
8. Chen, C.L., Tien, H.W., Chuang, C.H., Chen, Y.C., A comparison of the bone regeneration and soft-tissue-formation capabilities of various injectable-grafting materials in a rabbit calvarial defect model. *J. Biomed. Mater. Res. Part B*, 107, 3, 529–44, 2019. Epub 2018/05/04.
9. Uetanabaro, L.C., Claudino, M., Zancan, R., Zielak, J.C., Garlet, G.P., de Araujo, M.R., Osteoconductivity of Biphasic Calcium Phosphate Ceramic Improves New Bone Formation: A Histologic, Histomorphometric, Gene Expression, and Microcomputed Tomography Study. *Int. J. Oral Maxillofacial Implants*, 35, 1, 70–8, 2020. Epub 2020/01/11.
10. Huang, Y.C., Lew, W.Z., Feng, S.W., Lai, W.Y., Abiko, Y., Huang, H.M., Histomorphometric and transcriptome evaluation of early healing bone treated with a novel human particulate dentin powder. *Biomed. Mater. (Bristol England)*, 12, 1, 015004, 2016. Epub 2016/12/03.
11. Binsalah, M.A., Ramalingam, S., Alkindi, M., Nooh, N., Al-Hezaimi, K., Guided Bone Regeneration of Femoral Segmental Defects using Equine Bone Graft: An *In-Vivo* Micro-Computed Tomographic Study in Rats. *J. Invest. Surg. Off. J. Acad. Surg. Res.*, 32, 5, 456–66, 2019. Epub 2018/03/06.
12. Badwelan, M., Alkindi, M., Ramalingam, S., Nooh, N., Al Hezaimi, K., The Efficacy of Recombinant Platelet-Derived Growth Factor on Beta-Tricalcium Phosphate to Regenerate Femoral Critical Sized Segmental Defects: Longitudinal *In Vivo* Micro-CT Study in a Rat Model. *J. Invest. Surg. Off. J. Acad. Surg. Res.*, 33, 5, 476–88, 2020. Epub 2018/11/16.
13. Miquelestorena-Standley, E., Jourdan, M.L., Collin, C., Bouvier, C., Larousserie, F., Aubert, S., *et al.*, Effect of decalcification protocols on immunohistochemistry and molecular analyses of bone samples. *Mod. Pathol. an Off. J. U. States Can. Acad. Pathology Inc.*, 33, 8, 1505–17, 2020. Epub 2020/02/26.
14. Craig, J.C., Freeman, M., Walton, S., Rogers, D., Mehrad, M., Gordetsky, J.B., A Quality Analysis of Bony Specimens for Optimal Ethylenediaminetetraacetic Acid (EDTA) Decalcification. *Int. J. Surg. Pathol.*, 30, 8, 853–60, 2022. Epub 2022/03/29.

15. Charnwichai, P., Kitkumthorn, N., Ruangvejvorachai, P., Wongphoom, J., Meesakul, T., Tammachote, N., *et al.*, Rapid decalcification of articular cartilage and subchondral bone using an ultrasonic cleaner with EDTA. *Acta Histochem.*, 125, 2, 152009, 2023. Epub 2023/02/02.
16. Fretz, J.A. and Troiano, N.W., Optimized Methyl methacrylate embedding of small and large undecalcified bones. *MethodsX.*, 13, 103046, 2024. Epub 2024/12/05.
17. Roth, D.M., Puttagunta, L., Graf, D., Histological Techniques for Sectioning Bones of the Vertebrate Craniofacial Skeleton. *Methods Mol. Biol. (Clifton NJ)*, 2403, 187–200, 2022. Epub 2021/12/17.
18. Rentsch, C., Schneiders, W., Manthey, S., Rentsch, B., Rammelt, S., Comprehensive histological evaluation of bone implants. *Biomatter.*, 4, 2014. Epub 2014/02/08.
19. Agrawal, R.S., Bhavthankar, J.D., Mandale, M.S., Thakur, A., Bhagde, P.A., Salve, S., Histochemical characterization of bone and cementum using modified gallego's iron fuschin stain and van gieson stain and its application in fibro-osseous lesions. *Indian J. Dental Res. Off. Publ. Indian Soc. Dent. Res.*, 31, 6, 888–92, 2020. Epub 2021/03/24.
20. Peev, S., Parushev, I., Yotsova, R., A Modified Protocol for Staining of Undecalcified Bone Samples Using Toluidine Blue—A Histological Study in Rabbit Models. *Appl. Sci.*, 14, 1, 461, 2024.
21. Tebyanian, H., Norahan, M.H., Eyni, H., Movahedin, M., Mortazavi, S.J., Karami, A., *et al.*, Effects of collagen/β-tricalcium phosphate bone graft to regenerate bone in critically sized rabbit calvarial defects. *J. Appl. Biomater. Funct. Mater.*, 17, 1, 2280800018820490, 2019. Epub 2019/03/06.
22. Bernar, A., Gebetsberger, J.V., Bauer, M., Streif, W., Schirmer, M., Optimization of the Alizarin Red S Assay by Enhancing Mineralization of Osteoblasts. *Int. J. Mol. Sci.*, 24, 1, 2022. Epub 2023/01/09.
23. Nakamura, T., Kawaai, K., Kuroda, Y., Matsuo, K., Osteoclast visualization: Tartrate-resistant acid phosphatase activity staining using NewFuchsin compatible with non-aqueous mounting and tissue clearing. *MethodsX.*, 14, 103136, 2025.
24. Aludden, H., Mordenfeld, A., Dahlin, C., Hallman, M., Starch-Jensen, T., Histological and histomorphometrical outcome after lateral guided bone regeneration augmentation of the mandible with different ratios of deproteinized bovine bone mineral and autogenous bone. A preclinical *in vivo* study. *Clin. Oral Implants Res.*, 31, 10, 1025–36, 2020. Epub 2020/08/14.
25. Zampara, E., Alshammari, M., De Bortoli, J., Mullings, O., Gkisakis, I.G., Benalcázar Jalkh, E.B., *et al.*, A Histologic and Histomorphometric Evaluation of an Allograft, Xenograft, and Alloplast Graft for Alveolar Ridge Preservation in Humans: A Randomized Controlled Clinical Trial. *J. Oral Implantology*, 48, 6, 541–9, 2022. Epub 2022/04/22.

26. Aludden, H., Starch-Jensen, T., Dahlin, C., Sdik, J., Cederlund, A., Mordenfeld, A., Histological and radiological outcome after horizontal guided bone regeneration with bovine bone mineral alone or in combination with bone in edentulous atrophic maxilla: A randomized controlled trial. *Clin. Oral Implants Res.*, 35, 4, 396–406, 2024. Epub 2024/01/31.
27. Brent, M.B. and Emmanuel, T., Contemporary Advances in Computer-Assisted Bone Histomorphometry and Identification of Bone Cells in Culture. *Calcif. Tissue Int.*, 112, 1, 1–12, 2023. Epub 2022/10/31.
28. Dore B, F.P. and Masali, M., Histological techniques and microscopic analysis of biological agents for preservation of human bone remains. *Biotech. Histochemistry*, 76, 2, 89–95, 2001.
29. Dempster, D.W., Compston, J.E., Drezner, M.K., Glorieux, F.H., Kanis, J.A., Malluche, H., *et al.*, Standardized nomenclature, symbols, and units for bone histomorphometry: a 2012 update of the report of the ASBMR Histomorphometry Nomenclature Committee. *J. Bone Mineral Res. Off. J. Am. Soc. Bone Miner. Res.*, 28, 1, 2–17, 2013. Epub 2012/12/01.
30. Tizhoosh, H.R. and Pantanowitz, L., Artificial Intelligence and Digital Pathology: Challenges and Opportunities. *J. Pathol. Inf.*, 9, 38, 2018. Epub 2019/01/05.
31. Moreno-Jiménez, I., Garske, D.S., Lahr, C.A., Hutmacher, D.W., Cipitria, A., Targeted 2D histology and ultrastructural bone analysis based on 3D microCT anatomical locations. *MethodsX.*, 8, 101480, 2021.
32. Shah, F.A., Ruscsák, K., Palmquist, A., 50 years of scanning electron microscopy of bone—a comprehensive overview of the important discoveries made and insights gained into bone material properties in health, disease, and taphonomy. *Bone Res.*, 7, 1, 15, 2019.
33. Stan, E., Muresan, C.-O., Daescu, E., Dumache, R., Ciocan, V., Ungureanu, S., *et al.*, A Review of Histological Techniques for Differentiating Human Bone from Animal Bone. *Methods Protoc.*, 7, 4, 51, 2024.
34. Schmidlin, P.R., Nicholls, F., Kruse, A., Zwahlen, R.A., Weber, F.E., Evaluation of moldable, *in situ* hardening calcium phosphate bone graft substitutes. *Clin. Oral Implants Res.*, 24, 2, 149–57, 2013. Epub 2011/11/19.
35. Kucera, T., Sponer, P., Urban, K., Kohout, A., Histological assessment of tissue from large human bone defects repaired with β-tricalcium phosphate. *Eur. J. Orthopaedic Surg. Traumatology Orthopedie Traumatologie*, 24, 8, 1357–65, 2014. Epub 2013/10/05.
36. Al-Qutub, M.N., Al-Omar, N.A., Ramalingam, S., Javed, F., Al-Kindi, M., Ar-Rejaie, A., *et al.*, Guided Bone Regeneration Using Biphasic Calcium Phosphate With Adjunct Recombinant Human Bone Morphogenetic Protein-2 With and Without Collagen Membrane in Standardized Calvarial Defects in Rats: A Histologic and Biomechanical Analysis. *Int. J. Periodontics Restorative Dentistry*, 36 Suppl, s11–20, 2016. Epub 2016/04/01.

37. Pripatnanont, P., Praserttham, P., Suttapreyasri, S., Leepong, N., Monmaturapoj, N., Bone Regeneration Potential of Biphasic Nanocalcium Phosphate with High Hydroxyapatite/Tricalcium Phosphate Ratios in Rabbit Calvarial Defects. *Int. J. Oral Maxillofacial Implants*, 31, 2, 294–303, 2016. Epub 2016/03/24.
38. Miron, R.J., Sculean, A., Shuang, Y., Bosshardt, D.D., Gruber, R., Buser, D., *et al.*, Osteoinductive potential of a novel biphasic calcium phosphate bone graft in comparison with autographs, xenografts, and DFDBA. *Clin. Oral Implants Res.*, 27, 6, 668–75, 2016. Epub 2015/08/01.
39. Correia, F., Pozza, D.H., Gouveia, S., Felino, A.C., Faria-Almeida, R., Advantages of Porcine Xenograft over Autograft in Sinus Lift: A Randomised Clinical Trial. *Mater. (Basel Switzerland)*, 14, 12, 2021. Epub 2021/07/03.
40. Al-Askar, M., Javed, F., Al-Hezaimi, K., Al-Hamdan, K.S., Ramalingam, S., Aldahmash, A., *et al.*, Guided Bone Regeneration in Standardized Calvarial Defects in Rats Using Bio-Oss and β-Tricalcium Phosphate with Adjunct Platelet-Derived Growth Factor Therapy: A Real-Time *In Vivo* Microcomputed Tomographic, Biomechanical, and Histologic Analysis. *Int. J. Periodontics Restorative Dentistry*, 36 Suppl, s61–73, 2016. Epub 2016/04/01.
41. Nooh, N., Ramalingam, S., Al-Kindi, M., Al-Rasheed, A., Al-Hamdan, K.S., Al-Hezaimi, K., Real-Time Assessment of Guided Bone Regeneration in Standardized Calvarial Defects in Rats Using Bio-Oss With and Without Collagen Membrane: An *In Vivo* Microcomputed Tomographic and Histologic Experiment. *Int. J. Periodontics Restorative Dentistry*, 36 Suppl, s139–49, 2016. Epub 2016/04/01.
42. Benic, G.I., Thoma, D.S., Muñoz, F., Sanz Martin, I., Jung, R.E., Hämmerle, C.H., Guided bone regeneration of peri-implant defects with particulated and block xenogenic bone substitutes. *Clin. Oral Implants Res.*, 27, 5, 567–76, 2016. Epub 2015/06/16.
43. Sakaguchi, R., Xavier, S.P., Morinaga, K., Botticelli, D., Silva, E.R., Nakajima, Y., *et al.*, Histological Comparison of Collagenated Cancellous Equine Bone Blocks Used as Inlay or Onlay for Lateral Bone Augmentation in Rabbits. *Materials*, 16, 20, 6742, 2023.
44. Jafrani, A., Mehmood, H., Shaikh, M.S., Lone, M.A., Fareed, M.A., Zafar, M.S., A narrative review on the role of adipose-derived stem cells in periodontal regeneration. *J. Dent.*, 158, 105801, 2025.
45. Reinisch, K.B., Zuk, G., Raptis, D.A., Bueter, M., Guggenheim, M., Stasch, T., *et al.*, Autologous lipotransfer for bone defects secondary to osteomyelitis: A report of a novel method and systematic review of the literature. *Int. Wound J.*, 16, 4, 916–24, 2019. Epub 2019/03/28.
46. Alfotawi, R., Ahmed, R., Atteya, M., Mahmood, A., Siyal, A., AlHindi, M., *et al.*, Assessment of novel surgical procedures using decellularised muscle and bioactive ceramic: a histological analysis. *J. Mater. Sci. - Mater. Med.*, 32, 9, 113, 2021. Epub 2021/08/29.

47. Hakeem, L., Al-Kindi, M., AlMuraikhi, N., BinHamdan, S., Al-Zahrani, A., Evaluation of the regenerative potential of decellularized skeletal muscle seeded with mesenchymal stromal cells in critical-sized bone defect of rat models. *Saudi Dental J.*, 33, 5, 248–55, 2021. Epub 2021/07/02.
48. Sundar, R., Bhagavandas Rai, A., Naveen Kumar, J., Devang Divakar, D., The role of Vitamin D as an adjunct for bone regeneration: A systematic review of literature. *Saudi Dental J.*, 35, 3, 220–32, 2023. Epub 2023/04/24.
49. Elboraey, M.O., Alqutaibi, A.Y., Aboalrejal, A.N., Borzangy, S., Zafar, M.S., Al-Gabri, R., *et al.*, Regenerative approaches in alveolar bone augmentation for dental implant placement: Techniques, biomaterials, and clinical decision-making: A comprehensive review. *J. Dent.*, 154, 105612, 2025.
50. Su, W., Ma, X., Sun, Z., Yi, Z., Cui, X., Chen, G., *et al.*, RhBMP-2 and concomitant rapid material degradation synergistically promote bone repair and regeneration with collagen-hydroxyapatite nanocomposites. *J. Mater. Chem. B*, 6, 26, 4338–50, 2018. Epub 2018/07/14.
51. Sun, Y., Xu, C., Wang, M., Wei, L., Pieterse, H., Wu, Y., *et al.*, Radiographic and histological evaluation of bone formation induced by rhBMP-2-incorporated biomimetic calcium phosphate material in clinical alveolar sockets preservation. *Int. J. Implant Dentistry*, 9, 1, 37, 2023. Epub 2023/10/16.
52. Xu, L., Jacobs, R., Cao, Y., Sun, X., Qin, X., Tissue-engineered bone construct promotes early osseointegration of implants with low primary stability in oversized osteotomy. *BMC Oral Health*, 24, 1, 69, 2024. Epub 2024/01/11.
53. Alrasheed, A., Al-Ahmari, F., Ramalingam, S., Nooh, N., Wang, C.Y., Al-Hezaimi, K., Real-Time Assessment of Guided Bone Regeneration in Standardized Calvarial Defects Using a Combination of Bone Graft and Platelet-Derived Growth Factor With and Without Collagen Membrane: An *In Vivo* Microcomputed Tomographic and Histologic Experiment in Rats. *Int. J. Periodontics Restorative Dentistry*, 36 Suppl, s173–86, 2016. Epub 2016/04/01.
54. Kaigler, D., Avila, G., Wisner-Lynch, L., Nevins, M.L., Nevins, M., Rasperini, G., *et al.*, Platelet-derived growth factor applications in periodontal and peri-implant bone regeneration. *Expert Opin. Biol. Ther.*, 11, 3, 375–85, 2011. Epub 2011/02/04.
55. Novak, S., Madunic, J., Shum, L., Vucetic, M., Wang, X., Tanigawa, H., *et al.*, PDGF inhibits BMP2-induced bone healing. *npj Regener. Med.*, 8, 1, 3, 2023.
56. Zhang, M., Yu, W., Niibe, K., Zhang, W., Egusa, H., Tang, T., *et al.*, The Effects of Platelet-Derived Growth Factor-BB on Bone Marrow Stromal Cell-Mediated Vascularized Bone Regeneration. *Stem Cells Int.*, 2018, 3272098, 2018. Epub 2018/12/06.
57. Al-Ahmari, F., Al-Rasheed, A., Ramalingam, S., Aldahmash, A., Nooh, N., Wang, C.Y., *et al.*, Efficacy of Mesenchymal Stem Cells as Adjunct to Guided Bone Regeneration in Standardized Calvarial Defects in Rats: An *In Vivo* Microcomputed Tomographic and Histologic Analysis. *Int. J. Periodontics Restorative Dentistry*, 36 Suppl, s23–37, 2016. Epub 2016/04/01.

58. Al-Hezaimi, K., Ramalingam, S., Al-Askar, M., ArRejaie, A.S., Nooh, N., Jawad, F., *et al.*, Real-time-guided bone regeneration around standardized critical size calvarial defects using bone marrow-derived mesenchymal stem cells and collagen membrane with and without using tricalcium phosphate: an *in vivo* micro-computed tomographic and histologic experiment in rats. *Int. J. Oral Sci.*, 8, 1, 7–15, 2016. Epub 2016/03/31.
59. Shiu, S.T., Lee, W.F., Chen, S.M., Hao, L.T., Hung, Y.T., Lai, P.C., *et al.*, Effect of Different Bone Grafting Materials and Mesenchymal Stem Cells on Bone Regeneration: A Micro-Computed Tomography and Histomorphometric Study in a Rabbit Calvarial Defect Model. *Int. J. Mol. Sci.*, 22, 15, 2021. Epub 2021/08/08.
60. Muresan, G.C., Hedesiu, M., Lucaciu, O., Boca, S., Petrescu, N., Effect of Vitamin D on Bone Regeneration: A Review. *Med. (Kaunas Lithuania)*, 58, 10, 2022. Epub 2022/10/28.
61. Ye, S., Wen, J., Ye, W.-H., Li, Z., Huang, X., Chen, S., *et al.*, A facile and smart strategy to enhance bone regeneration with efficient vitamin D3 delivery through sterosome technology. *J. Controlled Release*, 370, 140–51, 2024.
62. Hacibektasoglu, M.S., Balcioglu, H.A., Uyanikgil, Y., Balcioglu, N.B., The Effects of Systemic Vitamin D Level on the Healing of Different Graft Materials: An Experimental Histological Study. *Appl. Sci.*, 14, 2, 939, 2024.
63. Łuczak, J.W., Palusińska, M., Matak, D., Pietrzak, D., Nakielski, P., Lewicki, S., *et al.*, The Future of Bone Repair: Emerging Technologies and Biomaterials in Bone Regeneration. *Int. J. Mol. Sci.*, 25, 23, 2024. Epub 2024/12/17.
64. Bahadir, C.D., Omar, M., Rosenthal, J., Marchionni, L., Liechty, B., Pisapia, D.J., *et al.*, Artificial intelligence applications in histopathology. *Nat. Rev. Electr. Eng.*, 1, 2, 93–108, 2024.

Index

Printed and bound by CPI Group (UK) Ltd, Croydon, CR0 4YY
17/09/2026
14964284-0001